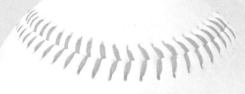 Portion Guide

These shapes will help you visualize portion sizes in *ChangeOne* meals.

Baseball
About 1 cup
Use for cereal, rice, pasta

Diner coffee cup
About 8 fluid ounces
Use for milk, yogurt, soups

Tennis ball
About ⅔ cup
Use for bread, rolls, potatoes, small starch portions

2 golf balls
About ½ cup
Use for beans, hot cereals

Deck of cards
About 3–4 ounces
Use for servings of beef, chicken, pork, salmon

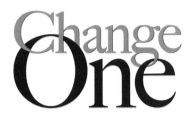

The **Breakthrough**
12-Week Eating Plan

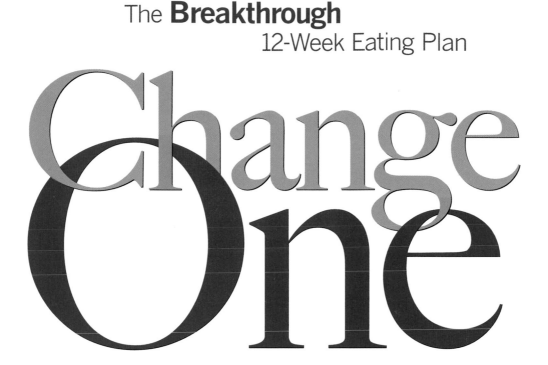

ChangeOne

Lose Weight
Simply, Safely, and
Forever

BY JOHN HASTINGS

With Peter Jaret and Mindy Hermann, R.D.

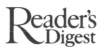

Reader's Digest

THE READER'S DIGEST ASSOCIATION
PLEASANTVILLE, NEW YORK / MONTREAL

ChangeOne is a registered trademark of The Reader's Digest Association, Inc.

Reader's Digest and the Pegasus logo are registered trademarks of The Reader's Digest Association, Inc.

Food photography by Elizabeth Watt
Exercise photography by Beth Bischoff
Portion guide photos by Christine Bronico
Portraits by George Kamper, except page 56 by Gary A. Morehouse
Cover photograph by Leland Bobbé

Address any comments about
ChangeOne to:
  Reader's Digest
  Editorial Director, Reader's Digest Health Publishing
  Reader's Digest Road
  Pleasantville, NY 10570-7000

Visit us on our Web site at: **changeone.com**

Library of Congress Cataloging-in-Publication Data

Hastings, John, 1962–
    ChangeOne : the breakthrough 12-week eating plan: lose weight simply, safely, and forever / by John Hastings, with Peter Jaret and Mindy Hermann.
      p. cm.
    Includes indexes.
ISBN 0-7621-0419-8
    1. Reducing diets. 2. Food habits. I. Title: Change one. II. Jaret, Peter. III. Hermann, Mindy. IV. Title.

    RM 222.2 .H276 2003
    613.2'5—dc21

        2002031927

Printed in the United States of America
  5 7 9 10 8 6 4
US 9100/IC

Note to our readers:
This publication is designed to provide useful information to the reader on the subjects of weight loss, healthy eating, and exercise. It should not be substituted for the advice of a physician or used to alter any medical therapy or programs prescribed to you by your doctor. Be sure to consult your doctor before proceeding with any weight-loss or exercise regimen. The use of specific products in this book does not constitute an endorsement by the author or the publisher. The author and the publisher disclaim any liability or loss, personal, financial, or otherwise, which may be claimed or incurred, directly or indirectly, resulting from the use and/or application of the content of this publication.

Acknowledgments

What you see on the pages of *ChangeOne* is a program that can help anyone achieve the weight and health they want and deserve. But *ChangeOne* began as a concept, and turning this concept into a book, a Web site, magazine articles, and more took a huge number of passionate, dedicated people. You know who you are; please accept my sincerest thanks. Several people warrant special note:

My co-authors, Peter Jaret and Mindy Hermann, brought formidable knowledge, prodigious talent, and great wit to this project. These brilliant collaborators worked tirelessly to make *ChangeOne* what it is.

Four of the top weight-loss researchers in the country played a key role in shaping the *ChangeOne* program: John Foreyt, Ph.D., Robert I. Berkowitz, M.D., Gary Foster, Ph.D, and Sachiko St. Jeor, Ph.D., R.D. To each of you, my deepest gratitude.

My main partners in building this book were Neil Wertheimer, the editor, and Susan Welt, the designer. They found a way to create a book that's both beautiful and readable. And thanks to Hannu Laakso for covering us.

While the theory and techniques behind *ChangeOne* have been proven successful many times over, we thought it crucial to give our program a rigorous test run before putting it in print. To the many test pilots of our 12-week program (several of whom you will meet inside this book), my thanks and congratulations.

My co-conspirators John Poppy and Edward S. McFadden supplied crucial input and direction.

Andrew Bein, Rachel Erickson-Hee, and Christine Many led the development of a companion Web site—**changeone.com**—that's an extraordinary tool for anyone wishing to lose weight the *ChangeOne* way.

An exceptional business team worked furiously to get *ChangeOne* into as many hands as possible. To Harold Clarke, Chris Reggio, Bill Adler, and Keira Krausz, many thanks.

I cannot overstate my gratitude to Eric W. Schrier, editor-in-chief of Reader's Digest Association Inc., who encouraged the creation of *ChangeOne* and helped put all of the company's resources behind it.

Finally, I thank my wife, Kathy, and my boys, Max, Cole, and Moses, for their patience, understanding, and love.

John Hastings

Contents

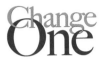

Part 1
The *ChangeOne* Program

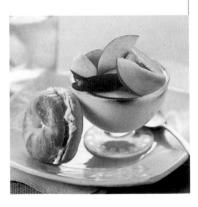
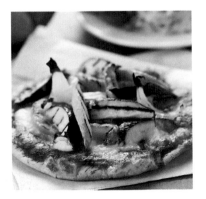
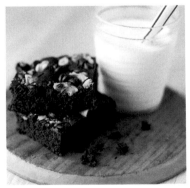

Part 1

Change One

The Program

Quick-Start Guide

ChangeOne Eating

The central theme of our 12-week program is that all foods are allowed in the appropriate amounts. Most people will eat about 1,300 calories a day on this plan. Larger or more active people can add roughly 300 calories through extra servings of grain or protein each day. Here's an overview of the first four weeks:

Week 1: Breakfast

Roughly 300 calories

Eat a healthy breakfast and love it, even if you don't normally eat anything.

The Basic Menu

- **One grain or starch**—roughly a cup (baseball) of ready-to-eat cereal, a slice of toast, or a roll (tennis ball).
- **One dairy or high-calcium food**—a cup of milk or a cup of yogurt.
- **Fruit**—one piece, or an equivalent amount of melon or berries.

Variations: Pancakes, champagne brunches, lox and bagels, even a parfait are fine if done the *ChangeOne* way.

Week 2: Lunch

Roughly 350 calories

You'll learn to recognize a sensible lunch that fits your lifestyle and tastes.

The Basic Menu

- **One grain or starch**—two slices of sandwich bread; a tennis ball-sized potato or roll, or serving of pasta or rice.
- **One protein**—thin palm-sized slice of cheese, a small burger patty, or three CD-sized pieces of lunch meat.
- **Fruit**—one piece, or an equivalent amount of melon or berries.
- **Vegetables**—as much as you want.

Variations: Soups, salads, wraps, even chili, done in sensible portion sizes.

Week 3: Snacks

Up to 200 calories

Yes, you can have cake and eat it, too. In fact, you get two snacks a day.

- **Salty**—a handful of chips, microwave popcorn, crackers, or nuts in the shell.
- **Sweet**—a palmful of M&Ms, jelly beans, malted-milk balls, raisins, or hard candy, or a mini candy bar.
- **Baked**—two small cookies, one mini cupcake, or a 2-inch-square brownie.
- **Frozen**—2 golf balls worth of frozen yogurt, sorbet, or Italian ices; half a tennis ball worth of regular ice cream; or a fudgsicle or juice bar.

Week 4: Dinner

Roughly 450 calories

A full day's worth of dieting begins this week, and you'll never look back.

The Basic Menu

- **One protein**—a tennis ball worth of shrimp, scallops, or crab; a deck of cards portion of chicken breast filet, beef, salmon, or tofu; a serving of light-flesh fish the size of a checkbook; 2 golf balls of beans.
- **One grain or starch**—a tennis ball serving of rice, pasta, noodles, or bread.
- **Vegetables**—as much as you want.

Variations: Pot roasts, Chinese buffets, shish kebabs, barbecue.

that merely shopping for food can be fattening. On a given weekend, for instance, you can sample more than 20 different "tastes" at the typical discount club and pile on hundreds of calories in the process. All this while you're being pitched the giant twin box of sugar-coated cereal and monster containers of mayonnaise.

It's time for Americans to regain control of what they eat. With *ChangeOne*, you don't have to give up the foods you love. You don't have to learn to like tofu. And you don't have to eat dry, tasteless snacks—what some dieters refer to as "roofing material." You just have to change one eating habit at a time, starting in Week 1 with breakfast. Then it's on to lunch, snacks, dinner, dining out, and beyond as you watch the weight melt away. Simple. Smart. Sensible.

Behind all the recipes, tips, and nutritional guidance is one very special idea: we'll be with you throughout this 12-week program. Every page of *ChangeOne* is designed to make it easy on you, answer your questions, and keep you motivated. Think of us as your diet buddy, a trusted friend who's been through it all before. And if you want to work privately online, we have built a companion Web site— **changeone.com**—that takes you every step of the way. It's also your place to post messages to one another, and to us. Please let us know if you feel healthier, have more energy, or have finally been able to fit into the clothes that make you feel like a million. We know you can do it. Make a change!

Jacqueline Leo

Jacqueline Leo
Editor-In-Chief, *Reader's Digest*

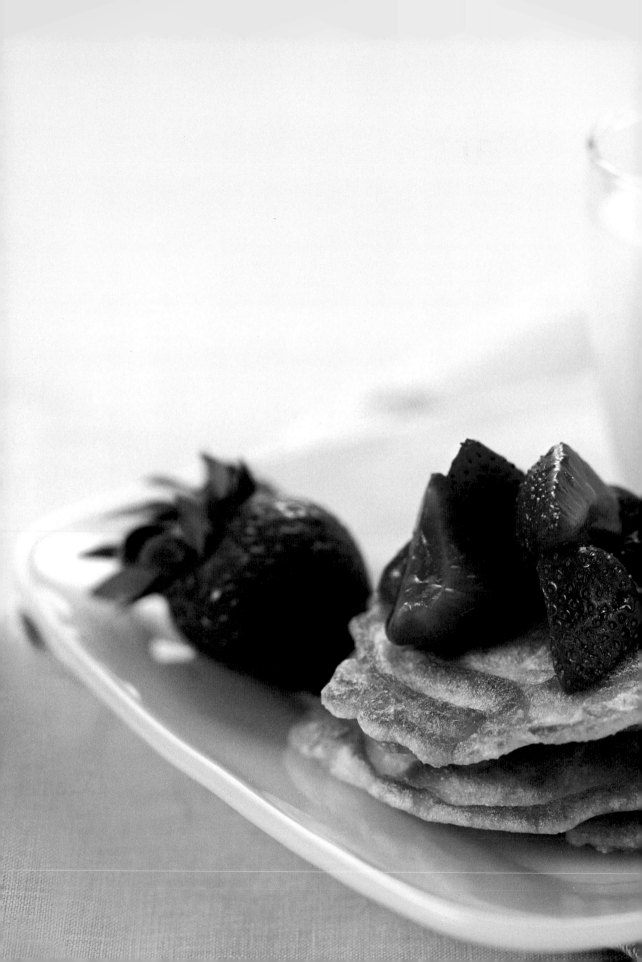

Part 2
ChangeOne Resources

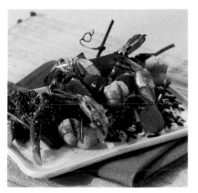

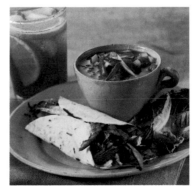

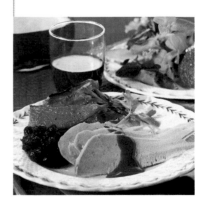

Winning at Losing

How many diet plans have you tried? High protein? High carbs? Low fat? Only eat things that are white? Don't eat anything white? Only eat grapefruit, or cabbage? You know the drill. For a few weeks the latest fad seems to be working. You lose a few pounds, feel better about yourself and life in general, and then boom—like a boomerang, the weight comes back and then some. Now you're left with two problems: you still have those pounds to lose, and you feel like a failure.

Well, *Reader's Digest* wants to help you. That's why, for the first time ever, we have created a diet of our own. You will lose weight without giving up the foods you love to eat. And you'll be stronger—in body and mind. We've tapped some of the country's top nutritionists and dietary specialists to come up with this completely new eating plan that takes the weight off ... and keeps it off. In only 12 weeks—with just one simple change each week—you will win the weight-loss battle. *ChangeOne* is easy. It's different. And thanks to the testing we've done, we know it works.

Regain control over your eating *without* giving up the foods you love.

There's so much more at stake than simply looking good. More than half of all U.S. adults are now overweight. According to David Satcher, former U.S. Surgeon General, obesity is now a national health crisis, causing nearly as much preventable disease and death as cigarette smoking. Scientists know that type II diabetes, for example, is on the rise thanks to obesity, and some 16 million Americans are at risk.

But that should be no surprise. Eating is our new national pastime. In big cities, you can find breakfast, lunch, and everything in between on the street from vendors who push calories on wheels. In the suburbs, go to the mall, where restaurants and retailers combine shopping and eating as a full-time sport. On the road, burger, taco, and pizza joints are more common than deer crossings. And let's not forget

The Key Principles

1. Make one change at a time. You can't become a new person overnight— lasting change requires a measured approach.
2. The secret to weight loss is understanding portion sizes, not math. If you don't want to count calories for the rest of your life, don't diet that way.
3. All foods are allowed. Let your meals be a source of healthy pleasure and never skimp on flavor or delight.
4. Eating for a healthy weight is the same as eating for health. Think of *ChangeOne* as a way of life, and this will be the *last* time you have to lose weight.

ChangeOne Living

While the first four weeks cover meals, the next eight weeks offer essential health lessons. Each week takes on an aspect of daily life that influences how you eat:

Week 5: Dining Out

We'll ask you to go out for meals at least twice this week (that's right, you'll *have* to visit restaurants) to practice ordering—and eating—only what you want.

Week 6: Weekends & Holidays

Plan meals or parties with family and friends; you'll not only enjoy yourself, you'll be able to resist temptation.

Week 7: Fixing Your Kitchen

Take a hard look at what's in your refrigerator and on your shelves. Is the food you see going to help you lose weight or undermine your best intentions?

Week 8: How Am I Doing?

Everybody take a deep breath. You're two months into the program, so it's time to assess your progress and clear any roadblocks.

Week 9: Stress Relief

Stress has a way of sneaking up on you, and eating often serves as a coping mechanism. We'll help you identify and relieve those hidden pressures.

Week 10: Staying Active for Success

C'mon, you knew you couldn't avoid exercise. This week you'll learn the only foolproof way to keep weight off.

Week 11: Keeping on Track

If the pounds start to return, they won't do it all at once. Your goal is to devise your own "First Alert" program that will help you contain the gain.

Week 12: *ChangeOne* for Life!

You made it! So don't let boredom ruin the new you. Here's how you can make great food an ongoing source of pleasure—and maintain your loss.

Welcome to
ChangeOne

You've opened this book for one simple reason: you want to lose weight. Maybe a little, maybe a lot. Maybe you'd like to improve the reflection looking back at you from the mirror. Maybe you're hoping to fit more easily into an old pair of slacks or jeans. Or perhaps you simply want to be healthier and feel better.

Whatever your goal, *ChangeOne* will help you lose weight—and keep it off.

That may sound like a big promise. But there's really no mystery to dieting, despite the bewildering number of plans out there. Want to know a little secret? They all can work. Only one thing matters in the weight-loss game: eat fewer calories than you burn. All diets, even the seemingly crazy ones, restrict your calories, and that's why you lose weight. Eat reasonable amounts of food and the pounds will melt away.

Honest, Sensible Weight Loss

You won't find any silly gimmicks in *ChangeOne*. We're not going to make you become a vegetarian, a strict carnivore, a caveman, or a goddess. But we're radically different in one crucial way: *ChangeOne* asks you to approach dieting one meal at a time, one week at a time. (*ChangeOne* means just that—one change at a time.) We won't overwhelm you on the first day. Most diets ask you to throw out the way you eat overnight and adopt a new plan. You might be Mary today, but tomorrow you're supposed to become Elle. The biggest problem with that kind of approach is people will eventually go back to their old ways—after all, you *are* Mary—and gain back the weight they lost.

Imagine a psychologist who expects depressed patients to be happy after one visit. Or a language teacher who announces on the first day of class that students will be able to speak French the next day. It sounds laughable because making a significant change takes time; new skills require practice. Yet instant change is what most diets ask for, and that may be why so many people end up regaining the weight they've lost.

ChangeOne slows dieting down so you can experiment and learn. (Don't worry, the pounds will start coming off right away.)

In the first week you'll make just one change to your diet: overhaul your breakfast, following one of the five suggested *ChangeOne* breakfast menus. We've counted the calories, so all you have to do is learn to recognize and eat reasonable portion sizes.

In the second week, while you stick with your new habit of eating a healthy, low-calorie breakfast, you'll move on to lunch. Again, we offer a

The *ChangeOne* Team

To put *ChangeOne* to the test, we recruited volunteers from around the country—people just like you, who wanted to lose weight and look and feel better. Many of our volunteers were here at Reader's Digest in Pleasantville, New York. When we offered people the opportunity to try out the program, the response was overwhelming. The results were equally gratifying. Over the 12-week program our volunteers lost an average of 17 pounds each. Just as important, they honed skills and strategies that have continued to help them keep the weight off. Throughout this book you'll hear first-hand how they shaped the *ChangeOne* approach to work for them. To read some of our volunteers' stories and see before-and-after photos, visit changeone.com.

variety of simple menu choices. All you do is choose one each day during the week.

In the third week you'll focus on snacks. What do snacks have to do with dieting? Plenty. Snacks will keep you from getting too hungry, thereby strengthening your willpower. We'll offer you a variety of satisfying choices that will help your diet, not derail it.

In the fourth week, with breakfast, lunch, and snacks up and running, you'll move on to what's typically the biggest meal of the day: dinner. You'll find a tantalizing variety of great-tasting dinner menus and tried-and-true strategies for keeping portion sizes under control.

Voilà. By the end of the fourth week you will have retooled your diet, reduced calories and fat, and discovered new ways to enjoy good nutrition and great-tasting food. And you'll be watching the pounds melt away.

This measured approach makes it easy to experiment with each meal, allowing you to incorporate the foods that you enjoy. By focusing on one meal at a time, you'll discover more about the way you eat. You may find that eating a reasonable breakfast and lunch is easy, but at dinner you break the bank; or maybe snacks are your biggest stumbling

Dieting as a Tennis Match

Reading the health sections of newspapers and magazines can make you feel like you're at Wimbledon. One day you'll read that carbohydrates are terrible and fat is fine; the next day you'll get the rebuttal. What's the real answer? It'll be years—even decades— before the scientific debate over low-carbo-hydrate and high-carbo-hydrate diets is resolved.

But maybe it doesn't matter. Consider a recent study that tested two very different diets. The first was low in carbo-hydrates and very high in fat; 15 percent of calories came from carbs, 53 percent from fat, and 32 percent from protein.

> Ultimately, the protein vs. carbs debate is missing the point.

The second diet was high in carbo-hydrates and low in fat; 45 percent of calories came from carbs, 26 percent from fat, and 20 percent from protein.

The only thing the diets had in common was that each one totaled 1,000 calories a day. When the two groups of volunteers stepped up to the scale after six weeks, guess what? On average, all of them had lost nearly the same amount of weight and body fat.

High fat, low fat, high protein, low protein—none of it made a whit of difference on the scale. What mattered was calorie intake. The key to losing weight is as simple as that.

Change One Quiz

Ready, Set ... Lose

Sure, you want to lose weight. But before you start, it's worth checking to make sure you've got what it takes to succeed. To test your readiness, answer these 10 questions by circling the appropriate number in the right-hand column.

1. **Which term best describes your attitude toward losing weight?**

Gung-ho	4
Positive	3
Lukewarm	2
Resigned	1

2. **How many pounds do you want to lose?**

10–20	4
21–40	3
41–60	2
More than 60	1

3. **How would you rate your odds of reaching your goal?**

Excellent	4
Very good	3
So-so	2
Poor	1

4. **How do you feel about being physically active?**

Enjoy it	3
Don't really mind it	2
Hate it	1

5. **Which of the following statements best describes you?**

Once I make up my mind to do something, I get it done	3
My intentions are good, but my willpower is sometimes weak	2
I tend to get discouraged easily	1

6. **How important is losing weight to your health?**

Very important	3
Somewhat important	2
Not very important at all	1

7. **How well do you deal with stresses and strains in your life?**

Very effectively	3
So-so	2
I get frazzled easily	1

8. **How much time do you spend in front of TV on a typical day?**

Less than an hour	4
One to two hours	3
Three to four hours	2
Four or more hours	1

9. **Which of these statements best describes your knowledge about how to lose weight and keep it off:**

I know what it takes	4
I'm pretty sure I know	3
I'm confused by conflicting advice and diet plans	2
I have no idea where to start	1

10. **Think about the people closest to you; how are they likely to react to your decision to diet?**

Very enthusiastically	4
Somewhat positively	3
Skeptically	2
Negatively	1

Turn to next page to tally your score.

Quiz Score

Now tally your score. A 22 or higher means you're good to go, but a lower score is no cause for alarm. Many dieters feel grim about their chances early on. Look for any 1's or 2's in your responses, and then read the answers below to boost your readiness.

1. Enthusiasm doesn't guarantee success, but it sure helps. If yours needs a tune-up, draw a line down the middle of a piece of paper. In the left-hand column, write all the benefits you expect to get from losing weight. In the right column, jot down all the obstacles you anticipate. Finally, begin thinking about ways you can get around those obstacles in order to achieve the benefits you've listed.

2. Experts say your first goal should be about 10 percent of your current weight. With a reasonable goal you're less likely to get discouraged before you reach the finish line. It may not seem like much, but people who lose 10 percent look better, feel more confident and energetic, and are ready to set their next goal.

3. Despite discouraging words to the contrary, many people do lose weight and keep it off. Researchers at the University of Colorado and the University of Pittsburgh have been keeping track, in the National Weight Control Registry, of people who succeed at weight loss. We'll share many of the strategies that work for these successful weight-losers.

4. Not everyone likes to break a sweat. But you'll stand a better chance of succeeding if you become more active—walking, playing tag or touch football with the kids, riding a bike around the neighborhood, swimming, taking the stairs instead of the elevator.

5. A lot of frustrated dieters want to put the blame on willpower failures. The surprising truth is that you don't need a rock-solid will to lose weight. You need strategies that will spare you from having to rely on willpower all the time. You'll find

them here: ways to ward off hunger, navigate restaurants, and satisfy your sweet tooth on fewer calories, for example.

6. Better health is a bonus for *everyone* who sheds excess pounds. Carrying around too much weight increases your risk of diabetes, heart disease, and some cancers. The changes in *ChangeOne* are designed not only to help you shed pounds but also to be healthier.

7. Too much stress can undermine even the most determined dieter's plan. All of us face stresses and strains in our lives. What matters is how you deal with them. In *ChangeOne* we'll introduce you to effective ways to take the sting out of stress—techniques that will help you get through even the rockiest times.

8. The more television people watch, studies show, the more they're likely to weigh. Ask yourself this: would you be willing to give up just half an hour of TV three times a week to lose weight and feel a whole lot better? If so, you've just jump-started your chances of success.

9. Feeling a little unsure of the facts? Don't worry. In *ChangeOne* we do more than just tell you what to do. We explain why you should do it, based on the latest research. The more you know about gaining and losing weight, the better your chances of meeting your goal.

10. The support of family and friends makes a big difference when you're trying to make a change for the better. But they may not be as supportive as you'd like. If that's true for you, remember that you are the only person whose opinion matters. You can do this on your own.

block. You'll also gain confidence as you succeed in getting each meal under control. And then in the following eight weeks you'll tackle the big issues dieters face, such as how to eat smartly at restaurants, manage stress, and exercise for long-term success. Best of all, you'll learn skills that will help you eat sanely for the rest of your life. Losing weight is something you want to do only once. With *ChangeOne* you'll take the time to get it right.

The Numbers Behind *ChangeOne*

The meals and menus you'll find in the following pages are more than just delicious. They've been designed to offer maximum nutrition with a sensible number of calories. That's important. When you're cutting back on calories, you certainly don't want to cut back on vitamins, minerals, fiber, and the other health benefits of good food. The beauty of *ChangeOne* is that you don't have to weigh every gram or calculate every calorie. We've done that for you.

The *ChangeOne* meal plans are designed to meet the following daily guidelines:

- **Calories:** from 1,300 to 1,600.
- **Calories from fat:** 30 to 35 percent.
- **Saturated and hydrogenated fats:** no more than 10 percent.
- **Fiber:** at least 25 grams.
- **Calcium:** about 1,000 milligrams.
- **Fruits and vegetables:** at least five servings a day.

The calorie target of 1,300 to 1,600 a day is the one used in most diet programs run by experts in the field of weight loss. Not everyone needs precisely the same number of calories, of course. A large person uses up more calories than a small one. A very active person uses more than someone who doesn't get around much. As you'll discover,

What You'll Find Inside

On the following pages you'll find regular features packed with helpful tips and advice based on the latest weight-loss research, including:

ChangeOne Menu
Meals and recipes that will help you cut calories without losing the pleasure of eating. And our photos are accurate—the portion sizes you see pictured reflect what you'll be eating.

Help!
Troubleshooting tips to help you overcome many of the most common obstacles on the path to successful weight loss.

First Person
Insights from people who have used the *ChangeOne* approach to shed pounds and keep them off.

Fast Track
Optional strategies to help you speed up your weight loss.

ChangeOne is designed to let you set your own calorie target and readjust it along the way to suit your needs.

You'll also notice that *ChangeOne* meals don't slash fat to unrealistically low levels. In fact, you may be surprised to find that some of our meal plans come in slightly higher than the American Heart Association's recommendation to get 30 percent of your daily calories from fat. The latest scientific studies show that diets with a decent amount of fat—the healthy kinds, of course—are actually more successful than diets that restrict fat to an absurd minimum.

ChangeOne is designed to help you slim down gradually, from one to three pounds a week. People who lose weight at a steady, moderate pace like this are the most likely to keep it off. But many dieters are impatient to slim down. If you are one of them, *ChangeOne* offers "Fast Track" features with suggestions to help you drop pounds faster.

Sound simple? We hope so. That's the *ChangeOne* goal—to take the mystery and frustration out of weight loss.

Water, Water...

What can you quench your thirst with? Here's the *ChangeOne* approach to drink:

- Coffee or tea is fine. If you take either with milk or sugar, choose skim or a non-dairy (low-calorie) creamer, and use an artificial sweetener.
- Drink water, and lots of it. Seltzer, mineral water, and diet sodas are also acceptable. All quench your thirst—and reduce appetite—at no additional calories.
- Avoid regular soda, with all its sugar and empty calories.
- Fruit juice is healthy, but adds calories without fiber, so you're better off with the whole fruit and a glass of water.
- One glass of wine or beer per day is acceptable. They add more than 100 calories to your day, but there's debate whether those calories will slow your weight loss.

Getting Started

The basic *ChangeOne* meal plans you'll find in this book contain about 1,300 calories a day.

That's a reasonable goal for many people who want to lose weight. But if you're very active or heavy, you may want to set your calorie target higher. People who are physically active burn more calories minute by minute than people who are not as active. And people who are heavy burn more calories than lighter people because they use more energy carrying around the extra weight.

What's the ideal target for you? Here's what we recommend:

Aim for 1,300 calories if:

- You're a woman who weighs less than 190 pounds and gets less than half an hour's worth of physical activity (including walking and other everyday activities) most days.

■ You're an inactive man and you weigh less than 190 pounds.

Aim for 1,600 calories if:

■ You get at least half an hour's worth of vigorous exercise most days of the week.

■ You weigh more than 190 pounds.

Keep in mind that you can always adjust your calorie target up or down during the program. If you aren't losing weight as quickly as you'd like, you can decrease your calorie level. (We don't recommend going below 1,300 calories a day, however, because a diet that skimpy is likely to fall short on vitamins, minerals, and other nutrients you need.) If you feel too hungry on most days, you can increase it. What's key is that you do *not* feel hungry. Researchers have found that dieters quickly adjust to a lower calorie level, so if after a few weeks you're still starving, eat a little more. Once you reach your weight goal, we'll help you find a calorie target that balances the energy you take in with the energy you burn. (For more help on this, check out **changeone.com**.)

Real Rewards

Most people on a diet want to see changes on the scale. That's natural. We recommend that you weigh yourself once a week, preferably every Monday (it will help you stay honest over the weekend). Use the same scale and choose the same time of day. Keep a log of your weight.

But remember, logging pounds on the scale is only one way to measure your progress, and not necessarily the best way. If you're losing fat and adding muscle, for instance, your weight may remain the same but you'll look and feel a lot better (and your waistline is likely to slim down). One of our *ChangeOne* volunteers actually stopped lifting weights when the numbers on the scale weren't dropping as fast as he would have liked. But he looked great, and the strength training had a lot to do with that. We convinced him to start exercising again and to pay less attention to the scale.

That's good advice for anyone beginning a diet. Keep an eye on your image in the mirror, your clothing size, your energy, and the notches on your belt, and you'll enjoy all the rewards of slimming down.

The 1,600 Club

If you opt for 1,600 calories a day instead of the *ChangeOne* basic plan of 1,300, don't worry about counting every extra calorie. Here's all you have to do:

■ At breakfast double your starch or grain serving.

■ At lunch or dinner double your portion of protein (that is, your meat, chicken, fish or tofu serving); *or*, at dinner double your portion of starch or grain again.

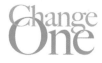

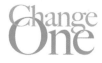

Week 1

Breakfast

How does this sound? This week you'll start *ChangeOne* by eating breakfast every morning.

Maybe you don't eat breakfast. Plenty of hopeful dieters forgo the first meal of the day. What better way to make my diet work, the thinking goes, than not eating? People figure they'll end up taking in fewer calories that way.

In fact, it works the other way around. People who skip breakfast often end up consuming *more* calories during the day. Those who start the day with a healthy meal, meanwhile, are more likely to stick to healthy eating throughout the day.

In this chapter you'll find several great breakfasts, along with simple ways to adapt them to your own tastes. Every day this week, help yourself to whichever *ChangeOne* breakfast strikes your fancy. Experiment—and don't worry if you try something that doesn't fill you up. The rest of the day you can eat the way you normally do. That's all there is to taking your first step toward losing weight— and keeping it off.

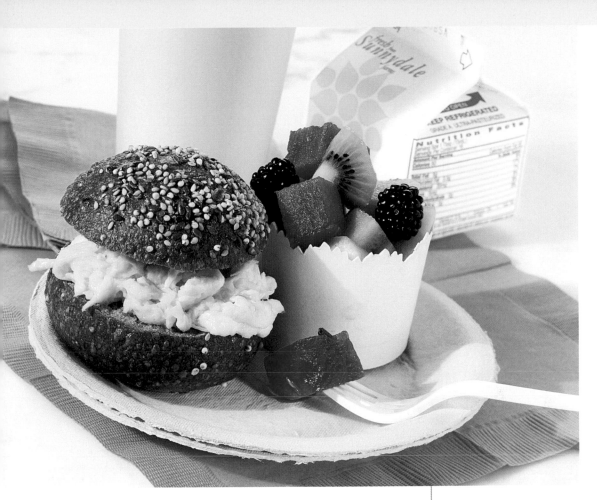

Egg on a Roll

1 egg, scrambled, poached, or hard cooked

1 small whole wheat roll (size of a tennis ball)

½ cup fresh fruit salad (2 golf balls)

1 half-pint (8 ounces) skim or low-fat (1 percent) milk

Calories 300, fat 8 g, saturated fat 2.5 g, cholesterol 215 mg, sodium 340 mg, carbohydrate 41 g, fiber 4 g, protein 19 g, calcium 400 mg.

Instead of	Try
1 egg	½ cup scrambled egg substitute, or ½ cup low-fat cottage cheese
1 small roll	1 English muffin 1 small pita 1 slice wheat toast
½ cup fruit salad	6 ounces orange juice 1 orange 1 banana 1 apple

Time-Saver

This is a breakfast you can make at home or buy on the road. If you have a favorite diner or coffee shop, let them know this is "the usual" and that you'll be by often to order it. Or ask a fast-food outlet such as McDonald's or Dunkin' Donuts to make it for you on an English muffin.

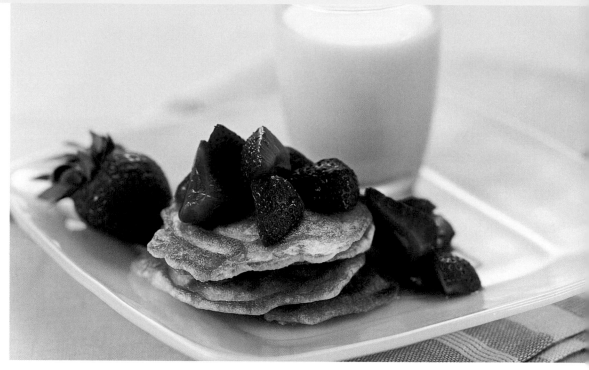

Pancakes to Start

4 silver dollar pancakes

1 tablespoon light maple or sugar-free strawberry or almond syrup (2 syrup bottle caps)

½ cup sliced strawberries (2 golf balls)

1 half-pint (8 ounces) skim or low-fat (1 percent) milk

Calories 280, fat 6 g, saturated fat 1.5 g, cholesterol 60 mg, sodium 530 mg, carbohydrate 41 g, fiber 2 g, protein 15 g, calcium 450 mg.

SILVER DOLLAR PANCAKES

Serves 4

  ½ **cup self-rising flour**
  ½ **tablespoon sugar**
  ¼ **teaspoon baking soda**
  ¾ **cup buttermilk**
  1 **tablespoon vegetable oil**
  1 **large egg**
  ½ **teaspoon vanilla extract**

1. Whisk flour, sugar, and baking soda in medium bowl. Make a well in center of mixture. In separate bowl whisk together buttermilk, oil, egg, and vanilla until blended. Pour this into well and whisk just until moistened. Let batter stand 5 minutes.

2. While the batter waits, coat large nonstick skillet with cooking spray and set over medium heat until hot, but not smoking.

3. For each pancake, pour 1 tablespoon batter into skillet. Cook until bubbles appear all over cakes and begin to burst, about 3 minutes. Turn and cook until undersides are golden, about 1 to 2 minutes longer. Makes 16 pancakes.

4. Make 4 pancakes for yourself. If not cooking for others, you can cover extra batter and refrigerate for the next day. Or cook entire recipe, wrap extra pancakes in foil, and refrigerate for a day or freeze for a week. To reheat, place wrapped pancakes in a 350°F oven for about 10 minutes.

Instead of	Try
4 silver dollar pancakes	1 waffle, 1 slice French toast, 1 slice cinnamon toast, or 1 crepe (about 7 inches)

Why Breakfast Is Key

If you usually skip the morning meal, you may need a little convincing to get you to eat it. Many of the volunteers who tested *ChangeOne* weren't breakfast eaters, either. What they discovered was that beginning the day with a healthy meal was the single most important change they made.
"I was amazed, really amazed," one *ChangeOne* volunteer told us. "Starting to eat breakfast changed the way I ate all day long. It really made the difference."

Don't just take our word for it. Scientific evidence comes from experiments like one conducted at Vanderbilt University in Nashville, Tennessee. Researchers recruited overweight women who typically missed breakfast. All the women were put on a 1,200-calorie-a-day diet. One group divided calories between just two meals, lunch and dinner. The second group ate those meals plus breakfast. Twelve weeks later the breakfast eaters had lost 17 pounds; the women who didn't eat breakfast had shed 13.

Wait a minute, you might say: weren't both groups consuming the same number of calories? No, the researchers concluded. The women who ate breakfast were better able to stick to the 1,200-calorie diet. Those who went hungry until lunch were more tempted to cheat a little.

Four out of five successful dieters eat breakfast every day of the week.

Breakfast Portions

To help you assess portion sizes, we use both standard measurements and the *ChangeOne* portion-size guide. Make it a point to get the items we use as guides and hold them in your hands to get a clear sense of correct portion sizes. In the breakfast portions below, members of the 1,600 Club can double the starch or grain serving.

Type of food	Example	Amount	*ChangeOne* guide
One starch or grain	Ready-to-eat cereal	1 cup	Baseball
	Hot cereal	½ cup	2 golf balls
	Toast	1 slice	
	Roll	Small	Tennis ball
One dairy or high-calcium food	Milk	1 cup	Diner coffee cup
	Yogurt	1 cup	
One piece of fruit	Orange, apple	1	
	Berries, cut fruit	½ cup	
Optional	Butter, jam	1 teaspoon	Thumb tip
	Nuts	1 tablespoon	Thumb

If you pass up breakfast, this study showed, you're likely to eat more, not less, than if you start the day with a meal.

The reason is pretty obvious when you think about it. The longer you go without eating, the hungrier you get. And the hungrier you get, the more likely you are to gobble down anything you can get your hands on. When you open the day with breakfast, you begin by taming the hungry beast inside and make it easier to keep cravings in check.

You'll also be starting your day with an easy success: of the three meals, a healthy, sensible breakfast is the simplest to pull off. That will help you stay on track for the day. Psychologists say that levels of two brain chemicals that give us a sense of control—cortisol and adrenaline—peak right after we get up. The confidence they provide may make it easier to stick to our good intentions, such as a healthier diet. These chemicals ebb later in the morning, so it can be tougher to say no to the donuts someone brings into the office—especially if you're starving because you skipped breakfast.

Here's a compelling argument: most successful dieters eat breakfast. Since 1993 researchers at the University of Colorado and the University of Pittsburgh have been gathering data on people who manage to lose 30 pounds or more and keep the weight off for at least one year. The project, called the National Weight Control Registry, is designed to learn—from the people who know best—what it takes to shed pounds permanently. Four out of five say they eat breakfast every day of the week.

Help!

"I'm just not hungry in the morning. Do I really have to force myself to eat if I'm not hungry?"

Give it a try. One reason you're not hungry may be that you're unaccustomed to eating so early. So try this: start off with a few bites of something that sounds appealing—toast, say, or a cereal bar—for five mornings in a row. After two or three mornings, you might start to notice your early-morning appetite increasing. Also, schedule dinner a little earlier than usual if you can, and eat only enough to feel satisfied without being stuffed. This will increase the chances of your appetite waking up when you do. If you're still struggling, eat just one item from a *ChangeOne* breakfast—a piece of fruit, for instance—and save the rest for a mid-morning mini-meal.

Making the Change

Choose a *ChangeOne* breakfast each day this week. Mix and match the meals any way you like. The important thing is to start your day with a good breakfast and then go on with life—and the rest of your day's regular meals. Don't worry that you'll end up consuming more calories than usual. Like a lot of breakfast converts, you're likely to feel less hungry in midmorning and at lunch time.

Don't let the morning rush get in the

Hoping to drop a size before your upcoming class reunion? Determined to cut a slimmer figure when you hit the beach come summer? To speed your progress, choose one or more of these Fast Track changes this week:

Eat breakfast twice

Instead of having your usual lunch, make your midday meal another *ChangeOne* breakfast. Eating breakfast twice during the day isn't our idea. Lately several big cereal manufacturers have been touting it as a novel weight-loss method.

Help yourself to a bowl of their flakes for breakfast and lunch, they promise, and you can have a full dinner and still shed pounds. It works, especially if high-calorie lunches are your downfall.

Turn downtime into activity

Add 15 minutes of extra physical activity to your schedule every day this week. Walking is fine: a brisk stroll in the neighborhood, a quick circuit of the office complex, or up and down a few flights of stairs if they're handy.

Aim for 15 minutes of activity every day when you would otherwise have been inactive. Here's why: if you weigh 180 pounds, for instance, you burn about 2.2 calories a minute sitting in a meeting or in front of the TV. Get up and walk and you more than double that number, to 4.7 calories. Quicken your pace to a brisk walk and your metabolism knocks off 7.2 calories a minute.

The benefits can add up fast. Sitting still you burn just 33 calories every 15 minutes. Brisk walking burns 108 in the same period.

Keep a food diary

People who are asked to keep close track of what they eat during the day, researchers have found, almost always begin to lose weight—even if they don't consciously go on a diet. There are several reasons for this.

When you're keeping a food diary, you become more aware of what you actually eat. And when you know you have to write down every nibble, you think twice before you grab a sweet roll during the morning coffee break or help yourself to a piece of chocolate decadence.

Keeping a food diary also reveals eating patterns you may not have been aware of—the fact that you snack more than you imagined, for instance, or that most of your eating occurs late in the day. Those insights can help you shape the best strategy for losing weight. You'll find a handy Food Diary form and instructions on page 307. Track your eating every day this week.

Speed up the program

Though our volunteers liked the week-by-week pace of *ChangeOne*, you could do the first four weeks' assignments in less time to speed your weight loss. For example, give yourself three days for breakfast, four days for lunch, three days for snacks, and four days for dinner.

That would get you through the first four weeks and have you dieting from breakfast to bedtime in two weeks, instead of the four we recommend. The tradeoff is that you won't have as much time to experiment with meals to find the foods that satisfy you, and you could miss out on the opportunity to discover—and solve—problems in your eating patterns. But if your goal is to look stunning for your beach vacation and you don't have a lot of time ...

way. Putting breakfast together doesn't have to require more time than it takes to put cereal in a bowl, scatter a little fruit over it, and pour the milk. If you're really in a hurry:

- Set the table for breakfast before going to bed. You'll save time, and the table will be a reminder when you get up.
- Take care of one or two morning chores the night before. Instead of deciding what to wear after you get up, for example, select the next day's outfit before bed.
- Prepare a fruit salad on Sunday so that you can quickly spoon up some every morning of the week.
- Set the alarm clock 10 minutes early.

If all else fails, keep a box of breakfast bars and plenty of fresh fruit around for a handy, easy-to-pack breakfast.

Behind the *ChangeOne* Breakfast Menu

Each *ChangeOne* breakfast is designed to contain 300 calories or less. That's enough energy to power your morning and still get you started on losing weight.

Help!

"What if I can't find a cup of yogurt with only 80 calories? Or a granola bar that has 120 calories? How exact do I have to be?"

Don't get too hung up on exact calorie counts. If you can come within 10 to 20 calories of the recommended amount in the target food, you'll be fine. Remember, the *ChangeOne* program is more about recognizing healthy foods and eating reasonable servings than it is about counting calories.

What's more, each *ChangeOne* breakfast includes at least one food that's high in fiber. There are several good reasons for this. The biggest shortfall in most people's diets is fiber, experts say. We should get about 25 to 30 grams a day to be our healthiest; we average a mere 15.

Fiber's an important defense against several common health problems. It's also a key player in a healthy weight-loss diet. Because it's filling, fiber makes a meal feel more satisfying on fewer calories. One form, called soluble fiber, absorbs water to form gels that slow digestion, so high-fiber foods stay with you longer than other kinds of food, keeping you from getting hungry. (For more on why high-fiber foods are so terrific, see "More Good Reasons to Fill Up on Fiber" on page 34.)

To test the hunger-taming effects of high-fiber foods, scientists at Australia's University of Sydney compared two seemingly similar breakfasts: a bowl of bran flakes, which are high in fiber, and a bowl of cornflakes, which are not. Volunteers in the bran group reported feeling less hungry later in the morning than those who ate cornflakes. In a

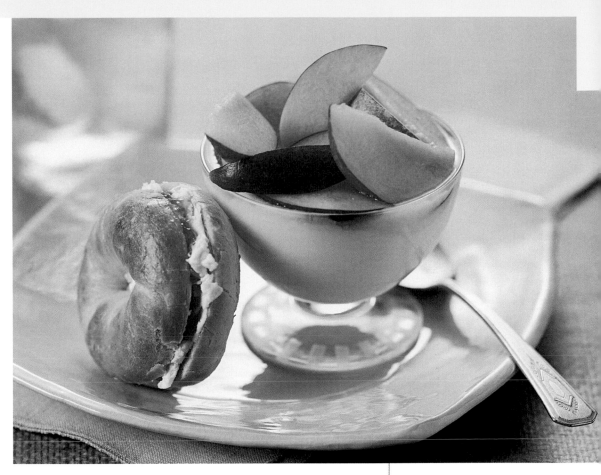

Bagel Delight

½ small (2-ounce) bagel or 1 mini-bagel

2 teaspoons cream cheese (2 thumb tips)
   or 1 tablespoon yogurt cheese (thumb)

1 teaspoon jam (thumb tip)

1 peach, sliced

1 cup artificially sweetened or plain nonfat
   yogurt (tennis ball)

Calories 301, fat 4.5 g, saturated fat 3 g, cholesterol 19 mg, sodium 336 mg,
carbohydrate 50 g, fiber 3 g, protein 17 g, calcium 500 mg.

Time-Saver
*Cut bagels into correct
portion size when you
bring them home from
the market, then freeze
them in a resealable
plastic bag.*

HOW TO MAKE YOGURT CHEESE

Line a drip-coffee basket with a coffee filter, and rest the filter
on a bowl or measuring cup. Put 1 cup plain nonfat or low-fat
yogurt (select a brand that does not contain gelatin) in the
filter. Cover and refrigerate for at least one hour. The liquid in
the yogurt drips out through the filter, allowing the yogurt to
thicken into a spread.

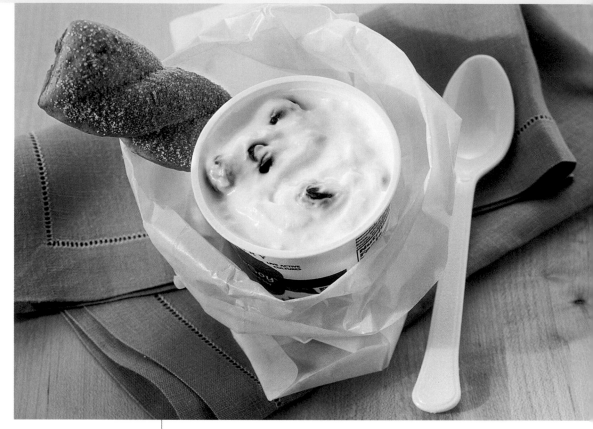

Time-Saver
Pack a portable break-fast in a bag the night before so you can grab it and go in the morning.

HEALTH TIP

A half cup of blue-berries contains 40 calories and 2 grams of fiber. For top flavor, swap the berries for a ½ cup of what's in season: apples (37 calories, 2 grams of fiber), oranges (42 calories, 2 grams of fiber), strawberries (25 calories, 2 grams of fiber), or plums (91 calories, 1 gram of fiber).

Breakfast on the Run

1 cereal bar, 120-140 calories

½ cup blueberries (2 golf balls)

1 cup artificially sweetened or plain nonfat yogurt

Calories 300, fat 3.5 g, saturated fat 0.5 g, cholesterol 0 mg, sodium 240 mg, carbohydrate 60 g, fiber 3 g, protein 9 g, calcium 600 mg.

ABOUT CEREAL BARS

Soft-textured "cereal bars" are generally lower in calories and fat than are traditional granola bars. Those at about 120 to 140 calories may be a bit tougher to find than their heavy-weight cousins, but with a bit of careful label reading you'll find flavors you like. Brands to try include Kellogg's Nutri-Grain and Nutri-Grain Twists, and Quaker Oats Fruit & Oat-meal. Look for a bar with at least 1 gram of fiber, but if you have a favorite that contains no fiber, go ahead and enjoy it—there's fiber in the fruit you eat with it.

similar experiment, researchers at the New York Obesity Research Center at St. Luke's-Roosevelt Hospital recently pitted a sugary, low-fiber breakfast cereal against oatmeal, among the highest-fiber cereals. When volunteers ate the sweetened flakes, they tended to eat as much at lunch as if they'd had nothing but a glass of water at breakfast. When they sat down to a bowl of oatmeal, they felt fuller longer and ate as much as 40 percent less for lunch.

Set the breakfast table the night before for easier mornings.

A Fruitful Choice

ChangeOne breakfasts also include at least one serving of fruit. Fruit, like whole grains, is a terrific source of fiber. One apple has almost six grams of fiber, which is 20 percent of the recommended daily amount. Also, the lion's share of people who hit the recommended goal of five servings of fruits and vegetables every day got at least one of those at breakfast.

When we say fruit, we mean fruit you can chew. Fruit juice is fine now and then, but many are surprisingly high in calories, especially if they've been sweetened. A cup of cranberry juice cocktail contains a hefty 140 calories. Even a cup of apple juice weighs in at 116 calories. Ounce for ounce that's more than cola. What's more, most fruit juices don't have nearly as much fiber as the fruit from which they're made. Compare three of the most popular:

Orange juice (1 cup)
Calories: 100
Vitamin C: 80 mg
Fiber: 0.4 g

An orange
Calories: 64
Vitamin C: 80 mg
Fiber: 3.3 g

Apple juice (1 cup)
Calories: 116
Vitamin C: 2.2 mg
Fiber: 0.2 g

An apple
Calories: 81
Vitamin C: 7 mg
Fiber: 4 g

Grapefruit juice (1 cup)
Calories: 115
Vitamin C: 67 mg
Fiber: 0.2 g

Half a grapefruit
Calories: 60
Vitamin C: 62 mg
Fiber: 1.3 g

ChangeOne encourages you to help yourself to fruit not only at breakfast but for snacking, too. We stop short of saying you can eat as much fruit as you want because most fruit contains a fair amount of sugar, which means it adds

Continued on page 34

The Cereal Story

A good bowl of cereal, cold or hot, is one of the smartest breakfast choices you can make, as long as you choose wisely. Try to find cereals with lots of dietary fiber—at least 3 grams per serving. And check the ingredients for whole grains like oats or wheat. Pictured at right are the most familiar breakfast cereals in portions that contain 100 calories. Add milk and fruit and you'll have a complete meal.

A PERFECT BOWL OF CEREAL

- ²⁄₃ **cup bran flakes**
- 2 **tablespoons raisins**
- 2 **teaspoons chopped nuts or sunflower seeds (optional, but adds 30 additional calories)**
- 1 **half pint (8 ounces) skim or low-fat (1 percent) milk**

Calories 260, fat 3 g, saturated fat 1.5 g, cholesterol 15 mg, sodium 360 mg, carbohydrate 51 g, fiber 5 g, protein 13 g, calcium 300 mg.

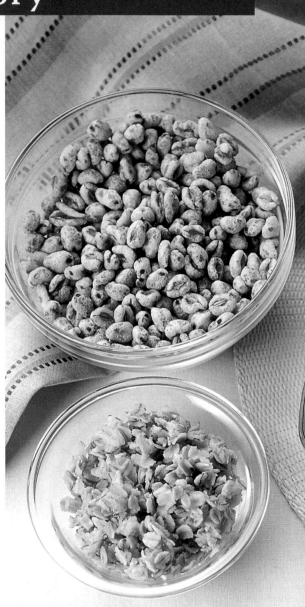

MAKE YOUR OWN

You can create your own signature breakfast cereal by mixing two or more different types. Here's a combination that will last for days:

- 4 cups puffed wheat cereal
- 1½ cups oat rings
- ½ cup low-fat granola
- 1½ cups bran flakes
- ½ cup sliced almonds

Mix and store in an air-tight container. One serving equals ¾ cup. You'll have a little left over after 10 servings.

Calories 130, fat 4 g, saturated fat 0 g, cholesterol 0 mg, sodium 115 mg, carbohydrate 21 g, fiber 3 g, protein 4 g, calcium 40 mg.

TIPS FOR TOPPINGS

Staring down the same old bowl of flakes can be daunting. Here are five toppings that can liven up your breakfast flakes for an additional 30 to 50 calories:

- 1 tablespoon shredded coconut
- 2 teaspoons chopped peanuts
- 1 teaspoon cinnamon-sugar
- ½ teaspoon cocoa powder
- 2 teaspoons mini chocolate chips

Clockwise from top left: 2 cups puffed wheat, ¾ cup corn flakes, 1 cup crispy rice, ¼ cup nuggets or low-fat granola, ⅔ cup wheat cereal (hot), ¾ cup oat rings, ½ cup sugar-coated flakes, ⅔ cup bran flakes, ⅔ cup oatmeal (hot).

HOT CEREALS

When it's cold outside there's nothing like a steaming bowl of hot cereal. Oatmeal and farina are classics, but there are many others to choose from:

- Cracked wheat*
- Cream of rice
- Grits
- Malt
- Maple wheat*
- Oat bran*

Extra high in fiber

ABOUT MILK

Still drinking whole milk? Now's the time to lighten up. Take it one change at a time: step down from whole milk to 2 percent, then from 2 percent to 1 percent. It won't take long before lower-fat milk tastes as good as what you were drinking before. Here's what you'll save in artery-clogging saturated fat and calories:

Type of milk	Saturated fat per cup	Calories
Whole (3.5% fat)	5 grams	149
Reduced fat (2%)	2.9 grams	122
Low fat (1%)	1.6 grams	102
Skim (nonfat)	0.3 grams	86

Continued from page 31
calories to your diet. But we've never met anyone who got fat eating too many mangoes. Certainly, if the choice is between a candy bar or a piece of fruit, reach for the fruit.

Weight Loss Secrets From the Dairy Case

Something else you'll notice about *ChangeOne* breakfasts: most of our meal plans include milk or yogurt. Nonfat or low-fat dairy products are a terrific low-calorie source of calcium, which you need for a key trio of health reasons: it helps keep bones strong, it reins in blood pressure, and recent studies suggest it may lower the risk of colon cancer.

Calcium also turns out to have a surprising weight-loss benefit. The evidence first showed up in a study designed to test whether men who added two cups of yogurt to their diet every day would lower their blood pressure; their read-

More Good Reasons to Fill Up on Fiber

With all the attention being given to carbohydrates, protein, and fat, it's easy to forget fiber. But when you're dieting, fiber could well be the part of food most worthy of focus.

Fiber, which is the indigestible part of food, gives whole grains, fruits, and vegetables their snap, crunch, and crispiness. And since your body can't digest fiber, it passes through without adding calories.

The research tells the story. In a 1999 study published in the *Journal of the American Medical Association*, scientists tracked the diets of 2,909 men and women over the course of 10 years. Those who chose high-fiber foods ended up weighing almost 10 pounds less, on average, than those who got very little fiber.

Chances are they scored in other ways, too. High-fiber foods have been shown to lower LDL cholesterol, the bad stuff. A study by University of Toronto researchers recently showed that a diet that gets more than one-third of its calories from high-fiber foods like fruit, vegetables, and nuts can lower LDL cholesterol by 33 percent. Volunteers on a high-fiber diet saw their LDL numbers drop within the first week.

Fiber eaters are also less likely to develop diabetes as adults. In two major studies conducted by researchers at the Harvard School of Public Health, people who ate the most fiber from whole grains had the lowest risk for type 2 diabetes: high-fiber grains cut their risk for the disease by 30 percent.

And here's one more reason to reach for whole grains, fruits, and vegetables: many studies show a lower risk of several kinds of cancer among people who include lots of fiber in their diets. By eating a healthier diet based on plant foods, most of us could cut our cancer risk by at least one-third, experts say.

> Fiber is the perfect diet food: no calories, and very filling.

Changing Time Zones

"Great," Walter Williams, 50, remembers thinking when he learned that the first step in *ChangeOne* was eating breakfast. "At last a diet that means I get to eat more, rather than less."

Like a lot of people, Williams, a systems engineer from Hartsdale, New York, mostly skipped the morning meal. By the time lunch rolled around, he remembers, he was ravenous.

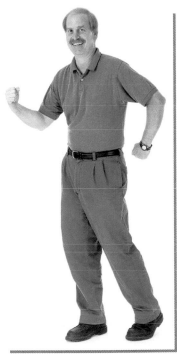

"I was so hungry I'd go through the lunch line at work and fill my tray as high as I could manage. Soup, an entrée, onion rings, french fries, a big glass of sweetened ice tea, dessert. Even after all that, when dinner time came along, I'd eat another giant meal. And often, at around nine in the evening, I'd make a sandwich or heat up a piece of pizza. I just seemed to be hungry all day."

At first Williams wasn't convinced that eating breakfast would help him get his appetite under control. Starting the day with a meal actually seemed to make him hungrier in the morning, he recalls. But he stuck with it, and after a week he noticed a change.

"At lunch, I felt less of an urge to eat everything in sight. Before long I was having a sandwich on whole wheat and maybe a piece of fruit. No french fries. No dessert. And that was enough to keep me satisfied through the afternoon."

Even at dinner, he found, he could eat less and still feel satisfied. He was also rarely tempted to fix a sandwich or pizza for the bedtime snack.

"Eating breakfast had the effect of time-shifting my appetite," he says. "I'm hungry in the morning now, and again at noon, and then at six for dinner. I'm eating earlier in the day. One effect has been to eliminate that big late-night snack I used to have. And I'm satisfied eating a much more reasonable lunch than before. All that from one simple change: eating breakfast."

Williams dropped 15 pounds on *ChangeOne*. His goal? Ten pounds.

ings did drop. They also lost weight—11 pounds in a year, on average. Another study showed that dieters who ate three to four servings of dairy products daily lost 70 percent more weight in six months than people on the same diet who were not eating dairy. And better still, those in the dairy group also lost more fat from around their middles.

The magic ingredient in dairy products seems to be calcium. One two-year study found that college-age women who ate a low-calcium diet gained weight; women who got plenty of calcium in their diets maintained a steady weight, or even lost a few pounds.

Pop a Pill

For years researchers were divided on the value of taking a multivitamin. Now there's a growing consensus that popping a one-a-day-type pill is a smart move.

In 2002, in fact, the *Journal of the American Medical Association* published a landmark article that recommended taking a multivitamin daily. We think that's especially smart advice when you're trying to cut back on calories. Even the best-planned diet, after all, can fall short on essential vitamins and minerals. A multivitamin will fill in any gaps.

Why? Experts have found that getting too little calcium triggers the release of a hormone called calcitriol, which tells the body to store fat rather than burn it. When calcium levels are high, calcitriol levels remain low, and the body burns fat instead of storing it. Calcium's not quite the whole story, since subjects who took a calcium supplement pill in the diet studies didn't lose quite as much weight as people who got the mineral in their meals. That finding suggests that something else in dairy products may help spur weight loss.

Okay, what if you're allergic to dairy? You're not alone. As many as 30 percent of people are lactose intolerant, which means they do not have enough of the lactase enzyme, crucial for the digestion of milk sugars. But even with low lactase, experts say, you may be able to digest milk with no stomach discomfort thanks to sugar-processing microbes we all carry in our intestines. If you're lactose intolerant and want to find out if these microbes will help your body tolerate dairy on a small level, try adding milk gradually to your diet, rather than all at once. Start with a half cup a day.

Of course, you don't have to drink milk or eat other dairy products to be healthy or lose weight. You can substitute low-fat soy milk or rice milk and get calcium other ways—from a supplement, for example, or in calcium-fortified foods. The *ChangeOne* menu includes several foods with added calcium to help you hit the target level. Other nondairy sources rich in calcium include tofu, oatmeal, beans, and dark leafy green vegetables like collards, spinach, and mustard greens.

Changes Ahead: Lunch

This week, while you focus on breakfast, keep an eye on what you eat for lunch. Don't change your lunch menu; we'll get to that next week. Eat the way you normally do for the rest of the day. Just keep track of where you have lunch and what you usually eat. Be aware of the choices you have: Eat out? At your desk? Cafeteria? Restaurant? Deli? And be alert to how you feel. Is lunch something you jam into the middle of a frantic day, for instance, or is it a time when you relax and recharge your batteries? On at least one day write down exactly what you have for lunch and estimate the serving sizes. If you have time, keep a small notebook handy and write down what you eat for lunch each day of the week.

More Breakfast Choices

Can't find something you like from among the five suggested breakfasts? Starting on page 252 you'll find more quick and delicious *ChangeOne* breakfasts. Here's a sampler:

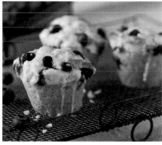

Blueberry Muffins with Lemon Glaze
page 252

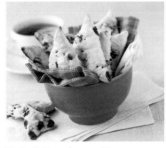

Dried Cranberry Scones with Orange Glaze
page 253

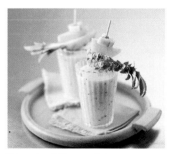

Tropical Smoothie
page 254

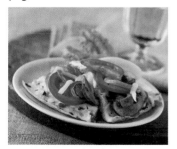

Vegetable Frittata
page 255

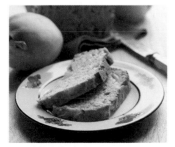

Peach Quick Bread
page 256

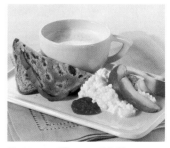

Cottage Cheese Melba
page 258

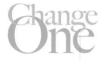

Week 2
Lunch

Contrary to what you've heard, the single biggest problem Americans face in the battle of the bulge isn't *what* they eat, it's *how much*. We now annually gobble up 140 pounds more food per person, on average, than we did in 1990. How is that possible? Take a look at lunch.

Giant cheeseburgers with strips of bacon, 64-ounce jumbo drinks, super-size fries: runaway inflation has hit the luncheon counter.

This week sanity prevails. You'll eat delicious lunches that satisfy without crazy excess.

For many people lunch presents the biggest challenge of the day. We grab our midday meals in the middle of crowded schedules, work, errands, and distractions. And because lunch is the meal we're least likely to eat at home, we typically have less control over what's on the menu.

But that's all the more reason for you to learn ways to make lunch a great-tasting, sensible meal. With some advance planning, and using the lunches in this chapter and on pages 259-267, you'll be able to keep your calories in line and still keep the midday meal an event to enjoy.

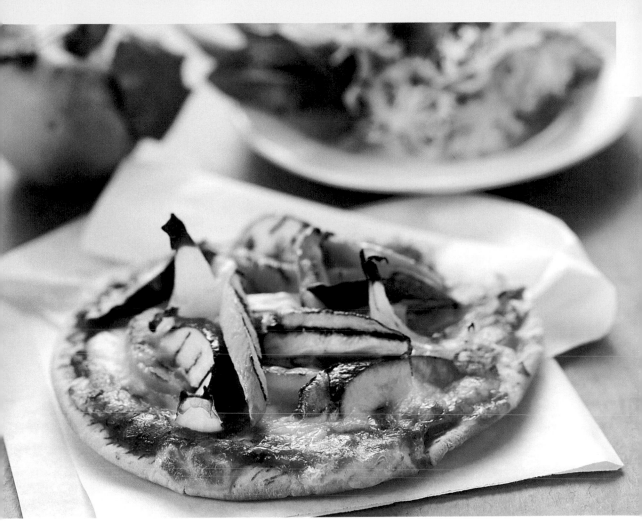

Pizza and Salad

Pita Pizza

- **1 2-ounce pita bread**
- **2 tablespoons tomato sauce**
- **¼ cup grated part-skim mozzarella**
  Grilled vegetables

1 green salad, unlimited, with 2 tablespoons fat-free dressing (2 salad dressing caps), or reduced-fat Italian dressing (adds about 30 calories)

1 apple

To prepare pizza:
Spread sauce on pita bread, sprinkle with cheese, top with grilled vegetables, and bake at 350ºF until cheese bubbles, about 5 minutes. For ham or pepperoni pizza, use half the amount of cheese and top with a couple of thin slices of the meat.

Calories 370, fat 11 g, saturated fat 3.5 g, cholesterol 15 mg, sodium 620 mg, carbohydrate 55 g, fiber 7 g, protein 15 g, calcium 300 mg.

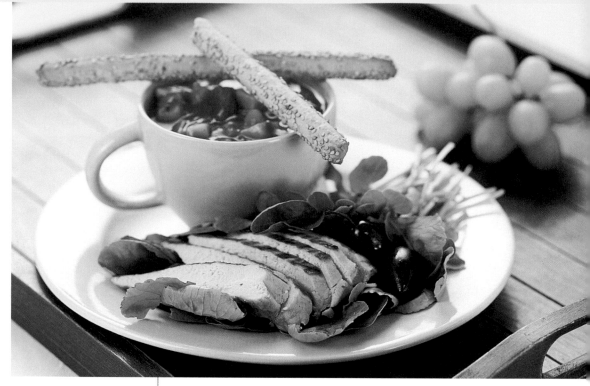

Soup and Salad

1 cup vegetable soup (diner coffee cup)

2 breadsticks, medium

1 green salad, unlimited, topped with:

>   **2 ounces grilled chicken**
>   **2 tablespoons olives,**
>   **or 1 tablespoon chopped nuts,**
>   **or 1 tablespoon grated cheese**
>   **2 tablespoons fat-free dressing** (2 salad dressing caps)**, or**
>   **reduced-fat Italian dressing (adds about 30 calories)**

½ cup grapes (cupped handful)

Calories 350, fat 10 g, saturated fat 2.5 g, cholesterol 60 mg, sodium 1,680 mg, carbohydrate 39 g, fiber 5 g, protein 26 g, calcium 100 mg.

ABOUT SOUP

Soup is great for staving off hunger. Researchers at Penn State University discovered that chicken rice soup was more filling than the same amount of chicken and rice with a glass of water. Why? Soup is satisfying because it brings out all the flavors of its ingredients. Also, it may linger longer in your stomach, which will keep you feeling full.

Instead of	Try
Vegetable soup (1 cup, 72 calories)	Gazpacho (1 cup, 46 calories)
	Beef barley (1 cup, 67 calories)
	Chicken noodle (1 cup, 75 calories)
	Manhattan clam chowder (1 cup, 78 calories)
	Minestrone (1 cup, 82 calories)
	Tomato (1 cup, 85 calories)

Don't Let Lunch Blindside You

Let's face it: food corporations have our number. Super-size it! Two sweet rolls for the price of one! A free bucket-sized soda when you order the giant fries!

We're conditioned to look for a good deal, and more food for less money sounds about as good as it gets.

But consider the numbers. A double cheeseburger with bacon weighs in at a massive 600 calories. Add on the large fries and you get another 500 calories. With a small drink—or what passes for small these days—you're up to about 1,300 calories.

That's the basic *ChangeOne* calorie target for a whole day, all in one meal!

Of course, most dieters know better than to order a huge, fatty meal. But even healthy-sounding lunch selections can hide a surprising number of calories. Crispy chicken? "I always thought chicken was the healthiest choice," one of our volunteers told us. Then she learned that at one leading restaurant chain, a single such serving packs 550 calories. An individual-size pizza? Throw on the toppings and the calories can exceed 800. Taco salad? Order one at another well-known lunch spot and you'll help yourself to more than 900 calories. You get the point.

Unless you have a clear idea of what to choose—and

Lunch Portions

These meal plans use both standard measurements and the *ChangeOne* portion-size guide. Here's what a standard serving looks like (members of the 1,600 Club can double your protein portion at lunch or dinner; *or* double your starch or grain at dinner):

Type of food	Example	Amount	*ChangeOne* guide
One starch or grain	Potato	Medium	Tennis ball
	Roll	2 ounces	Tennis ball
	Pasta, rice	⅔ cup	Tennis ball
One protein	Cheese	¼ cup grated	Palmful
	Lunch meat	2–3 ounces	2–3 CDs
One fruit	Orange, apple	1	
	Berries, cut fruit	½ cup	Cupped handful
Vegetables		Unlimited	

make sure that you can get it—you could find yourself having to pick between going hungry during the day or going overboard on calories.

Making the Change

This week, while you keep up the good work at breakfast, help yourself to your choice of the *ChangeOne* lunches pictured on the pages of this chapter. *ChangeOne* lunches contain about 350 calories. That includes everything—eats and drinks. Compare that to the calories in most fast-food and deli meals and you'll see why sticking to the *ChangeOne* menu will speed your weight loss.

The meal plans you'll find here include lunches you can make at home, lunches you can pack, lunches you can order at a good deli or sandwich shop that's willing to do it your way, and even a fast-food meal that will work for you. Mix and match them any way you like. If you prefer to have pretty much the same lunch every day, go for it. If variety is the spice of your life, there are plenty of options here. What matters is sticking as closely as you can to the *ChangeOne* lunch plan every day this coming week.

As much as possible, decide in advance what and where you're going to eat. Right off the bat you're in control. No more putting yourself at the mercy of the burger hut because it's the only thing you can find. No more searching the vending machine for something, anything, that looks halfway healthy. No more raiding that bag of tortilla chips because you're famished and it's the only edible item in the drawer.

Instead, consider some other options.

If you eat most of your lunches out: Make a list of the *ChangeOne* lunches that you'll be able to order at your favorite lunch spot or company cafeteria. Try to choose a place that really will do it your way, including keeping por-

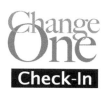

Check-In

Over the past week you began to take control of breakfast. If you weren't a breakfast eater before, you've become one. If you were already sitting down to the breakfast table, you've started helping yourself to healthier choices or more sensible portions. Don't sweat it if you ended up grabbing a sweet roll one morning on the way into work. The important thing is not to fall into the trap of thinking you failed just because you had a misstep. What matters is that you're finding time to sit down first thing in the morning to a breakfast that starts your new healthy diet off on the right track. If you're not quite there yet, consider taking another week to get breakfast under control. With the confidence that comes with making just this one change for the better, you'll find it will be easier to move forward with the next change. If you feel comfortable with breakfast, you're ready to move on to lunch.

Change One Fast Track

If you're anxious to speed your progress, choose one or two of the following Fast Track changes and you're likely to see pounds melt away faster:

Turn off the TV

At least three times this week, turn off the television and walk for half an hour when you would otherwise have sat in front of the tube. It doesn't take a genius to figure out that sitting around watching television is bad for anyone's waistline. Yet even researchers have been surprised by the link between TV viewing and tubbiness.

Women who watch three hours of television a day have an average body mass index (BMI) that is 1.8 points higher than those who watch just one hour a day, according to a recent study by University of Utah researchers. For a 5-foot-7-inch woman, that's an extra 12 pounds. (To calculate your BMI, check out page 311.)

Hate to miss your favorite shows? Tape the ones you really want to see. By fast-forwarding through the commercials you'll save at least eight minutes per half-hour show—extra minutes you can grab to do something active and keep off the couch.

Put down your fork

When you eat too fast, you deny your body the time it needs to signal that you're full. Experts say it takes about 20 minutes from the time you start eating for your stomach and brain to coordinate on these so-called satiety signals.

This week during lunch and dinner, lay your utensils down between each bite. Take notice of what happens when you slow down. Savor what you're eating. And try another tactic: the minute you feel satisfied, get up from the table. Quit eating, even if there's still food on your plate.

Pour it on

This week carry a bottle of water with you and take a swig whenever you feel thirsty. That way you'll be less tempted to grab a sugary, calorie-filled drink. And drink one eight-ounce glass of water with lunch and dinner. When you include a glass of water with your meal, you get some calorie-free help on quenching your hunger along with your thirst.

Use the 50-percent solution

Dinner portions, like lunch, are often bigger than most of us want or need. And since dinner's usually the biggest meal of the day, giant portions can really pile on the calories. This week downsize your dinner entrées. Serve up half of what you normally would eat. After you're done take a few minutes to relax and savor the meal. If you're still hungry, help yourself to half of what's left over. Otherwise, get up from the table.

Create a diversion

Identify one time of the day when you're eating for no other reason than because that's when you typically eat. This wouldn't be a regular mealtime, but perhaps a midmorning coffee break, afternoon snack, or late-evening splurge.

Now instead of eating at that time, do something else—something that really appeals to you. Read the paper, take a brief stroll, pursue a hobby, call a friend—anything that gets you through that period. You may find that the reason you ate at that time was habit, not hunger. Develop a habit that doesn't involve food and you could cut more than 100 calories a day.

Chef's Salad

Time-Saver

Purchase a quarter pound at a time of different thin-sliced lunch meats. Roll up each meat and slice crosswise into fourths. When making your salad, top with one piece each of three different meats.

Salad greens, unlimited, topped with:

> **1 ounce turkey breast**
> **1 ounce deli ham**
> **¾ ounce cheese**
> **2 tablespoons fat-free dressing** (2 salad dressing caps)**, or reduced-fat Italian dressing (adds about 30 calories)**

1 **medium whole grain roll (2 ounces)** (tennis ball)

½ **cup cantaloupe** (cupped handful)

Calories 340, fat 10 g, saturated fat 4.5 g, cholesterol 40 mg, sodium 1,620 mg, carbohydrate 45 g, fiber 7 g, protein 22 g, calcium 250 mg.

TIPS FOR TOPPINGS

Combine any three of these to top your salad. Serving size for each is 1 ounce (the size of a CD, or as indicated), slightly less for cheese:

- Turkey breast
- Chicken breast
- Lean roast beef
- Shredded chicken
- Deli ham

- Canned tuna (in water)
- Swiss cheese
- Cheddar cheese
- Smoked gouda
- Grated parmesan, ¼ cup (palmful)

- Tofu cubes (thumb)
- Kidney or other beans, 2 tablespoons (2 thumbs)
- Chopped nuts, 1 tablespoon (thumb)

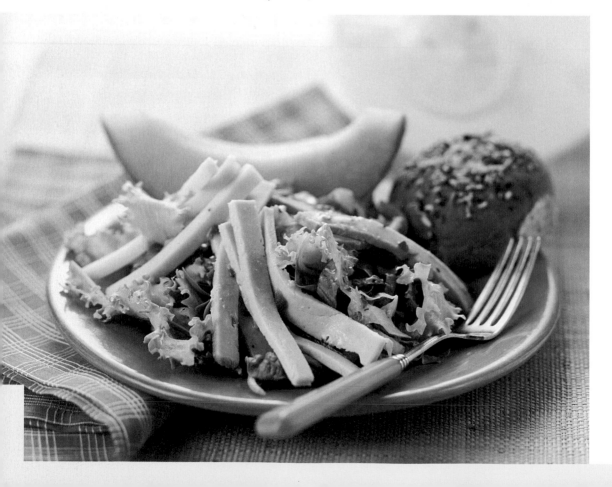

tion sizes under control. When in doubt, eyeball the serving sizes in this chapter for a rough idea of what a *ChangeOne* lunch should look like. Keep the handy visual equivalents in mind. Before you dig into lunch, make sure that what's on your plate matches up. At some lunch places, you may end up eating just half of what you're served and taking the rest home. Ask for a to-go container when you place your order, and enjoy what's left over tomorrow. Think of it as two meals for the price of one. Now that's a bargain.

If you usually eat at home: Choose the meals you think you'll like the best from the *ChangeOne* lunch suggestions. Or try a different one each day this week. You may find that something you wouldn't normally eat tastes great and really fills you up. Remember, there's little risk. If you feel ravenous by midafternoon, you can have a snack and your usual dinner later. Eventually you may want to stick to one or two particular meals (See "Keep It Simple," below). If you end up going for a wide variety, consider writing each day's lunch menu on your calendar the way fine restaurants post their menu *du jour*. When you begin to feel hungry as the noon hour approaches, you'll know exactly what's coming

If you plan to pack a sack: Make up your shopping list and buy what you'll need at the beginning of the week. Don't forget lunch bags and storage containers. If your early mornings are crazy, do as much preparation as you can the night before; until you get in the swing of packing your lunch, it's easy to rush out the door empty-handed. Write "Got Lunch?" on a note and stick it on the refrigerator or front door to make sure you won't forget.

Keep It Simple

Many people prefer not having to decide every day what they're going to eat. They find it comforting to open up the lunch sack to the same peanut butter and jelly sandwich with an apple and an oatmeal raisin cookie. And talk about being in control: if you eat the same lunch every day, you never have to wonder about how many calories you're get-

Help!

"I don't have a refrigerator at work to store my sack lunch. Should I worry about food going bad?"

No. The packable lunches on the *ChangeOne* menu will keep just fine for five hours in a coolish spot on a shelf or in a desk drawer. To be on the safe side, try a few simple preparation tips:

- Freeze a small plastic bottle of water to use as a sandwich chiller, and then as a drink.
- Use a refreezable ice pack.
- Buy an insulated lunch box.
- Peel eggs only when you're ready to eat them.

ting. Some diet experts even recommend monotonous meals. In one study volunteers who were offered a four-course meal consumed 44 percent more calories than those offered just one course.

Still, not everyone wants to sit down to the same thing every day. And variety will give you this: by trying out several *ChangeOne* lunch options, you'll find the ones that work best for you. All that really matters is arriving at a plan for lunch that you can stick with.

Behind the *ChangeOne* Lunch Menu

You may be surprised by some of the choices you find on the *ChangeOne* lunch menu. Like avocado slices. Peanut butter. Cheese. Nuts. None of these would make its way into a low-fat diet. Yet we've included them in *ChangeOne* for a very good reason. The latest evidence demonstrates that you don't have to cut way back on fat to lose weight. New data even show that most people shed pounds more successfully on diets containing moderate amounts of fat than they do on very low-fat regimens.

Surprised? For years nutritionists have told us to cut back on fat—all fat. Too much fat on the menu makes people fat, they said. Gram for gram, fat contains twice as many calories as protein or carbohydrates. Just as bad, it puts our hearts and arteries at risk by increasing cholesterol. Or so the experts said.

And we listened. Over the past three decades the total percent of calories from fat in the American diet has fallen by a remarkable six percent.

But now, in a stunning reversal, the experts are offering very different advice. Some fats are actually good for our hearts, they say. What's more, slashing fat from your diet, rather than helping you lose weight, may actually make it harder to maintain a healthy weight. Very low-fat diets could even be unhealthy.

Good Fat, Bad Fat

Truth is, experts have long known that there are various kinds of fat. The two main categories are saturated fat and unsaturated fat. Saturated fat comes mainly from animals,

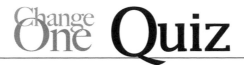

Ready For Lunch?

Thinking over the food choices you made last week will help you find the best ways to master the midday meal this week. Complete these nine questions by circling the number to the right of the appropriate answer.

1. **Last week how often did you know in the morning what you'd have for lunch?**

Never	1
A few days	2
Most days	3
Every day	4

2. **How often did you know at least where you would have lunch?**

Never	1
A few days	2
Most days	3
Every day	4

3. **How often did you grab whatever happened to be handy?**

Most days	1
Several days	2
Rarely or never	3

4. **Which phrase best describes the choices available to you at lunch?**

Very little choice	1
Some choice—same three or four things	2
Ample choice—varied and interesting	3

5. **How would you rate your typical lunch?**

Not very healthy	1
Healthy enough	2
Very healthy	3

6. **How many servings of vegetables did you typically eat at lunch? (French fries don't count.)**

None	1
1	2
2 or more	3

7. **What was your usual choice for a sandwich bread?**

White or French roll	1
Whole wheat, rye, or other dark brown bread	2
Seven-grain or other whole-grain bread	3

8. **How often did you eat lunch at home this past week or bring lunch to work?**

Never	1
1-2 times	2
3-4 times	3
5-7 times	4

9. **What was your usual beverage at lunch?**

Regular soft drink	1
Sweetened fruit drink	2
Milk, sugar-free soft drink, or water	3

Turn to next page to tally your score.

47

Quiz Score

Add up the numbers you've circled in the right-hand column.
A score of 24-30: You're already well on your way to eating a good lunch.
A score of 19-23: A few simple strategy changes could help make the switch to a *ChangeOne* lunch easier.
A score of 9-18: Okay, you've got serious work to do. By improving your lunches, you can take a giant step toward trimming calories and slimming your waistline. Put checks beside questions that scored a 1 or 2. Then look for the corresponding answers in the key below for tips that will help you this coming week.

1, 2, 3. If you have no idea where you'll have lunch—or what you'll choose—you're at risk of grabbing whatever's handy when lunchtime rolls around. That could spell trouble for your diet. Study the tips on pages 42 and 45 to master lunch by planning ahead.

Of course not all of us always know ahead of time where we'll eat lunch. If that sounds like you, then it's time to keep a very close watch on portion sizes, wherever lunch hour finds you.

4. When your choices are limited, your best option may be to bag it—lunch, that is. You'll find several tasty packable lunches in the *ChangeOne* menus. If you're pressed for time in the morning, put your lunch together the night before.

5. Is your lunch falling short on good nutrition? Most of what's available at fast-food restaurants and other lunch spots is high in saturated fat and sugar and low in fiber and nutrients. If your typical lunch rarely sees a green vegetable, it needs work. If there's a huge cheeseburger on your lunch tray—well, you already know there's work to do. If the lunch spots available don't offer much choice, your best bet is to bring your own meal.

6. What, no vegetables? You're missing out on one of the best health and diet foods around. Follow the *ChangeOne* menu this week and you'll get at least one serving at lunch, usually two.

7. Breaking the white bread habit can be tough, but you'll get more nutrients—and feel fuller longer—when you eat breads that are made from whole wheat or rye flour. You'll get even more fiber, plus healthful vitamins and minerals, from breads that contain whole grains like oats.

8. Don't dismiss the idea of brown-bagging your lunch. This week give it a try for a day or two. There's no better way to control exactly what and how much you eat. Many people find that packing a lunch relieves them of the pressure of having to choose the food they'll have when they're hungry. Not to mention the fact that it will save you a *lot* of money.

9. Sugary soft drinks and fruit-based beverages pack a load of calories. Some experts place much of the blame for the country's growing weight problems on the popularity of colas. No wonder: the sugar and corn syrup in soft drinks, added to juices and laced in sports drinks, now supply more than 10 percent of our total calories.

That's an awful lot of calories from foods that don't supply much else in the way of nutrition. Switch to a sugar-free beverage or help yourself to a glass of plain or sparkling water, and you'll shave 150 calories from your diet just like that.

Nonfat or low-fat milk, a great source of calcium, is another smart choice. Sure, milk contains calories, but it's also loaded with protein and calcium. Calcium is essential for healthy bones. And as you discovered last week, there's new evidence that it also helps speed weight loss by encouraging your body to burn more fat.

either in the form of meat or the fat in cheese, milk, and other dairy. Unsaturated fat comes mainly from plants and fish. One of the biggest sources in our diets is vegetable oils such as corn, safflower, olive, peanut, and canola.

When it comes to heart disease, the culprit is saturated fat. Because of its chemical makeup, saturated fat causes the body to churn out extra LDL cholesterol, the harmful, artery-clogging kind.

Unsaturated fat, in contrast, has been shown to lower LDL. Further, it can also raise HDL cholesterol, the friendly form that removes dangerous cholesterol from the body. Remarkably, getting plenty of unsaturated fat actually protects your arteries from hardening. Studies around the world bear it out: the less saturated fat and the more unsaturated fat people eat, the lower their risk of heart disease.

So why did so many nutritionists recommend cutting back on all fat? Because some of them thought the good fat/bad fat message was too complicated for people to understand. By telling people to cut back on all fat, the thinking went, saturated fat levels would fall. And with the nation's waistline expanding, cutting back on total fat didn't seem like such a bad idea.

A diet too low in fat may actually make it harder to lose weight.

Carbohydrates Aren't So Simple

When we dutifully cut back on fat, we replaced it largely with carbohydrates, mostly the simple kind found in French fries, white bread, crackers, and sugar. That's bad news for two reasons. First, it turns out that a high-carbohydrate, low-fat diet of this kind increases levels of triglycerides, a form of fat in the blood. Higher triglyceride levels are strongly linked to a greater danger of heart disease.

Second, a diet low in fat and high in simple carbohydrates may actually make it harder, rather than easier, to lose weight. Simple carbohydrates, because they are so easy for the body to digest, send blood sugar levels spiking up. The surge in blood sugar triggers a surge in insulin from the pancreas. That's normal. One of insulin's jobs is to move blood sugar into muscles, where it provides fuel for movement. But another of its roles is to prompt the body to store excess energy as fat. That's normal, too. But if blood sugar and insulin levels continually spike and then drop, it can

Friendly Fast-Food

1 regular hamburger, with desired condiments

1 green salad, unlimited, topped with chopped vegetables (tomato, red cabbage, green pepper)

2 tablespoons fat-free dressing (2 salad dressing caps), or reduced-fat Italian dressing (adds about 30 calories)

Calories 310, fat 14 g, saturated fat 4 g, cholesterol 30 mg, sodium 660 mg, carbohydrate 36 g, fiber 3 g, protein 14 g, calcium 150 mg.

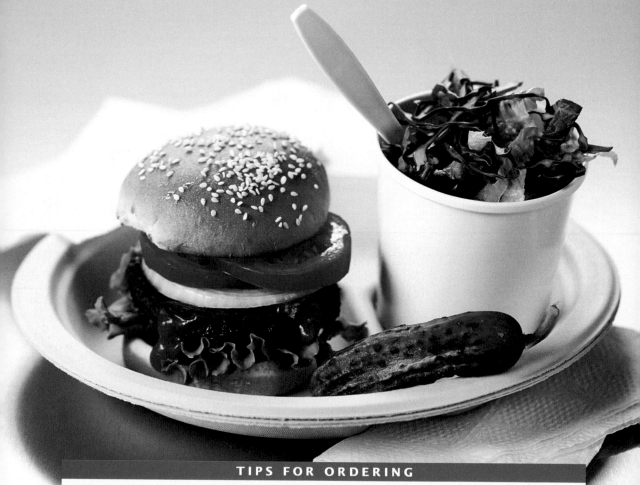

TIPS FOR ORDERING

The nation's favorite fast-food chains offer some lower-calorie picks. Ask the restaurant where they've posted their nutrition information. Be sure to choose entrées that fall between 260 and 310 calories. Here are some safe choices:

Taco Bell: Tostada, Gordita Supreme, Soft Taco Supreme
Burger King: Hamburger, Whopper Jr. (no mayo)
McDonald's: Hamburger, chicken McGrill (no mayo), any salad (fat-free dressing)
Wendy's: Jr. hamburger, grilled chicken sandwich, small chili with cheese
Subway: Any "7 Under 6" sandwich

spell trouble. And that's what seems to happen when you eat a lot of simple, easy-to-digest carbohydrates. When blood sugar slumps, we feel hungry. Naturally, we reach for something to eat. And if that something is another simple carbohydrate, up go the blood sugar levels. The resulting roller coaster, researchers are beginning to think, makes people hungry more often during the day, and the surges of insulin prime the body to store fat.

There's still much unresolved about the roles of carbohydrates, insulin, and blood sugar levels. But one thing is certain: cutting back on total fat and filling up on simple carbohydrates like low-fat crackers and cakes hasn't made us thinner. We're fatter than ever. And evidence is accumulating that a diet with moderate amounts of fat in it may make it easier to shed pounds.

Eat Fat, Get Slim

Consider the surprising results of an experiment conducted at Brigham and Women's Hospital in Boston. Thirty overweight people followed a low-fat diet. Another group of 31 people followed a diet with a moderate amount of fat—very much like the *ChangeOne* diet. The total calorie target was the same for both groups. Six months later volunteers in the two groups had lost the same amount of weight. But after 18 months a telltale difference surfaced: only 20 percent of the people in the low-fat group were still following the diet, compared to 54 percent of those in the moderate-fat group. What's more, the moderate-fat dieters, as a group, had lost more body fat and slimmed their waistlines more than the low-fat dieters.

Why? One reason, researchers say, is that a diet with moderate amounts of fat is simply more satisfying than a harsh low-fat regimen. It's a healthy diet people can live

Continued on page 54

Help!

"Last week I was so hungry by the middle of the morning that I felt almost light-headed. Is that normal?"

Well, the light-headed part is. Hunger can make you feel woozy. It can also make you feel distracted or grumpy. If you get that hungry, however—at any time of the day—it's time to eat something. If you're especially heavy or active, you may simply need more calories. Your body is burning more to keep you moving.

We're not talking about scarfing down donut holes. In a reduced-calorie diet like *ChangeOne*, it's important to make every calorie count for nourishment. Choose snacks that do what they're supposed to do: take the edge off hunger. Next week we'll take a closer look at snacks. For now, consider helping yourself to one of the following if hunger threatens:

■ A piece of fruit
■ A handful of nuts (about one ounce)
■ All the celery or carrot sticks you like
■ As big a glass of tomato or vegetable juice as you want
■ Popcorn (skip the butter and you can help yourself to 2 cups worth)
■ A cup of chicken or miso soup
■ A cup of nonfat or low-fat milk, or a cup of nonfat or low-fat yogurt

Don't be afraid to reach for a snack. One recent survey found that snacking wasn't the downfall of most failed dieters; what got most of them into trouble was losing control at one of the three big meals of the day. Tame your hunger and you'll stay in control.

Build a Better Sandwich

A deli can be a dieter's best friend, believe it or not. The options are endless, and if you're vigilant, you can craft a satisfying and sensible sandwich.

But whether you're ordering over the counter or making your own, keep an eye on what's in even the supposed lightweight choices—turkey, tuna, even meatless options. You can easily overstuff a sandwich with 5 to 8 ounces of meat (twice as much as it's smart to swallow in a meal) or drown it with mayonnaise (as much as 700 calories worth in a tuna salad sandwich).

What you get, the experts point out, can be a day's worth of calories between two slices of bread. Not only will that blow your diet, it will also put you to sleep by midafternoon.

What you want is what you see here. Check out these *ChangeOne* tips for building a better sandwich.

THE PERFECT DELI LUNCH

Turkey and Swiss cheese sandwich

> **2 slices whole wheat bread**
> **2 ounces deli turkey breast**
> **2/3 ounce Swiss cheese**
> **Lettuce, tomato, pickles, mustard, onion, peppers, unlimited**

½ cup Italian pickled vegetable salad (cupped handful)

½ cup melon

Calories 330, fat 10 g, saturated fat 4 g, cholesterol 40 mg, sodium 1,750 mg, carbohydrate 43 g, fiber 7 g, protein 23 g, calcium 250 mg.

Bread
- Whole grain roll (tennis ball)
- Rye bread, 2 slices
- Pumpernickel bread, 2 slices
- Italian, French, or sourdough bread, 2 slices
- Tortilla, medium
- Sub roll, 3 inches

Meats
- Turkey, 2 ounces (2 CDs)
- Deli ham, 2 ounces
- Lean roast beef, 2 ounces
- Corned beef, 1½ ounces
- Tuna salad (with low-fat mayo), ½ cup (2 golf balls)

Meat alternatives
- 2 tablespoons peanut butter (2 thumbs)
- 2 tablespoons soy nut butter
- 2 tablespoons tofu cream cheese
- 3 tablespoons hummus (3 thumbs)
- ¼ avocado, sliced

Complements
- Reduced-fat cheddar or jack cheese, ⅔ ounce (palmful)
- Lettuce, tomato, grilled vegetables, unlimited
- Spinach, arugula, watercress leaves, unlimited
- Thinly sliced apple, 3 slices
- Jam for peanut butter, 2 teaspoons (2 thumb tips)
- Hummus, 1 tablespoon (thumb)
- Pickles, unlimited

Okay, you can enjoy your deli favorites if you keep to a modest 2 ounces of filling (2 CDs). That said, here are popular lunch meats ranked from best to "wurst" based on calories and artery-clogging fat. There's no harm in enjoying them once in a while, but keep in mind that they're all higher in calories than leaner fillings like turkey breast.

- Prosciutto di Parma
- Turkey salami
- Beer salami
- Corned beef
- Beef salami
- Cotto salami
- Beef bologna
- Liverwurst
- Beef pastrami
- Genoa salami
- Dry salami

Dressings
- Yellow mustard, unlimited
- Dijon mustard, unlimited
- Honey mustard, 2 teaspoons (2 thumb tips)
- Low-fat mayonnaise, 1 tablespoon (thumb)
- Apple butter, 2 teaspoons (2 thumb tips)
- Fat-free salad dressing, 2 tablespoons (2 salad dressing caps), or reduced-fat dressing (adds about 30 calories)

Continued from page 51
with. And that's the only kind of diet that really works over the long term. Another reason may be that people consuming moderate amounts of fat are less likely to overdo simple carbohydrates and will find it easier to keep hunger in check.

The new advice is the same whether you hope to protect your heart or shed excess weight. Replace saturated fat with unsaturated fat wherever you can. Switch from butter to olive or canola oil, for instance, and eat less meat and more fish. (Fish is abundant in polyunsaturated fats, particularly a form that contains omega-3 fatty acids, which have been shown to protect the heart.) Keep portion sizes under control so you don't overdo calories. And steer your diet away from simple carbohydrates like sugar and white bread and toward more complex carbohydrates like those in whole-grain breads and cereals. These recommendations are the basis of the *ChangeOne* menu because they are the surest strategy for slimming down and keeping pounds off—not just for a few weeks, but for good.

Sandwich Sides

Stumped by side salads? Choose one of these—and keep in mind that pickles are freebies:

- Green salad topped with chopped veggies (tomato, cucumber, peppers, broccoli, etc.), two tablespoons sliced olives, a couple shakes of olive oil, and vinegar
- "Clear" coleslaw, made with vinegar and a touch of sugar rather than mayo, ½ cup
- Three-bean salad, ½ cup
- Italian-style pickled vegetables, unlimited
- Grilled vegetables, unlimited (but not too oily)
- Sliced or diced tomato, unlimited

The Perfect Diet Food

Something else you'll notice about the *ChangeOne* lunch menu: it features plenty of vegetables. Every meal includes at least one serving, often two. No other food fills you up on fewer calories while delivering more nutrients. Vegetables are rich not only in fiber but also in disease-fighting antioxidants. They're mostly complex carbohydrates, the kind that keep blood sugar levels off the roller coaster. Vegetables are so good in so many ways that they're free on *ChangeOne*—with the exception of potatoes, which are high in simple carbohydrates.

And as any chef will tell you, nothing brightens up a plate like dark leafy greens, red or yellow peppers, a luscious ripe tomato, or rich orange carrot slices. On the *ChangeOne* lunch menu, you'll find plenty of clever ways to add a serving or two of vegetables to your favorite sandwiches and soups to make them not only more filling, but more flavorful . . . without piling on calories.

Burrito to Go

1 medium tortilla (7-8 inches), filled with:

   2 ounces grilled chicken
   1 tablespoon refried beans
   1 tablespoon guacamole
   1 tablespoon shredded cheese
   Salsa, unlimited
   Shredded lettuce and diced tomato, unlimited

1 orange

To prepare a burrito:

Place chicken, beans, and cheese on tortilla. Microwave for
30 seconds, or until filling is warm. Add remaining ingredients,
roll up, and eat.

Calories 370, fat 8 g, saturated fat 3 g, cholesterol 55 mg, sodium 510 mg,
carbohydrate 49 g, fiber 7 g, protein 26 g, calcium 200 mg.

Time-Saver
*Purchase cheese that is
already shredded,
possibly seasoned,
and sold in a resealable
plastic bag.*

ABOUT TORTILLAS

Choose a small- to
medium-sized tor-
tilla—corn or flour—
to keep calories in
check. A large flour
tortilla has as many
calories as four
slices of bread.

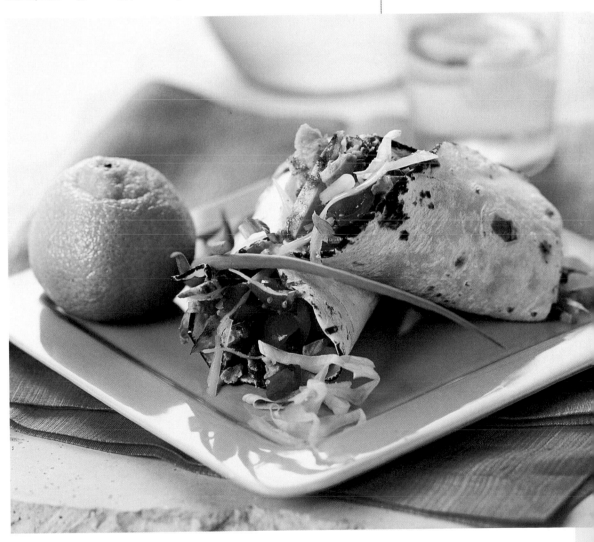

Change One First Person

In the Groove

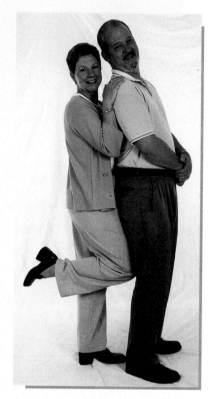

"It's gotten to be a joke around our household," says Sue Licher, a university administrator who lives in Cedar Rapids, Iowa. **"Every day my husband fixes the same sandwich. Turkey on whole wheat. An apple. Carrot sticks. Baked potato chips. Every day.**

"I try to throw in a little variety myself. A different sandwich. A salad. A cup of yogurt. For both of us, packing a lunch has made a big difference. Before that we pretty much ate whatever happened to be around at work."

Mark Licher had never dieted before he and his wife started *ChangeOne*. "The first time we went shopping for the breakfast week, I remember kidding around and saying, 'My life as I knew it is over.' But it's funny the way it works. I didn't eat breakfast before we started *ChangeOne*, except a sweet roll sometimes. Now I eat melon and a piece of toast, and I'm not tempted to eat the pastries people bring into the office. I'm just not hungry for them. And now that I'm packing a lunch, I'm fine through the afternoon. Sure, it's the same lunch every day. But the truth is, I was always eating exactly the same lunch every day before I started *ChangeOne*. It just happened to be a fast-food cheeseburger with fries. I guess I like the routine. My lunch now is a whole lot healthier than it was before."

What his wife likes best is feeling in control. "Breakfast and lunch are the easiest for me. It's easy to get into a routine during the weekdays. Since both of us have our work routines, fitting *ChangeOne* in was a cinch. And once you've got the first two meals of the day under control, the rest of the day begins to feel manageable."

Five weeks into the program, Sue Licher has lost 15 pounds. Mark is down 11, and on a roll. "I'm really in the groove right now. It's strange to say it, but I actually find myself thinking about and enjoying food much more than I did before we started. And I'm losing weight. Go figure."

Changes Ahead: Snacks

While you're settling on your *ChangeOne* meals for breakfast and lunch, be aware of times during the day when you have a snack attack—and what you typically do about it. Don't feel like you have to change anything about your snacks just yet. But be aware of how you feel, the choices you've given yourself, and what you usually do to satisfy the munchies or a sweet tooth. If you have time, keep track of all the snacks you eat and about how much of each you eat. In Week 3 we'll take a closer look at hunger and the best ways to satisfy it.

More Lunch Choices

Can't find something you like from the six suggested lunches in this chapter? Starting on page 259 you'll find more quick and delicious *ChangeOne* lunches. Here's a sampler:

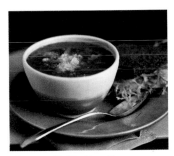

Hearty Split-Pea Soup
page 260

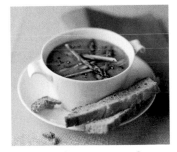

Cream of Asparagus Soup
page 261

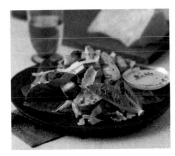

Grilled Turkey Caesar Salad
page 263

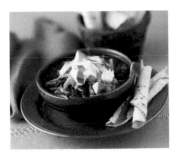

Meatless Chili Pots con Queso
page 265

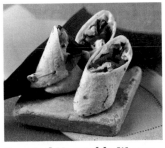

Roasted Vegetable Wraps with Chive Sauce
page 266

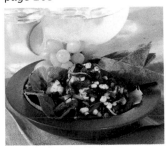

Pete's Chopped Salad
page 267

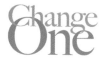

Week 3

Snacks

An entire chapter on snacks? In a book about losing weight? Are we serious? You bet we are.

Over the next several days you'll learn how to use two snacks a day to take the edge off hunger and make losing weight *easier*.

We think you'll be surprised at what you'll learn. In fact, one of the dieters in our *ChangeOne* pilot group asked to repeat the snacks week. "It wasn't until I filled in a food diary that I realized how often I snacked during the day," he explained. "And it wasn't until we tackled snacks that I saw how often I grabbed something when I wasn't even all that hungry." After two weeks of focusing on munchies, he really began to drop the pounds.

The same may be true for you. For years nutritionists wagged their fingers and told us not to eat between meals. Snacks seemed like the enemy. But now a new way of thinking about snacks has emerged. The two snacks a day you get on *ChangeOne* will help you stay on track. Eating something between meals, many experts say, can be one of a dieter's smartest strategies.

Nuts & Seeds

Nuts and seeds are filled with proteins and good fats, making them healthy but dense in calories. They are also filling, so it doesn't take too many to quell hunger. All of the snacks in this chapter equal about 100 calories (the size that *ChangeOne* recommends), starting with this selection:

- **Pistachios,** in shells, 30 (handful)
- **Pumpkin seeds** (handful)
- **Peanuts,** in shells, 10 (handful)
- **Almonds,** 16 to 20 (palmful)
- **Sunflower seeds,** in shells (palmful)
- **Peanut butter,** 1 tablespoon (thumb)

HEALTH TIP

Buy your nuts with their shells still on. Opening them takes time, so you're less likely to eat too many. And for many people, the mindless play of cracking, splitting, picking, and sorting is as satisfying as eating the nuts themselves.

ABOUT PEANUTS

Peanuts—actually a legume rather than a true nut—and peanut butter have become a trendy diet food. A Harvard University study showed that dieters eating peanuts and peanut butter found it easier to stick to their diets. More good news—peanuts may also be good for your heart.

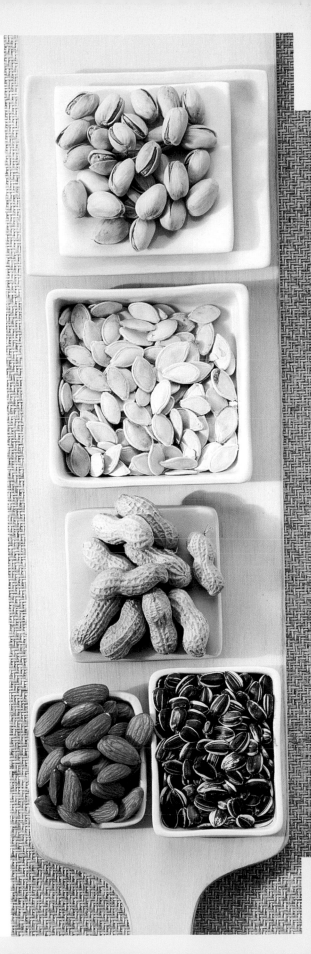

From top: pistachios, pumpkin seeds, peanuts, almonds (left), and sunflower seeds.

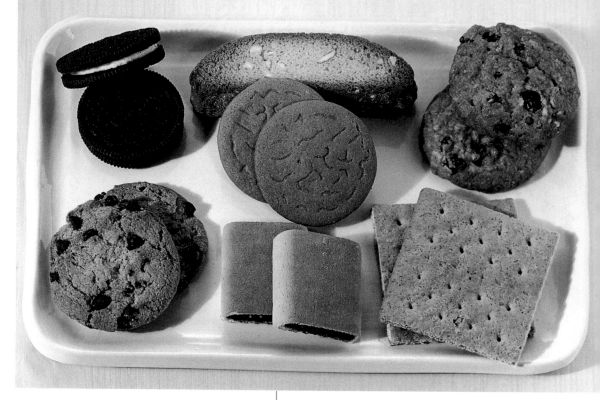

Cookies

Cookies are a special treat, whether homemade or store-bought. Here are 100-calorie portions that work for snacks or desserts:

- **Chocolate chip,** two 2-inch cookies
- **Oatmeal raisin,** two 2-inch cookies
- **Cream-filled sandwich cookie,** two 2-inch cookies
- **Fig bars** (like Fig Newtons), two
- **Graham crackers,** two squares
- **Ginger snaps,** two 2-inch cookies
- **Biscotti,** one

For more about cookies—and some tasty recipes—see pages 286–287.

Clockwise from top left: cream-filled sandwich cookies, biscotti, oatmeal raisin cookies, graham crackers, fig bars, chocolate chip cookies, ginger snaps (center).

TIPS FOR BUYING COOKIES

Don't rush to buy fat-free versions of regular cookies: they just don't taste as good, they tend to cost more, and most shave off few if any calories. And be careful of portion sizes when it comes to cookies bought at bakeries—not only are they huge in circumference, but they are often thicker than a normal cookie. One-third of a large cookie is all you need; save the rest or share.

HEALTH TIP

You can trim calories off your favorite cookie recipes—just take out a third of the sugar and butter or margarine; if the recipe calls for 1 cup, use 2/3 cup instead. Or look for recipes that call for light margarine, applesauce, and other calorie-lowering ingredients.

Make Snacks Work for You

When we asked the *ChangeOne* volunteers to describe the single biggest fear they faced in dieting, many of them listed "hunger." That's not surprising. Dieters often think they have to resist hunger in order to lose weight. This week we want you to pay close attention to hunger cues. And instead of resisting them, we want you to feed them . . . with a healthy snack. Here's why:

Hunger is an extremely powerful force. Getting enough fuel for our bodies is essential to survival. It is a matter of life and death, literally, so the body has a variety of internal signals that alert it when its energy stores are dipping low. Some come from the belly. Some originate in the brain.

The longer we go without eating, the more powerful those signals become. It doesn't take long before they're so urgent that almost all we can think about is food. As hunger intensifies, willpower weakens. If you get hungry enough, you'll reach for anything.

That's where smart snacking comes in. Help yourself to something sensible when you feel hungry, and in doing so you'll help ensure that hunger doesn't rise up and devour your determination to lose weight.

Worried that snacking will make it harder to lose weight? Worry not. Surprisingly, several large studies have found no link at all between how many snacks people eat and how much they weigh. Even people who snack before bedtime—once considered a big diet taboo—don't seem to be any more likely to be overweight than people who skip late snacks.

Eating more often than just three times a day might actually have advantages over the three-meals-a-day pattern when it comes to health. In a study at St. Michael's Hospital at the University of Toronto, researchers tested two nutritionally identical diets. One group of volunteers ate their allotted food in three square meals. The others ate the same food in the

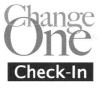

Check-In

Last week you added lunch to your *ChangeOne* menu. If you went off the plan for a day or two, don't worry. Change takes time. People sometimes take two steps forward and one step back. That's no cause to get discouraged. Take a deep breath, remind yourself of what matters most to you, then resolve to take two more steps forward starting tomorrow. This is an approach to eating that will last your entire life, so messing up a day or two is no big deal over the long run. If you feel frustrated because you don't quite have breakfast and lunch under control, consider taking another week with them before moving on.

same amounts but divided it among 17 snacks. Compared to the three-meals-a-day group, the snackers actually saw their cholesterol levels drop. Eating smaller meals more frequently, the experts concluded, kept blood sugar and insulin levels down, which in turn reduced the body's output of cholesterol. That's good, of course, and for anyone who wants to lose weight those results hint at even more good news: holding blood sugar and insulin levels steady can also keep hunger in check.

How We Snack

Almost everyone grabs at least one snack a day. Half of the people in a survey conducted by Columbia University researcher Audrey Cross snacked two to four times a day. Afternoons were their favorite snack time, when they were most likely to reach for something salty. The next favorite was before bedtime, when many people's taste buds yearn for something sweet, like chocolate or ice cream.

While eating 17 snacks might be going a bit overboard, one or two during the day is vital to weight loss. Just ask the successful dieters in the National Weight Control Registry. A majority of them report they eat five times a day: three small main meals and two snacks.

This week help yourself to a snack when you feel hungry. But before you reach for it, we're going to ask you to do one simple thing: make sure you're really hungry.

Learn to Spot Hunger Cues

In this chapter we've grouped snacks and desserts together. One of our reasons is that the same foods often serve both purposes—frozen yogurt, fruit, a piece of chocolate, an oatmeal cookie—depending on when we eat them. Another reason is that most of us think of snacks and desserts as optional foods, a treat that's not part of our basic diet. On *ChangeOne* we welcome you to help yourself to sensible portions of snacks and desserts. All we ask is that you reach for them to satisfy genuine hunger.

Isn't that the reason most of us eat in the first place? Surprisingly, no. Weight-loss experts say we typically eat for reasons that have nothing to do with genuine physical hunger. We take a tub of buttered popcorn or a box of chocolate-covered raisins to our seat at the movies simply because that's what we've always done. We eat because someone just brought a coffee cake into the office, and who can resist? Often we take up our forks simply because it's meal time, or because everyone else is eating.

Continued on page 66

Change One · Fast Track

To speed your progress, choose one or two of the following optional Fast Track changes this week.

Downsize your dishes

Portion sizes aren't the only things that have grown bigger in recent years. So have the sizes of the plates and bowls on which those portions are being served. If you have a tendency to pile your plate high and finish it all, try switching to smaller dinnerware.

Use a bread plate instead of a dinner plate for your entree. Ditch the giant pasta bowls and use a smaller cereal bowl to serve spaghetti. If the plates you already have won't do, buy an inexpensive set of downsized plates and bowls for everyday use. Another clever way to make a little less food seem like more: try using a salad fork instead of a regular fork at your next meal, and a teaspoon instead of a tablespoon for your soup and cereal.

Slim your sips

Plenty of people look to a cola for a pick-me-up in the midafternoon. If you're still reaching for soft drinks or other beverages sweetened with sugar, you're drinking a lot of calories that aren't doing much to satisfy hunger.

Studies show that beverages slip right down without triggering fullness signals. If you drink a 16-ounce cola you'll consume 160 calories or more before you know it. This week switch to sugar-free versions of your favorite beverages. Or try sparkling water flavored with a squeeze of lemon or lime.

Go for the gold

If you're a walker, increase your pace this week. On Day One walk at your normal pace and keep track of how long it takes you to do your normal circuit. On Day Two try shaving a minute off your time. Be aware of how you feel. A good brisk walk should leave you feeling winded but not gasping for air.

The quicker your pace, the more calories you burn each minute. A 180-pound person burns 4.7 calories per minute walking at a leisurely 20-minute-mile pace (three miles per hour). Speeding up to a 15-minute mile (four miles per hour, about as fast as most people can walk comfortably) increases the number of calories burned to 7.2 per minute.

You'll also increase your fitness level, which will translate into more stamina and energy. If you swim, jog, bicycle, exercise at a gym, or do another kind of activity, nudge your workout a bit this week by putting in a little more time or pushing the intensity a little harder.

And disregard the fitness advice about slowing down to burn more fat. Research has proven that's a myth.

Hold the butter

Accustomed to slathering butter on bread or dinner rolls? One pat of butter contains a whopping 36 calories and four grams of fat, most of it saturated. If you smear a bunch on bread, you can easily tally up 120 or more calories on butter alone.

This week enjoy the unadulterated flavor of bread without all those extra fat-laden calories. Choose whole grain varieties of breads and rolls. The extra fiber these contain will slow digestion and make you feel fuller, and you'll get so much extra flavor that you may not even miss that butter—at least not terribly.

Salty Snacks

Lusting for potato chips? Then have some—just not too many. The following lists show you 100-calorie portions for some favorite snacks:

Chips

- **Potato chips,** 12
- **Tortilla chips,** 8
- **Baked tortilla chips,** 10
- **Corn chips,** 15
  (If you can't bear counting, serving size for all is roughly a handful)

Crackers

- **Ak-Mak,** 4
- **Rye wafers** (such as Ryvita), 4
- **Wheat Thins** (reduced fat), 15
- **Ritz Bits,** 25
- **Triscuits,** 4
- **Peanut butter-filled crackers,** 2 sandwiches
- **Rice cakes,** 2 regular size

Pretzels

- **Pretzels,** 20 thin sticks
- **Soft pretzel,** about ⅓ of a pretzel
- **Peanut butter-filled pretzel nuggets,** 6

Popcorn

- **Air-popped popcorn or popcorn popped in a pot,** 3 cups (three handfuls)
- **Microwave popcorn** (butter flavor), 1 cup (handful)
- **Cheddar cheese popcorn,** 1 cup
- **Popcorn cakes,** 2

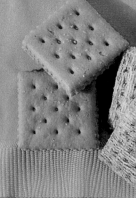

Clockwise from top left: peanut butter-filled crackers, Triscuits, baked tortilla chips, thin-stick pretzels, potato chips, popcorn popped in a pot, Ak-Mak crackers, Ritz Bits.

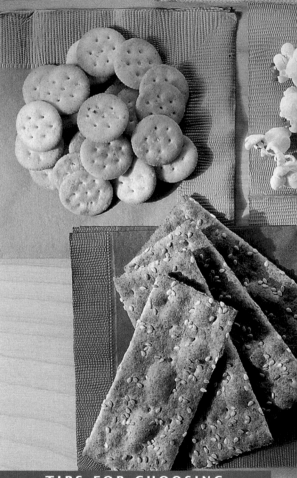

TIPS FOR CHOOSING CRACKERS

Looking for great taste *and* the benefits of fiber and low fat? Try Ak-Mak, lavosh, or rye wafers. Generally of Scandinavian or Middle Eastern origin, these are made with whole wheat or rye, meaning there's more fiber to fill you up and very little fat. Enjoy them plain or topped with hummus, roasted pepper dip, peanut butter, or reduced-fat cheese.

SPICING UP POPCORN

First, pop it on the stove or in a regular corn popper, adding a couple of tablespoons of vegetable oil to help heat up the kernels and prevent them from burning. Most of the oil stays behind in the pot, but enough gets onto the kernels to help salt and other seasonings stick. Next, sprinkle lightly with salt (if desired) and your choice of seasonings. Try chili powder, Italian seasoning, or a sprinkle of Parmesan cheese, or create your own flavor combos. One *ChangeOne* fan likes a light sprinkle of tamari (soy) sauce instead of salt. Devoted to your air-popper? Coat popped kernels very lightly with oil or cooking spray and then toss with seasonings.

BAKED VS. FRIED

Many brands of crackers and potato chips boast that they're "baked, not fried." The implication, of course, is fewer calories. But the calorie difference isn't always that great. The baked brands still use some fat, and their calorie count is often close to the fried products. So don't simply buy because the label says "baked." Look for brands that supply at least 1 gram of fiber and less than 3 grams of fat per serving.

Continued from page 62

The experts call these reasons for eating environmental cues. Something in our surroundings gives us the urge to eat. You may not be hungry in the sense that your body is running short of fuel. In fact, you may have just finished a big, filling meal. But the sight, smell, or memory of past occasions prompts the urge to eat, and you help yourself, often without thinking.

Emotional Eating

Environmental cues are just some of the reasons we eat when we're not really hungry. Many of us eat for emotional reasons, too. After all, food can be comforting. It's an integral part of being sociable. Getting together over a meal with friends or family can be a pleasant way to relax after a long day. And there's no need to get too fancy about it: food simply tastes good.

Food provides consolation, comfort, and calm. Unfortunately, none of those has anything to do with nutrition.

Pleasure we get from food has a biochemical basis, researchers say. When we eat something delicious, the experience triggers the release of endorphins in the brain, the same feel-good chemicals once associated with "runner's high." Certain foods may have their own mood-enhancing effects. Carbohydrates are thought to increase the absorption of an amino acid called tryptophan, which in turn boosts levels of serotonin, another brain chemical associated with mental well-being.

There are other reasons why eating is linked to emotions. If your parents comforted you or rewarded you with food, for instance, you may tend to reach for something to eat when you're feeling low or want to give yourself something for a job well done. If you get into the habit of eating something when you're feeling bored, you'll find yourself feeling hungry every time boredom strikes.

The same can be true for those feeling lonely. "I'd get home from work at the end of a long day, which was a hard time for me anyway after being divorced," a *ChangeOne* volunteer recalled. "I'd have dinner. And then, maybe because I was feeling lonely, I'd just go on eating and eating. Dessert. Cookies. I wasn't hungry. Somehow it just seemed to make me feel better. Recognizing that pattern made a big difference for me."

The problem with environmental and emotional eating is obvious. If you eat when you're not genuinely hungry, you'll

The Hungry I

What drives your snacking—emotions, environment, or just plain old hunger? Check only the shapes with the statements that apply to you.

○ When I go to the movies or a concert, I almost always get popcorn, candy, or some other treat.

☐ When I'm very busy, I sometimes don't even notice that I'm hungry.

◇ On stressful days, I often find it relaxing to eat something.

◇ If I'm bored and there's food around, I'll eat it.

☐ It's no big deal for me to say no to treats if I'm not really hungry.

◇ There are certain foods I really crave, like chocolate or salty snacks.

☐ I like the feeling of being really hungry when I sit down to a meal.

○ I have a tendency to clean my plate even if I'm not really that hungry.

◇ If I'm feeling a little down or blue, eating something can really help.

○ If there's a plate full of cookies or chips in front of me, I won't be able to resist taking some.

○ I have to be careful about having junk food around the house. If it's there, I'll eat it.

☐ My way of dealing with stress is to get up and do something.

☐ As long as I know I'll be sitting down to a meal soon, I can deal with feeling hungry.

○ Dinner just doesn't seem to be dinner without dessert.

◇ I definitely don't like the feeling of being hungry.

Turn to next page to tally your score.

almost certainly consume more calories than your body needs. There are healthier ways than overeating to deal with stress, boredom, or loneliness. Simply distracting yourself by doing something else you enjoy—listening to music, calling a friend, reading a book, watching a movie, going for a walk, or doing a crossword puzzle—often works. So how do you know if environmental or emotional cues are controlling when and how much you eat? The first step is paying attention to what genuine hunger feels like.

Last week you began to be more aware of times during the day when you felt hungry between meals—and what you did about it. Using what you learned, take the "Hungry I" quiz on this page to learn more about your own hunger profile.

Quiz Score

Tally up the number of colored shapes you checked according to color.

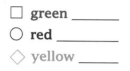

☐ green _____

◯ red _____

◇ yellow _____

What your score means:

☐ If you checked mostly green boxes, at least you're not snacking because you're bored or stressed. This week choose from among the recommended *ChangeOne* snacks and you'll keep calories under control.

◯ If you checked mostly red circles, you tend to be an "on cue" snacker. You reach for a snack not necessarily because you're hungry but because of cues in the environment around you.

Recognizing those cues—and asking yourself if you're really hungry—could help you avoid gobbling up calories you don't really want.

◇ If you checked mostly yellow diamonds, you tend to be an "emotional" snacker. You have the urge to eat something when you're feeling anxious, sad, lonely, or under stress. Many people do. Recognizing what real hunger feels like—and finding ways other than eating to deal with your emotions—will help you control calories and eat more healthfully.

If your score was divided evenly among greens, reds, and yellows, you're halfway to becoming a smart snacker. The tips in this chapter will guide you the rest of the way there.

Knowing When You're Genuinely Hungry

One day early this week try a simple experiment. If you typically have either a midmorning or midafternoon snack, skip it. Push the next meal about an hour later than usual. Then pay attention to how you feel. After you've gone four or five hours without eating anything, your body will begin to send out physical hunger cues. Some of these come from a part of the brain called the hypothalamus. When blood sugar levels fall, the hypothalamus senses an impending energy crisis and begins to issue "feed me" orders by way of the central nervous system. Your stomach growls. Your thoughts zero in on food. You may find yourself getting cranky.

This physical hunger is different from the emotional or

environmental kind, and it is not the same as a food craving. Food cravings target specific foods. You may crave chocolate when you're feeling lonely. You may find yourself craving a fast-food hamburger when you're on a car trip. Cravings are almost always responses to emotional or environmental cues.

Physical hunger isn't so specific. When your body needs more energy in the form of food, you don't focus on the taste of a particular food. What you want is food to fill you up. Any food at all.

Two Essential Questions

As part of your hunger test this week, try another experiment. When you finally sit down to eat, make a point of slowing down and paying close attention to how you feel as you eat. Notice what it feels like as your hunger sensation gives way to a feeling of satisfaction.

During the rest of this week, each time you feel the urge to grab a snack between meals, pause for as long as it takes to ask yourself these two simple questions: Am I really hungry? Can I wait until my next meal to eat?

If the answers are a resounding "Yes!" and "No!" help yourself to a snack. But if your answer is a lukewarm "Well, maybe," take five—get up and change what you're doing. Some options:

■ Take a quick stroll.

■ Drink a tall glass of water.

■ Make a phone call.

■ Complete a chore that needs doing—dusting, tidying up, pushing papers.

■ Wash your face or hands.

■ Brush your teeth.

■ Practice a relaxation technique like deep breathing.

■ Work on a crossword puzzle.

■ Page through a magazine.

With any luck you'll be distracted enough that, if you

Continued on page 73

Calcium Choices

Not only does calcium build strong bones, now there's research that shows it also helps the body burn fat. Some favorite calcium-rich snacks, in 100-calorie portions, include:

■ Low-fat or nonfat yogurt, plain or artificially sweetened (one cup)

■ Yogurt smoothie: In a blender, mix ½ cup yogurt, ½ cup skim or low-fat milk, and one cup frozen unsweetened strawberries until mixture is smooth

■ Low-fat or skim milk (one cup)

■ Skim or low-fat milk flavored with sugar-free syrup (one cup)

■ Reduced-fat cheese

■ Skim or low-fat latte (medium size)

■ Hot cocoa made with skim or low-fat milk (one cup)

■ Calcium-fortified orange juice (one cup)

■ Juice pop made with calcium-fortified juice

■ Sugar-free pudding made with skim or low-fat milk (one cup)

Sweet Snacks

Love sugary sweetness? As long as you trust your willpower enough to stick to our portion sizes, then *ChangeOne* has some sweets for you. Here are 100-calorie helpings of some favorites:

Sweets

- **Cracker Jack,** ⅓ cup (palmful)
- **M&Ms,** plain, 30 (palmful)
- **M&Ms,** with peanuts, 10 (palmful)
- **Caramel-peanut chocolate bar,** trick-or-treat size, 1
- **Chocolate and wafer bar,** trick-or-treat size, 2
- **Flaky peanut butter chocolate bar,** trick-or-treat size, 2
- **Mini rice cakes,** caramel corn flavor, 10
- **Raisins,** 3 tablespoons (palmful)
- **Jelly beans,** 25 (palmful)
- **Licorice,** 3 twists
- **Marshmallows,** large, 5
- **Marshmallows,** mini, 40 (palmful)
- **Chocolate-covered raisins,** 20 (palmful)
- **Malted-milk balls,** 7 (palmful)
- **Yogurt-covered raisins,** 2 tablespoons (2 thumbs)
- **Hard candy,** 4 pieces

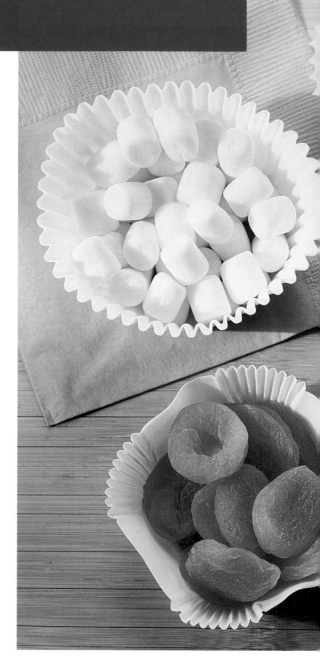

Fruit

There's no denying that fruit is good for you. The calories in fruit, however, can add up. We recommend getting small or medium fruit when possible, but having a portion that's a bit larger won't undo your *ChangeOne* plan.

- **Dried apricots,** about 6 to 8 (palmful)
- **Raisins,** 3 tablespoons (3 thumbs)
- **Grapes,** ¾ cup (tennis ball)
- **Apple,** 1
- **Orange,** 1
- **Fruit cocktail in juice,** ½ cup
- **Banana,** 1
- **Melon balls,** 1 cup (baseball)
- **Pineapple chunks,** ½ cup (2 golf balls)

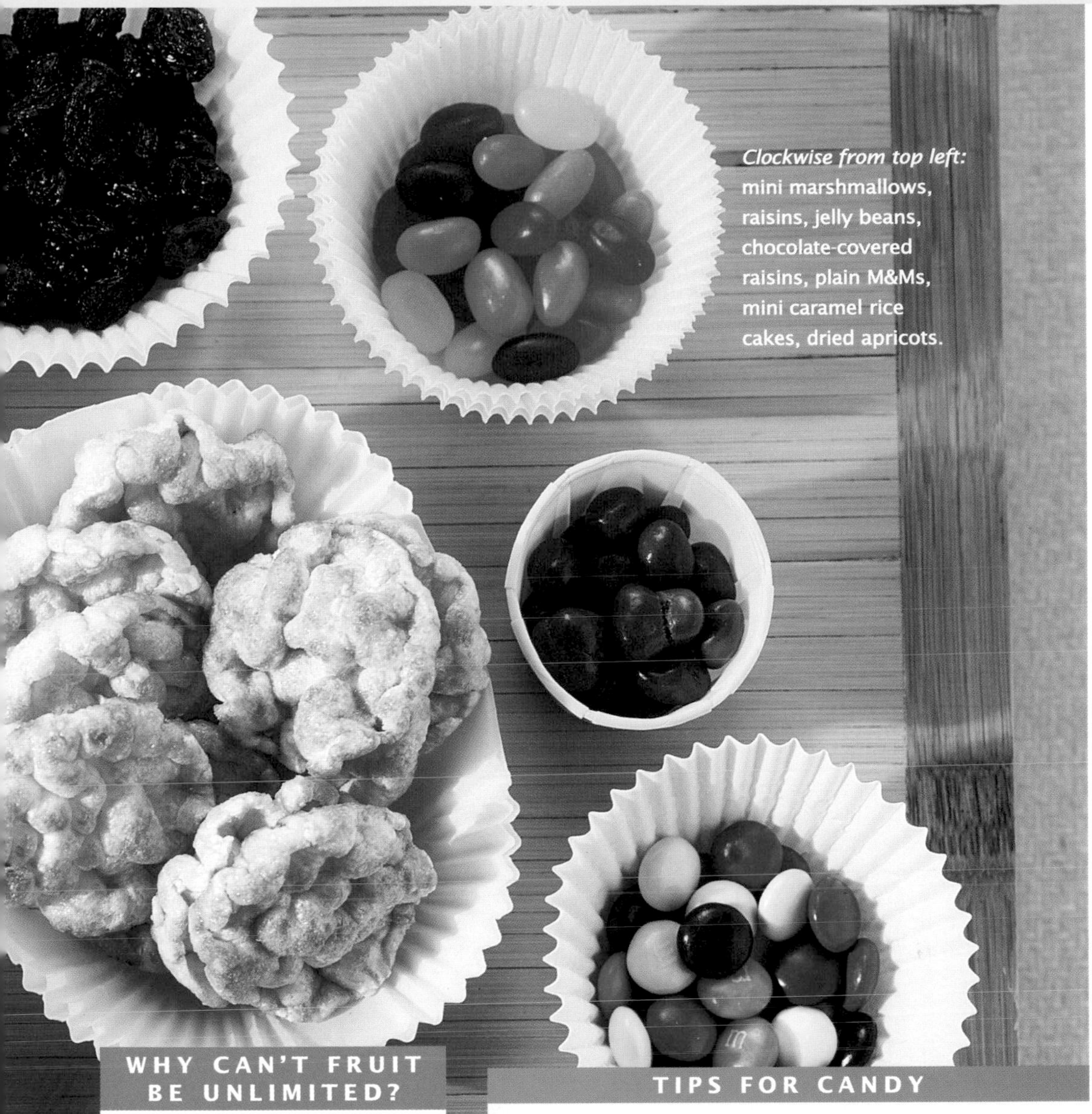

Clockwise from top left: mini marshmallows, raisins, jelly beans, chocolate-covered raisins, plain M&Ms, mini caramel rice cakes, dried apricots.

WHY CAN'T FRUIT BE UNLIMITED?

It's good and good for you, so why can't you eat unlimited quantities of fruit? Because the natural sugar content of fruit gives it more calories than most vegetables. *ChangeOne* suggests two servings of fruit, one at breakfast and one at lunch, along with the option of a third for a snack. Eating more than that is good for general nutrition, but keep in mind that the extra calories could slow down your weight-loss efforts.

TIPS FOR CANDY

When nothing but candy will do:

Minis are in. Buy the smallest pieces you can find. From the label figure out how many pieces equal 80 to 100 calories (or about 2/3 ounce). Eat them one by one, taking time between bites to enjoy each one.

Trick or treat year-round. Bags of fun- and bite-size candies are easy to find any month of the year. A portion is one or two pieces. Put them in an awkward, out-of-the-way spot—say, high in a cupboard behind the wineglasses—and then go there only to take out what you'll eat for the day. If you have to pull out some wineglasses before you can get a treat, you'll have time to reconsider your need.

Buy high-quality treats or candy that you really like. When the flavor is intense or when you're eating a favorite, you'll be satisfied with less.

71

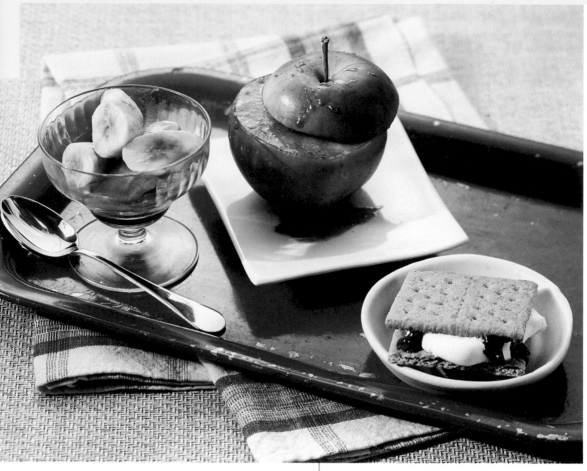

Baked Desserts

A baked dessert is a time-honored tradition. Here are 100-calorie portions for several popular choices, plus three make-your-own ideas:

- **Angel food cake,** 1 slice, or about $\frac{1}{12}$ of the cake

- **Fruit pie** (apple, berry, strawberry, etc.), as thin as you can slice it and still see it, about 4 forkfuls

- **Brownie,** 2-inch square

- **Chocolate cake with frosting,** 1 slice about $\frac{1}{2}$-inch thick

- **Cupcake with frosting,** 1 mini, half-dollar size across

- **Pumpkin pie filling,** without crust, $\frac{1}{3}$ cup, about 5 forkfuls

From left: Bananas Foster, Baked Apple, Microwave S'mores.

Bananas Foster
Slice a small banana into 1-inch pieces. Sprinkle with $\frac{1}{2}$ teaspoon brown sugar and add $\frac{1}{2}$ teaspoon butter. Microwave until bubbly, about 1 minute.

Baked Apple
Core a medium-size apple (not a Red Delicious—it gets too watery). Sprinkle inside with cinnamon and sugar. Cover and microwave for 3 minutes, or until soft.

Microwave S'mores
On each of two graham cracker squares, place 5 chocolate chips and 1 large marshmallow. Microwave for 10-15 seconds, until marshmallow gets puffy.

Continued from page 69

weren't hungry, you'll forget about snacking. Food cravings typically disappear as quickly as they come, and hunger from environmental or emotional cues lasts only as long as the cues are right in front of you.

But if after five minutes or so you're still hungry, then by all means, it's time for a snack.

Reach For a Snack That Satisfies

Snacks seem to be everywhere these days. Vending machines are crammed with them. Grocery stores have entire aisles devoted to them. There are snacks at the check-out counter, at the movie theater, where you pump gas—snacks almost wherever you turn.

And like so much else on the food landscape, many of these so-called snacks are oversized, fat-laden, calorie extravaganzas. The cookies on sale at delis these days are the size of saucers. Family-size bags of potato or tortilla chips could feed a village. And as the Tufts University *Health & Fitness Letter* discovered, even the venerable *Joy of Cooking* has felt the pressure. In the 1960s and 1970s, the book's recipe for brownies suggested 30 servings; in the latest edition the exact same recipe now suggests 16 servings. The fact is, even what passes for an individual-sized portion these days can spell big trouble when you're trying to lose weight. A seven-ounce package of tortilla chips can easily contain more than 1,000 calories. And sure, you could stop eating when you start feeling satisfied. But who among us can do that with these nutritional booby traps?

Nibblers, take heart. We've put together a menu of good-tasting, low-calorie snacks that will tame your hunger without scuttling your diet. Of course you'll find carrot and celery sticks on the list, simply because they make terrific

Continued on page 77

Help!

"My husband lost five pounds in two weeks. I've barely lost one. And we seem to be eating the same amount of food. What gives?"

You're different people. Some people can eliminate one thing from their diet—sugary colas, for instance—and begin dropping pounds immediately. Others have to watch everything they eat, and still the progress seems slow. There are many reasons. Some people's metabolic rates are higher than average, so they burn more calories even when they're just sitting around. Some people do a lot of fidgeting during the day, which also burns calories. One study found that fidgeters can burn more than 500 calories a day jiggling their legs or pacing around. If you're feeling frustrated by the pace of your weight loss, consider making an additional Fast Track change. (You'll find Fast Track suggestions on page 63.) And hang in there. Remember the tortoise and the hare. Even with weight loss, slow starters can be the first ones across the finish line.

Frozen Desserts

In summertime or any time, everyone loves a frozen treat. Here are lots of 100-calorie choices. The trick is to indulge and enjoy, without going overboard. Remember, it's a treat.

Cold and creamy treats

- **Nonfat frozen yogurt,** ½ cup (2 golf balls)
- **Light or fat-free ice cream,** ½ cup
- **No-sugar-added ice cream,** ½ cup
- **Italian ice,** ½ cup
- **Chocolate ice cream,** ⅓ cup (½ tennis ball)
- **Super premium chocolate ice cream,** 4 tablespoons (golf ball)
- **Sorbet,** ½ cup
- **Fudgsicle**

Frozen fruits

- **Frozen grapes,** ¾ cup (tennis ball)
- **Frozen banana**
- **Frozen strawberries,** 1 cup (baseball)
- **Fruit/juice pop,** 1
- **Homemade sorbet,** 1 cup

To make sorbet:

1. Freeze an entire can of fruit packed in heavy syrup.

2. Take out of the freezer 30 minutes ahead of time and place on the counter. After 30 minutes open the can on both ends and push out contents into a food processor. Add ½ cup apple juice and process until smooth.

3. Serve soft, or refreeze. One portion is ½ cup.

Clockwise from far left: nonfat frozen yogurt in a cone, fudgsicle, sorbet, Italian ice, chocolate ice cream, juice bars.

TIPS ON TOPPINGS

If you could have a tablespoon of topping on your ice cream, what would you choose? Here are tasty picks rated from lowest to highest in calories per tablespoon. Those over 50 calories are pushing out your second snack of the day.

Whipped cream	10
Raisins	27
Granola	28
Chocolate syrup	41
Chopped almonds	47
Butterscotch topping	52
Chocolate chips	52
Strawberry topping	53
Hot fudge topping	70
M&M candies	71
Chocolate sprinkles	72
Peanut butter candies	75

CHOOSING FLAVORS

Ice cream fruit flavors—strawberry and peach, for example—are lowest in calories because the fruit takes the place of higher-calorie, higher-fat ingredients such as whole milk and cream. Highest-calorie ice creams are vanilla, French vanilla, and varieties with mix-ins such as cookie pieces or nuts.

ABOUT FREEZING FRUIT

Fruit is easy to freeze and refreshing to eat. Start with your choice of ripe fruit—grapes, bananas, berries, melon, pineapple, peaches, mangoes, nectarines, plums—whatever you like. Cut whole fruit into bite-size pieces. Place on a baking sheet and freeze until firm. Remove from sheet and place in a resealable plastic bag or container. Store in freezer until needed.

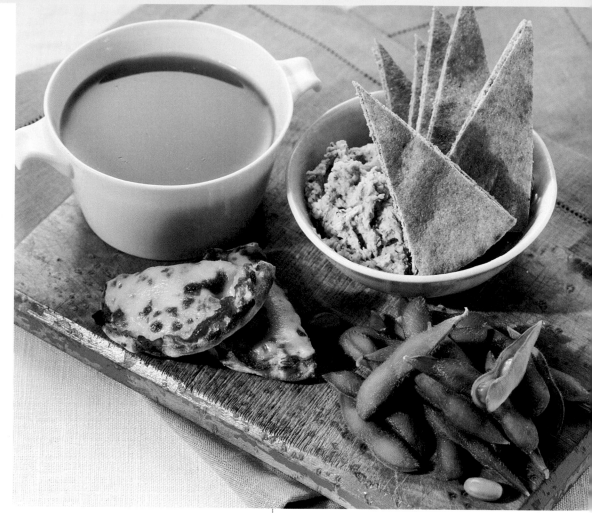

Savory Surprises

Break out of snacking boredom with these 100-calorie change-of-pace foods:

Unusual snacks that are healthy and delicious *(clockwise from top left):* tomato soup, hummus and pita, edamame, English muffin pizza.

- **Soup** (minestrone, vegetable, tomato, chicken noodle), 1 cup (diner coffee cup)
- **Edamame** (soybeans ready to eat from the shell), 4 ounces (deck of cards)
- **V8 juice,** up to 2 cups
- **Three-bean salad,** ½ cup (2 golf balls)
- **Hard cooked egg,** 1
- **Beef jerky,** 1 ounce (a 1-by-6-inch piece)
- **String cheese,** low fat, 1 piece
- **Hard cheese,** ⅔ ounce (thumb)

- **Peanut butter**, 1 tablespoon (thumb), on a regular size rice cake
- **Corn tortilla** topped with grated, reduced-fat cheese, 2 tablespoons (2 thumbs)
- **Hummus,** 2 tablespoons (2 thumbs), and ½ pita, cut into wedges
- **English muffin pizza:** half muffin spread with 1 tablespoon pasta sauce and 2 tablespoons grated cheese, baked at 350ºF until cheese bubbles.

Continued from page 73

munchies. But you'll also find some surprises, like wheat crackers with hummus, fudgsicles, a melted-cheese tortilla, pistachios, and even s'mores.

Behind *ChangeOne* Snacks

Every *ChangeOne* snack contains about 100 calories—enough to ease hunger pangs and still keep you within your calorie guidelines. We've chosen snacks that offer plenty of flavor. It may be a no-brainer, but it's worth repeating: if something doesn't taste good, don't eat it. Why waste calories on a fat-free cracker that tastes like sawdust when you can help yourself to a handful of rich-tasting nuts or a piece of pita with sizzling salsa?

Beyond good taste, a snack worth its calories should also be satisfying in other ways. If it's 95 degrees in the shade, you want something cool and refreshing, like a real fruit sorbet. If you're just in from shoveling snow, hot chocolate might be the pick. Naturally, a snack should also satisfy your hunger long enough to tide you over until the next meal. Research shows that snacks that take up a lot of volume per calorie—popcorn or fruit-and-yogurt smoothies, for instance—tend to make people feel fuller on fewer calories.

Snacks that pack a lot of nutrition also turn out to be more satisfying and filling than those with a lot of empty calories. Remember the nuts we mentioned earlier? One recent study found that snacking on nuts may actually help people keep their weight down. The reason: nuts are loaded with protein, vitamins, and, yes, fat. With all of that content, it doesn't take very many of them to satisfy your appetite.

Munch on low-fat crackers, which are made up mostly of simple carbohydrates, and you can go on eating and eating, hoping you'll find some flavor in the next bite, piling on calories before you begin to feel satisfied. A few nuts, on the other hand, can give you that satisfaction.

Choosing a nutritious snack is important for another reason: when you're on a low-calorie diet, it's just good sense to

Unlimited Snacks

Some foods are so low in calories that you can help yourself to as much as you want. Here are a few:

- Sugar-free popsicle
- Jicama slices
- Raw bell pepper slices
- Cherry tomatoes
- Carrot and celery sticks
- Sugar-free Jell-O

make those calories count. As we've said, a lot of us tend to think of snacks as a little something extra—a treat we allow ourselves that isn't really part of our diet. We're kidding ourselves. In fact, treats are a surprisingly big part of what we eat during the day. According to one survey, about 20 percent of our total calories on average comes from snacks—all the more reason to make sure those calories deliver essential nutrients as well as good taste.

8 Tips to Control Hunger Cues

1. Instead of buying snacks at a movie, a ball game, or other event, chew a stick of sugar-free gum. Pretty soon you'll associate the taste of gum, rather than high-calorie food, with that setting.
2. At parties stand as far away as you can from the bowls of chips, dips, and other munchies.
3. On car trips plan ahead by bringing a few *ChangeOne* snacks. If you have a tendency to munch in the car, bring just a single serving, not the whole box. Put the rest in the trunk.
4. Buy snacks in small packs. If you buy the giant size to economize, divide it into single-serving bags or containers as soon as you get home.
5. Put the healthiest snacks where you'll see them when you first open a kitchen cabinet or the refrigerator. Hide the others behind them.
6. Don't snack in your office. (And definitely don't keep bags of chips or pretzels in your desk drawer.) Go somewhere else—kitchen, cafeteria, lounge, or outside. That way you won't associate your office with food.
7. At home enjoy your snacks in the kitchen—and nowhere else.
8. Don't eat to relax. Relax, then eat. Stress is such a big factor in diet that we've devoted a whole chapter to it. Look ahead to Week 9, which begins on page 180, for stress-busting tips.

On *ChangeOne* snacks will make up about 15 percent of your total calorie intake. Naturally, since no one expects a snack to be a balanced meal, we're including some less-nutritious favorites just because they taste good. After all, it's not about avoiding candy, cookies, and other treats for good. It's more about eating them less often and in reasonable portions—and learning to enjoy them more.

Fitting Snacks Into Your *ChangeOne* Program

You can choose two snacks, a snack and a dessert, or two desserts during the day. You can also serve up slightly larger portions of food at your meals, especially if you find yourself getting too hungry. As often as possible, try to make sure that one selection comes from the "Calcium Choices" on page 69. You already know the evidence linking calcium to weight loss. And getting enough calcium is important for strong bones.

Use snacks this week to help manage your hunger. If you get ravenous in the morning, it's okay to munch on something. If your appetite roars to life in the midafternoon, then grab a snack. But before you do, remember to take the hunger test. Ask yourself: Am I really hungry? Can I wait until my next meal?

No More Open-Ended Snacking

"I realize now that I was simply setting myself up for trouble," says **Michael Krauss, an Internet designer. "I had all kinds of snacks around the house. I'd open a bag of chips and just start in on them without even thinking about what they tasted like. I never even took time to think about whether I was hungry. It was a habit I picked up in college, I think.**

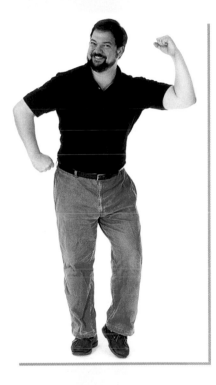

"On *ChangeOne*, it didn't take me long to realize that snacking was my biggest problem. That was really where the calories were coming from. I ended up putting off the dinner week and taking two weeks to get snacks under control. But once I did, I started to see results on the scale right away."

One of the first improvements Krauss made was to do away with what he calls open-ended snacking: that usually meant digging into a big bag of chips and eating with no end in sight. "Now when I get hungry for a snack, I decide how much I want, and I put that amount out and seal up the rest. Instead of digging into a bag of pretzels, I take two or three pretzels. It sounds simple, but it's made a huge difference for me."

Another change that helped was slowing down to taste what he was eating. "As soon as I began paying attention to flavor and texture, I began to make a kind of cost-benefit analysis. I'd think, 'Okay, do I really like this well enough to justify the calories?' And for the first time I found myself thinking, 'Gee, these chips are pretty greasy tasting. Or these cookies aren't really that good. Certainly not good enough to waste 200 calories on.'"

Before long, Krauss found himself snacking less often, but enjoying it more. He also started seeing the pounds fall off fast. His Week Four tally: down 13 pounds.

More Snack Choices

Need some more snacking options? No problem. Here are some of the additional *ChangeOne* snacks that you'll find starting on page 284.

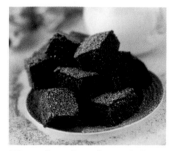

Chocolate Snacking Cake
page 284

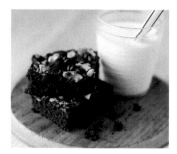

Brownie Bites
page 285

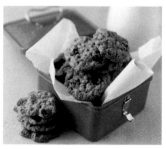

Chocolate Chip Oatmeal Cookies
page 286

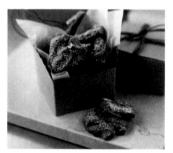

Meringue Nut Cookies
page 287

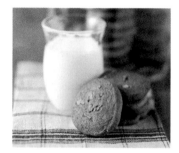

Pecan Icebox Cookies
page 287

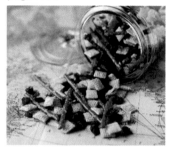

Ruby-Studded Trail Mix
page 288

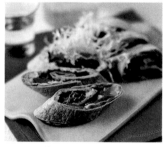

Roasted Pepper Pinwheels
page 288

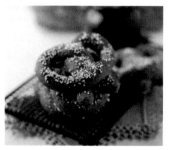

Multigrain Soft Pretzels
page 289

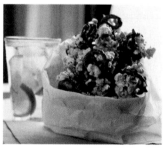

Sweet and Spicy Snack Mix
page 289

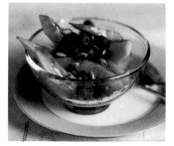

Cantaloupe Salad with Raspberry Vinaigrette
page 290

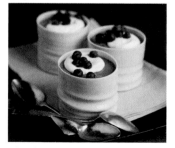

Blueberry Bonanza
page 291

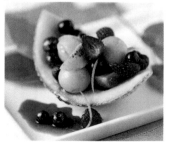

Fruit Boats with Orange-Balsamic Glaze
page 292

Changes Ahead: Dinner

This week, while you focus on snacking, start paying attention to what you have for dinner. Don't change what you eat, just notice what it is. Also be aware of how much time you spend eating dinner. Log how many nights you eat in and how many nights you eat out at restaurants or friends' houses. If you have time, keep a food diary of your dinners for the week, listing the foods in them and about how much you ate (you'll find an easy-to-use form on page 307). Pay attention to how you experience hunger and fullness, too. Those sensations can be a useful guide when it comes to eating sensible-sized portions.

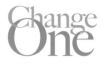

Week 4

Dinner

Pull a chair up to the table. It's dinner time.

For most of us dinner comes at the end of a long day of work or errands. It's the time we relax and reward our-selves. If you've been following *ChangeOne* week by week, this chapter will complete a month of determination and healthy changes. Good going! You've taken control of breakfast, lunch, and snacks.

This week we'll show you how to make dinner a daily celebration. You'll slow down, savor the flavors, and enjoy the company. And by doing so, you'll actually eat less.

Dinners are typically the biggest meal of the day and the source of the most calories. That's why taking charge of dinner can have the biggest weight-loss payoff. Many of our *ChangeOne* volunteers saw their weight loss accelerate when they got dinner in shape. By being sensible about portions, and using the meals in this chapter and on pages 268–283 as a guide, you'll discover that you, too, can enjoy delicious dinners while melting the pounds away.

Slow Down. Relax. Enjoy.

On the following pages you'll find a tantalizing selection of *ChangeOne* dinner suggestions, with plenty of ways to tailor them to your own tastes. We've made the menus as varied as possible to take advantage of the extraordinary culinary diversity available to us—from Chinese stir-fries to Italian pasta dishes to good old American beef on a bun. Of all the meals of the day, dinner is the one that most reflects our family history, culture, and special tastes.

(If you eat a lot of dinners out, you may want to glance ahead to Week 5, in which we take a look at strategies you can use to eat smart at restaurants. But first take a few minutes to look over the dinner meal plans on these pages. They'll give you a good idea of what a *ChangeOne* dinner contains and what sensible portion sizes look like.)

When you sit down to dinner this week, there's one simple change you'll want to make no matter what's on the table: slow down and savor the meal. Too often these days we're doing a mad dash from here to there, gobbling down meals without really taking the time to taste what's in front

Dinner Portions

These meal plans use both standard measurements and those from the *ChangeOne* portion-size guide; members of the 1,600 Club can add an extra serving of starch or grain here, *or* double your protein portion at lunch or dinner:

Type of food	Example	Amount	*ChangeOne* portion
One starch	Rice, pasta, noodles	⅔–1 cup	Tennis ball–baseball
or one grain	Roll	Medium	Tennis ball
One protein	Chicken, beef	3–4 ounces	Deck of cards
	Tofu	3–4 ounces	Deck of cards
	Light-flesh fish	6 ounces	Checkbook
	Salmon, shellfish	3–4 ounces	Deck of cards
	Beans	½ cup	2 golf balls
Vegetables		Unlimited	

of us. And eating too quickly is one reason so many of us find ourselves struggling with weight.

So this week give dinner your attention. Set aside enough time that you don't feel rushed. You may not be able to treat yourself to a leisurely dinner every night, but if you can make sure you enjoy an unhurried dinner at least three times during the coming week, you'll begin to see why savoring a meal is one of the simplest and smartest dieting strategies around.

Here's why: just as a body sends signals for hunger, research shows, it also signals when it's had enough food. Those cues, called satiety signals, are the body's way of balancing calories we consume with calories we burn. They work effectively as long as we take the time to notice them.

If you've ever stood up from a holiday feast feeling as if you're as stuffed as the dinner bird, though, you know that it's easy to eat more than you really need—sometimes a lot more. Studies show that it takes up to 20 minutes after food reaches your stomach for satiety signals to kick in.

It takes up to 20 minutes after food reaches your stomach for satiety signals to kick in.

Hence the problem with fast-food, and fast eating in general, regardless of what's on the menu. Scarf down food in a big hurry and you don't give your body time to tell you, "Hey, all right already, I've had enough!" You can end up consuming way more calories than you need or even want.

"I realize now I was like a feeding machine," one of our volunteers told us. "Hand to mouth, hand to mouth—I never paused. I just plowed through whatever was in front of me. I never stopped to think about what it tasted like. Or how I felt. The change that made the biggest difference for me was learning to put my fork down every few bites and just stop for a minute." As she learned, a leisurely meal gives your body and brain time to catch up with your fork. Slow down and you will end up feeling satisfied on far fewer calories than if you rushed through dinner.

Making the Change

We know, we know: given how crowded life is for many of us, taking time for dinner isn't always easy. You may have to rearrange your schedule a bit. You may need to let that rerun of *Frasier* or *Friends* wait for later. You may have to reschedule an appointment or two.

Even so, give it a try. Make it a goal that everyone in your house who plans to eat dinner sits down together. You'll find it's worth the effort, not only for the opportunity to relax and savor the meal but also for the new chance to spend time with your friends and family. If you're used to an eat-and-run approach to dinner, you can rediscover its pleasures—and make yourself a smarter eater—with these seven simple changes:

1. Arrange your schedule so you have at least 30 quiet minutes for dinner.

2. When you have dinner at home, always have it in your dining area. That way you won't associate food with other parts of the house—the couch in front of the television, for instance.

3. If the menu allows, divide your meal into courses—for instance, main course and vegetables, salad, and dessert. Choose the order that works best for you.

4. Make the meal the focus of dinnertime. Turn off the television. Put away the newspaper. Let the answering machine take your calls. A little dinner music is fine, as long as it doesn't distract you from the meal.

5. Serve an eight-ounce glass of water with dinner. Between each bite, put down your fork and take a small sip of water. Sipping water forces you to slow down. Water with dinner also makes a meal more filling without adding any calories. Many people find that it helps them clear their palate and more fully experience the flavors in a meal.

6. Pay attention to how the food tastes. Notice how the flavors complement or contrast with one another. Take small bites and let them linger in your mouth long enough so that the full flavor is released.

7. Between courses take a minute or two to relax, chat, and savor what you've just eaten. It may sound paradoxical, but lingering over dinner could help you drop pounds and maintain a healthy weight.

Change One
Check-In

Last week you added snacks to your *ChangeOne* menu. You'll find that low-cal snacks help you manage hunger and stay in control of what you eat. Still mastering the art of snacking? Struggling with breakfast or lunch? Then by all means, take another week. If you find yourself too rushed in the morning to put together a *ChangeOne* breakfast, look back to Week 1 for some time-saving tips. If you're having trouble controlling portion sizes when you go out to lunch, try packing it a few times this week. Still grabbing a candy bar from the vending machine when you suffer a midafternoon snack attack? Select a smarter snack from the *ChangeOne* suggestions in Week 3 or from the additional ideas on pages 284–292. And plan ahead to make sure the snack is handy when hunger strikes.

Change One Fast Track

In a hurry to see more pounds come off? Choose one or two of the following Fast Track changes to speed your progress:

Turn in early

Surprisingly, insomnia, or even chronically falling short on sleep by an hour or two, may keep you from reaching your goal. Some researchers suspect that overtired people unwittingly compensate for their lack of energy by eating more.

Coming up short on sleep can also make people more susceptible to stress, and thus more likely to overeat. Whatever the reason, weight-loss experts recommend trying to get seven or eight hours of sleep every night.

If you've been burning the candle at both ends lately, say good night to late nights a little early this week. If you find yourself repeatedly waking up in the night no matter when you go to bed—especially if you're a heavy snorer—talk to your doctor. You could have sleep apnea, a common problem that can be treated easily. Being overweight is a common risk factor for this condition.

Have some fun

This weekend set aside time to do something fun that also involves moving around. Hiking, badminton, touch football, gardening—anything that strikes your fancy, as long as it's active. Make it a family outing, if you'd like. Invite a friend. Or choose something you want to do just for yourself. Set aside at least an hour for activity.

Open your diary

Keep a food diary, again or for the first time. We've recommended it before, and we're recommending it again for one simple reason: it's the single best way to jumpstart your diet, research shows.

Now that you're adding dinner to the other *ChangeOne* meals, keeping a log of what you eat will help you see how far you've come in changing your diet. It's also a great way to spot trouble: certain times of the day when you eat more than you'd like, or certain situations that trigger hunger cues. You'll find a sample food diary form on page 307.

Chew on this

Pick up some packs of sugarless gum and place them everywhere: your kitchen, your desk, your car, your purse. When you're tempted to reach for a snack, grab a piece of gum instead. You may find that the act of chewing relieves your snacking impulses. Also, try chewing a stick while you're cooking meals—there's no way you can sample your wares while you're blowing bubbles.

Take the fitness challenge

Cutting back on calories is the quickest way to start losing pounds. But the best way to keep those pounds off, studies show, is to increase the number of calories you burn by becoming more active. Exercise will also help you replace fat with muscle, and that will make you look and feel trimmer.

If you aren't as active as you'd like to be, start the *ChangeOne* eight-week fitness challenge this week—details begin on page 236. This week-by-week plan offers a simple and easy way to ease yourself into a more active lifestyle.

Knowing When Enough is Enough

Paying attention to satiety signals is just one more way to make sure that you keep portion sizes under control. And in the end, portion size is really the key to the success of any diet. Some dieters discover that once they learn to stop eating when they're no longer hungry—before they're too full—they automatically eat reasonable portions.

Learning the art of knowing when you're satisfied takes time, though. And it doesn't work for everyone. So practice memorizing those portion sizes. We've suggested everyday objects for comparison, but another way to get a sense of how much a cup or an ounce contains is to prepare meals at home as often as you can this week.

To follow the *ChangeOne* recipes you won't need anything more exotic than a set of measuring cups and spoons. If you want to get fancy, invest in a kitchen scale that can be adjusted to zero after you place a bowl or plate on it. A scale makes it quick and easy to weigh three-ounce portions of pasta, for instance, or five ounces of fish. But it's not essential. You can also divvy up a 12-ounce package of pasta into four equal servings. A variety of individual portion-sized storage containers will also come in handy. (For more on helpful kitchen tools, check out pages 302–303.)

> **Vegetables are so low in calories, you can consider them "free" foods.**

Behind the *ChangeOne* Dinner Menu

Each of the suggested *ChangeOne* dinners contains between 400 and 460 calories. By following *ChangeOne* breakfast, lunch, snack, and dinner recommendations, you'll tally roughly 1,300—or 1,600—calories a day. As we promised before, that's a level that will guarantee you'll lose weight at a reasonable, healthy pace.

How can *ChangeOne* dinners be so thrifty with calories? A big reason is that each dinner includes at least two servings of vegetables. Vegetables are so low in calories—a half-cup of spinach contains only 27, for instance, and the same

Continued on page 94

Shish Kebabs

The name is Turkish, but shish kebabs—by any name—are a worldwide favorite.
Marinated meats and vegetables get grilled to perfection in eye-catching portions.

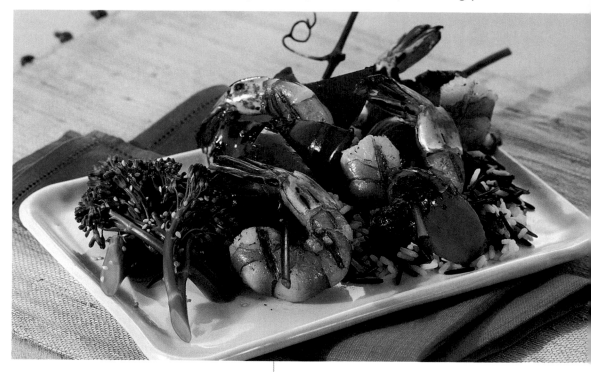

Shrimp Kebab Feast

2 skewers Shrimp and Pepper Kebabs

1 cup Wild and White rice (baseball)

½ cup Sesame Broccoli (2 golf balls)

Calories 430, fat 9 g, saturated fat 1.5 g, cholesterol
170 mg, sodium 220 mg, carbohydrate 55 g, fiber 7 g,
protein 34 g, calcium 150 mg.

SHRIMP AND PEPPER KEBABS

Serves 4

1 **pound shrimp, marinated for at
least 1 hour in the refrigerator
(see facing page for marinade ideas)**

1 **green and 1 red pepper, cut into
1-inch squares**

2 **teaspoons olive oil**

8 **skewers**

1. Microwave peppers 1 minute, or until soft.

2. Thread shrimp and pepper onto skewers.
Brush with olive oil.

3. Grill or oven-broil until shrimp are cooked
(turning pink), about 5 to 7 minutes.

Portion bonus: Add extra peppers and
vegetables to make 3 or 4 more skewers,
and help yourself to another skewer.

WILD AND WHITE RICE

Serves 4

2 ⅔ **cups water
Pinch of salt**

⅔ **cup wild rice, dry**

⅔ **cup long-grain white rice, dry**

1. In a medium pot with a lid, bring water,
salt, and wild rice to a boil. Cover, lower
heat, and simmer for about 20 minutes.

2. Add white rice, stir to combine, cover,
and simmer for an additional 20 minutes,
until rices are cooked.

3. Before serving divide into 4 equal portions and refrigerate extra.

SESAME BROCCOLI

Serves 4

    2 **cups broccoli florets**
    4 **tablespoons chicken stock or broth**
    2 **teaspoons sesame oil**
 1½ **tablespoons sesame seeds**

1. Place a medium-size nonstick pan on medium heat until warm.

2. Add vegetables and broth, and sauté until vegetables are soft, 7 to 10 minutes. Remove from heat.

3. Drizzle with sesame oil and sprinkle with sesame seeds.

Portion bonus: Add extra broccoli and stock.

Instead of Shrimp

- Firm-flesh fish like monkfish or salmon
- Skinless chicken breast
- Skinless chicken thigh meat
- Flank steak
- Lamb
- Extra-firm tofu

Instead of Peppers

- Eggplant, cut into 1-inch cubes, sprinkle with salt, rinse after 15 minutes, and spray with cooking spray
- Button (white) mushrooms
- Portobello mushrooms, ¼-inch thick
- Cherry tomatoes
- Pearl onions*
- Red onion, cut into wedges*
- Garlic cloves
- Zucchini, ¼-inch thick slices
- Carrots, cut into 1-inch pieces*

* Microwave for a couple of minutes to soften before grilling

TIPS FOR GRILLING KEBABS

Let your imagination run wild with kebabs. The combinations of seafood, meat, poultry, and vegetables are virtually endless. If you're grilling for a crowd, make all-vegetable and all-meat kebabs before you combine them. They'll cook more evenly.

- Brush kebabs with fresh marinade during cooking for more intense flavor; remember not to use the sauce you soaked them in. If you're using a sweetened marinade, move kebabs away from direct heat to prevent the sugar from burning.
- Turn kebabs over so that both sides cook evenly.
- Cover the ends of wooden skewers with foil to prevent burning, or invest in a set of metal skewers.

ABOUT MARINADES

A marinade is a seasoned liquid used to flavor, tenderize, and moisten food (typically meat, fish, or poultry). Marinades often contain ingredients such as oil, vinegar, lemon or fruit juice, yogurt, herbs, and spices. Marinating imparts great flavor without many calories. It also may fend off the cancer-promoting compounds that form on meat and other animal proteins grilled at high temperatures. Most grocers stock a wide selection of marinades, but as always, check the label to make sure the calorie and fat counts aren't exorbitant. Or make your own, using your favorite flavors.

To marinate, place food in a bowl or resealable plastic bag. Pour in about ¼ cup of your favorite marinade—teriyaki, lemon-pepper, lime-ginger—and mix well. Refrigerate for at least one hour. To ensure food safety, discard the remaining marinade after removing the food from the bag.

Stir-Fry

This cooking method is among the fastest, healthiest, and easiest around. Blend vegetables and meats for a fast sauté, and then create sauces as you go.

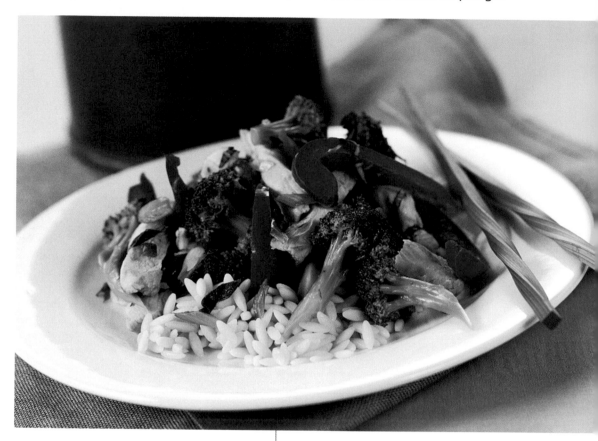

Italian-Style Stir-Fry

2 cups Chicken and Broccoli Stir-Fry (2 baseballs)

1 cup orzo (baseball)

Calories 420, fat 10 g, saturated fat 1.5 g, cholesterol 50 mg, sodium 350 mg, carbohydrate 53 g, fiber 8 g, protein 33 g, calcium 100 mg.

CHICKEN AND BROCCOLI STIR-FRY

Serves 4

- **3 teaspoons peanut oil**
- **3 scallions, thinly sliced**
- **3/4 pound skinless, boneless chicken breasts, cut across the grain into 1/2-inch wide pieces**

- **1 1/2 pounds broccoli florets**
- **1 cup diced red pepper**
- **1/2 cup chicken broth**
- **1/2 teaspoon grated lemon peel**
- **1/2 teaspoon salt**
- **1/2 cup water**
- **1 teaspoon cornstarch blended with 1 tablespoon water**
- **1 tablespoon olive oil**
- **1/2 cup slivered basil or 1/2 teaspoon dried basil**

1. In a large nonstick (or coated with cooking spray) wok or skillet, heat 2 teaspoons oil over medium heat. Add the scallions and sauté for 1 minute or until wilted. Add chicken and sauté for 3 minutes, or until it is no longer pink.

2. Add the remaining 1 teaspoon oil and the broccoli, and sauté for 2 minutes.

3. Add the red pepper, broth, lemon peel, salt, and ½ cup water, and bring to a boil. Reduce to a simmer and cook uncovered for 2 minutes or until the chicken and broccoli are just cooked through.

4. Stir in the cornstarch mixture, olive oil, and basil and cook, stirring, for 1 minute or until the sauce is lightly thickened.

5. Before serving divide into 4 equal portions and refrigerate extra.

Portion bonus: Use more scallions, broccoli, red pepper.

To make orzo:

Prepare 1⅓ cups orzo according to directions on package. Divide into four equal portions and refrigerate extra.

Instead of Chicken

You can use one of the following in the above recipe for about the same number of calories:

- Salmon filet, 9 ounces
- Pork tenderloin, 10 ounces
- Firm tofu, 9 ounces
- Beef tenderloin, 8 ounces
- Boneless leg of lamb, 8 ounces
- Cashews, ½ cup

ABOUT WOKS

If you don't have a wok, is it worth getting one? Absolutely. A wok is perfectly designed for low-calorie cooking, using little oil and cooking vegetables and meats so quickly that they stay tasty and keep their flavor and nutrition. A wok is not just for Asian cooking. Use it anytime you need to sauté something quickly. When shopping for a wok, you'll have several choices:

- **Nonstick, flat bottom:** Our favorite because it fits on any stove and clean-up is a breeze. Downside: it doesn't conduct heat as well as traditional steel woks do.
- **Traditional steel:** This version conducts heat extremely well, and the concave design makes it simple to keep the food cooking evenly. Downside: it requires regular seasoning with oil and careful drying after each use to avoid rust.
- **Grill-top:** Made from coated steel, this wok has small holes all over it so that smoky flavor penetrates the food. Downside: foods can overcook or burn easily.

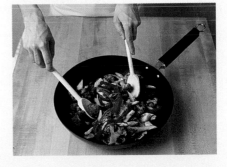

TIPS FOR STIR-FRY

Most of us associate stir-frying with Chinese cooking, but this low-fat cooking method can be used to create healthful meals with flavors from around the world. Use the above dinner's Italian-themed stir-fry recipe to create other international delights:

Cuisine	Instead of broccoli/red pepper	Instead of olive oil/basil
Mexican	Assorted peppers, corn	Squeeze of lime juice, ¼ cup cilantro
Chinese	Green beans, mushrooms	1 tablespoon soy sauce, ½ teaspoon sesame oil
Thai	Unchanged	2 tablespoons lime juice and peanut butter
Greek	Eggplant, assorted peppers	2 tablespoons lemon juice and olives

Stew

Every culture in the world has a recipe for slow cooking chunks of meat with vegetables, and this hearty American stew is one of the classics.

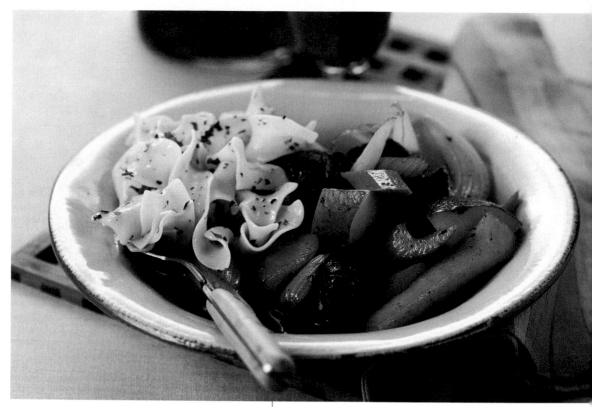

Beef Stew Dinner

2 cups Beef Stew (2 baseballs)

1 cup egg noodles (baseball)

Calories 420, fat 12 g, saturated fat 3.5 g, cholesterol 90 mg, sodium 170 mg, carbohydrate 52 g, fiber 7 g, protein 26 g, calcium 80 mg.

BEEF STEW

Serves 4

- 1 **tablespoon olive oil**
- 12 **ounces lean stew beef, cubed**
- 2 **cups carrots, cut into 1-inch pieces**
- 2 **medium onions, cut into quarters**
- 1 **cup parsnips, cut into 1-inch pieces**
- 1 **cup celery, cut into 1-inch pieces**
- 1 **cup potatoes, cut into 1-inch pieces**
- 1/2 **teaspoon dried thyme**
   Salt and pepper to taste
- 2 **cups beef broth or stock**

1. Heat oil over medium heat in a pot or casserole large enough to hold all ingredients. Brown beef cubes; drain excess fat.

2. Add remaining ingredients, cover, and simmer until beef and vegetables are cooked, about 45 minutes.

3. If using a crock pot, follow cooking directions for your crock pot.

4. Before serving divide into 4 equal portions and refrigerate extra. Serve over egg noodles.

Portion bonus: Increase stock and all vegetables, except potatoes.

To make egg noodles:
Prepare 4 cups dry egg noodles according to directions on package. Divide into four equal portions and refrigerate extra.

Stew meats—chuck, rump, round, brisket, and shoulder—are flavorful, less expensive, and tougher cuts that soften when cooked slowly with liquid. All are similar in calories and nutrition. It's best to buy a whole piece of chuck meat—it's the moistest of the stew meats—and cut it up yourself. Browning stew meat in a small amount of oil (and then draining the extra fat) before adding liquid caramelizes the surface of the meat and adds a richer flavor to your stew.

Instead of Egg Noodles

Egg noodles don't have that much cholesterol—35 milligrams, compared to the recommended daily limit of 300 milligrams. But if you'd prefer pasta without cholesterol, here are a few suggestions:

- "Yolk-less" egg noodles: made with whites only
- Egg-less noodles: broad, made without eggs
- Farfalle: bow-ties
- Fettuccine: flat ribbons

TIPS ON ROOT VEGETABLES

Carrots, parsnips ("blond" carrots), turnips, onions, and potatoes are particularly well suited for stewing. Their fibrous flesh stays firm during the stewing process. They are abundant in the winter months when fresh, locally grown vegetables may be in short supply. All supply fiber, along with an assortment of vitamins and minerals. Try these ways to prepare root vegetables:

- **Roast:** Cut into 1-inch chunks, toss with a bit of olive oil, and roast in a shallow pan at 450ºF until soft, about 30 to 45 minutes.
- **Puree:** Cut into 1-inch chunks, boil or microwave for 3 to 5 minutes or until soft, then mash or puree with a little milk or broth, a pinch of salt, fresh ground black pepper, and a teaspoon of butter, until smooth.
- **Braise:** Cut into 1-inch chunks, place in a pot with enough stock or broth to cover, simmer covered until the liquid is absorbed and the vegetables are soft, about 15 minutes.

ABOUT STOCK AND BROTH

Stock and broth are must-have ingredients for healthful cooking. They add lots of flavor and moisture, with very few calories.

- Stock, made by simmering bones (chicken, beef, veal, or fish stock), shells (fish stock), or vegetables in just enough water to cover them, has a rich flavor and texture. Concentrated stock can be purchased at many grocers and specialty food stores, and most general cookbooks will have standard stock recipes.
- Best vegetables for stock include carrots, onions, leeks, celery, and garlic. Avoid cabbage, broccoli, and other members of the cabbage family; they will make the stock bitter.
- Broth often is made by adding water and seasonings—salt, herbs, black pepper—to stock. Because it is more watery than stock, the flavor is less intense.
- When buying broth, look for canned varieties that are reduced in sodium, as regular canned broths are often quite salty.

Continued from page 87

amount of sliced carrots just 30—that you can think of them as "free" foods and help yourself to as much as you want.

One exception is vegetables that are creamed or sautéed in butter or oil. Another is fried vegetables. In these cases you do need to pay attention to serving sizes. Ounce for ounce, the fat in butter, cream, or cooking oil has more than twice as many calories as either protein or carbohydrates. So even small amounts can drive up the calorie total fast. A teaspoon of butter packs 34 calories. A teaspoon of cooking oil contains 40.

While the *ChangeOne* menus on these pages are relatively low in fat, we've been careful to include some fats, especially the unsaturated kinds that can improve cholesterol levels. Fat adds flavor and enjoyment to food. Diets with a moderate amount of fat offer much more variety and flexibility than strict low-fat diets. As long as you keep portion sizes under control, you can eat any kind of food you enjoy, even if it contains fat.

Remember, new research findings show that when you're trying to lose weight, diets with moderate amounts of fat work the best. Sure, it's wise to eliminate fatty foods that you don't really like or want. It's smart, too, to replace saturated fat with unsaturated fat. You can do this easily by using olive oil or canola oil instead of butter, for instance, and choosing a mayonnaise made with canola oil. But don't get hung up on fat. Managing portion sizes is a much smarter way to keep calories under control.

Help!

"I often don't get home from work until late—which means I eat dinner just before going to bed. I've heard eating before bedtime causes food to go right to fat. Is that true?"

Worry not. As long as you eat sensible portions at dinner, it won't magically appear on your thighs tomorrow. Despite what some fad diets tell you, the timing of meals makes almost no difference in whether the calories are burned up or stored as fat. It's the number of calories a meal contains that matters, not what time you eat.

Of course, many people don't like the feeling of going to bed on a full stomach. If you're one of them, try moving your dinner schedule up an hour. Choose meals that take a little less time to prepare. Do as much advance preparation as you can, either the day before or over the preceding weekend. After dinner take a walk. Many people find that walking helps them digest a meal and encourages sounder sleep.

About Those High-Protein Diets

We've all heard the buzz over high-protein diets. It's easy to see why they've proven so popular. Any diet that invites you to live on steak and eggs is going to attract attention.

But most doctors remain very skeptical of high-protein diets. It's not that these regimens don't help people lose weight. They do. A study by Arizona State University scientists published in 2002 showed that young women who ate a meal high in protein burned more calories during the next several hours than women who ate a high-carbohydrate, low-fat meal. The reason, researchers surmise: protein requires more energy to digest than carbohydrates do. That extra energy consumption showed up in slightly elevated body temperatures for the women consuming high-protein meals. Another study, this one from 1999, found that volunteers were more satisfied after eating a meal with 29 percent of its calories from protein than after a meal with only 9 percent of its calories from protein. They also burned more calories to digest the higher-protein meal.

Before you get too excited, though, keep this in mind: you'll burn a lot more calories by taking a 15-minute walk after dinner than you will consuming extra protein. And while it's true that high-protein foods seem to satisfy hunger well, complex carbohydrates do the same, often with fewer calories.

High-protein diets may also pose long-term risks if you don't choose the foods in them wisely. Many foods high in protein, like meat, are also high in saturated fat, which can be rough on your arteries. Probably more important when you're controlling calories is the fact that overloading your diet with protein raises the risk that you'll come up short on other nutrients, such as the essential vitamins, minerals, and fiber in vegetables. Over the long haul, a very high-protein diet could lead to nutritional deficiencies.

The watchword is moderation. Familiar? Sure. But it's still the best advice around. Protein, carbohydrates, and fat—you need them all. Tipping your diet too far in the direction of one or another forces you to cut way back on the variety of foods you get to eat, which makes it harder to stick to a diet. And by loading up on one constituent of food, you'll inevitably fall short on another that may

What If I'm Losing Weight Too Fast?

Yes, it sounds crazy—everyone on a diet wants this problem. But there's a danger to dropping pounds too fast. Experts recommend losing no more than three pounds a week.

Why? Because losing weight faster than that means you're burning off muscle as well as fat. Losing muscle tissue will leave you weaker than when you began your diet. It can also lower your basal metabolic rate—the rate at which your body burns fuel to sustain itself—because muscle tissue requires more calories for maintenance than does fat. The result: the less muscle, the fewer calories you'll burn, and the harder it will be to maintain weight loss.

If you've lost a lot more than three pounds a week on average—more than 10 pounds in your first three weeks—it's time to slow down. Add 200 to 300 calories to your diet by eating an extra snack or two, or increasing portion sizes slightly. And to make sure you don't lose muscle tissue, increase your exercise. You'll find details about an easy eight-week fitness program beginning on page 236.

Change One First Person

Slowly But Surely

"I was losing weight, a little every week. In the beginning I didn't think I was losing it fast enough. But the pounds were coming off, and that was great," says Barbara Deem, a tax accountant who lives in Ridgefield, Connecticut.

"Starting to eat breakfast helped. I hadn't been a breakfast eater before. Watching portion sizes at lunch also made a difference. But the biggest thing for me was dinner. It's not what I was eating, it's how much I was eating. That was the big revelation for me. As soon as I began to pay attention to portion sizes, I began to realize, 'Hey, I don't have to eat that much food to feel satisfied.'"

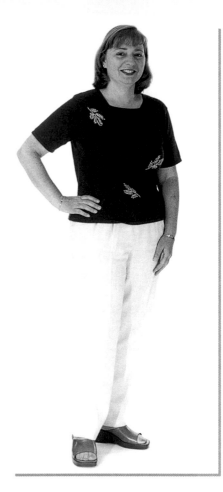

During her first month on *ChangeOne*, Deem did a lot of measuring in the kitchen. "You think you know, but you don't," she says. But soon she began to get a feel for what a reasonable portion should look like—and that also helped a lot when she and her husband went out for dinner.

By following her good example, Deem's husband lost four pounds during the first week of *ChangeOne*. Her own progress has been slower—one to two pounds a week— but steady. By the end of the fifth week she was down 11 pounds. "I still have a ways to go. But now I actually like the slower pace. I'm starting to feel a difference in how my clothes fit. I'm starting to feel a lot more confident that the changes I'm making are changes I can live with."

be just as important. We've made sure that the *ChangeOne* plan contains all the protein you need to be healthy and feel satisfied after a meal, but not so much that it bumps other essential components of a healthy diet off the menu.

Cutting back on calories is what really matters when you're trying to lose weight, after all. For most of us, that simply means eating less. That's all there is to it. No magic. Just good common sense about portions.

Goal-Setting: It's Finally Time

Chances are you had in mind the number of pounds you wanted to drop back when you started *ChangeOne*. That's great. In fact, this week we want you to put your goal in writing—and sign your name to it.

Now it might seem puzzling that we have waited until the fourth week of the program to get to the topic of goals. But there are two reasons we waited.

First is that it is impossible to set a reasonable goal when you are just embarking on a new skill. If you never played golf, for example, how can you predict how good a golfer you can be in 12 weeks? You need to learn some of the skills and practice them before assessing that. Only then can you determine a reasonable path to success.

The same is true for *ChangeOne*. These first four weeks you have been learning new skills and practicing them every day. We assume you have been losing weight and also reaping other personal rewards. Now that you know your weight-loss strengths and weaknesses, isn't it a smarter time to set a realistic goal?

The second reason for the delay is that goal-setting is

Continued on page 104

Help!

"I've been putting in lots of time being active, and I haven't seen big results on the scale. What's wrong?"

Nothing. By being as active as you can, you're doing the right thing. The frustrating fact is that it takes a lot of exercise to lose even a small amount of weight. The average weight loss most people can expect from exercise alone is about one-third of a pound a week.

So why bother? Here are three very good reasons:

1. Physical activity does burn calories—and those extra calories will help you lose weight over time.

2. You'll be much more likely to keep the weight off. Almost all the successful dieters in the National Weight Control Registry say that a big part of their success comes from exercise. On average they burn an extra 2,500 calories a week doing physical activities.

3. Being physically active has been shown to improve people's mental outlook and boost their self-confidence—two changes that can make it much easier to stick to a diet.

Don't stop exercising because you're not losing weight. Stay active and take another look at your diet. Make sure you're not consuming a lot of empty calories in the form of sweetened beverages, including sports drinks or sugary ice teas. Recalibrate portion sizes to make sure yours are still within the *ChangeOne* guidelines.

Pasta

What kid (grown up or otherwise) doesn't love the taste and feel of spaghetti? Our advice: skip the jarred tomato sauce and experiment for fun and flavor.

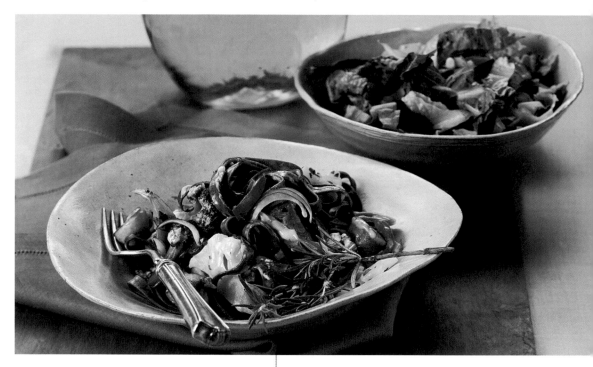

Pasta Primavera

2 cups Pasta Primavera (2 baseballs)

3 cups Italian Salad (3 baseballs)

Calories 410, fat 13 g, saturated fat 3 g, cholesterol 5 mg, sodium 690 mg, carbohydrate 60 g, fiber 10 g, protein 20 g, calcium 250 mg.

PASTA PRIMAVERA

Serves 4

- 1⅓ **cups small cauliflower florets**
- 1⅓ **cups small broccoli florets**
- 7 **ounces plain or spinach fettuccine**
- 2 **teaspoons olive oil**
- 1 **small red onion, diced**
- 2 **cloves garlic, minced**
- ½ **pound mushrooms, thinly sliced**
- ½ **teaspoon salt**
- ½ **teaspoon dried rosemary, crumbled**
- 1 **medium tomato, in ½-inch cubes**
- 2 **teaspoons flour**
- 1 **cup skim or low-fat milk**
- ¼ **cup grated parmesan cheese**
- ¼ **cup parsley**

1. In a large pot of boiling water, cook the cauliflower and broccoli for 2 minutes to blanch. With a slotted spoon, transfer the vegetables to a plate.

2. Add the fettuccine to the boiling water and cook according to package directions. Drain and transfer to a large serving bowl.

3. While fettuccine cooks, heat 1 teaspoon of oil in a large nonstick skillet over moderate heat. Add the onion and garlic and sauté for 5 minutes or until tender. Add the mushrooms and sauté 3 minutes or until softened.

4. Add the remaining 1 teaspoon of oil to the pan. Return the cauliflower and broccoli to the pan, sprinkle with the salt and rosemary, and sauté for 1 minute or until the vegetables are heated through. Add the tomato and cook for 3 minutes, or until softened.

5. Sprinkle the flour over the vegetables, stirring to coat. Add the milk and bring to a boil. Reduce to a simmer and cook, stirring, for 3 minutes or until slightly thickened. Stir in the cheese and parsley. Add to the hot pasta, tossing until combined.

6. Before serving divide into 4 equal portions and refrigerate extra.

ITALIAN SALAD

Serves 4

    1 **head romaine lettuce, torn into bite-size pieces**
    ½ **cup chopped olives**
    ⅔ **cup diced red peppers**
    ⅔ **cup diced green peppers**
    ¼ **cup pine nuts**
    ½ **cup canned or boiled chickpeas**

1. Toss all ingredients together in a large salad bowl. Dress with 2 tablespoons fat-free Italian dressing, or reduced-fat dressing (adds about 30 calories per serving).

TIPS FOR COOKING PASTA

The biggest challenge in cooking pasta is preventing it from sticking together. Follow this advice for perfect pasta:

- Use a large pot—big enough to hold 3 quarts of water per 8 ounces of dry pasta.
- Bring water to a roiling boil before adding pasta; salting is optional. Adding oil will not prevent sticking.
- Make sure the water continues to boil gently after pasta is added, and stir the pasta often.
- Cook until done (see package for suggested time). Reserve about ½ cup of cooking water. Drain pasta in a colander; do not rinse.
- Toss with sauce immediately, or place in a bowl with reserved cooking water and cover until ready to serve.

Instead of Primavera

Although primavera means springtime pasta, this dish is delicious year-round. What makes it so versatile is that you can mix and match ingredients almost any way you like.

Instead of	Try	Why
Fresh cauliflower and broccoli	Frozen vegetable combos	Always in season
Milk	1 cup part-skim ricotta cheese	Creamier
	Tomato sauce	Kids may prefer it
Dried rosemary	Dried oregano	More familiar flavor
	Fresh basil	Lighter, fresher flavor
Parmesan cheese	Romano cheese	Sharper flavor
Fettuccine	Pizzoccheri (buckwheat pasta)	More fiber

ABOUT PASTA PRIMAVERA

With so many vegetables, pasta primavera can be wonderfully healthful:

- Our version supplies 25 percent of your vitamin A, 90 percent of your vitamin C, and 15 percent of your iron for the entire day.
- To add more fiber, make this dish with whole wheat or buckwheat pasta.

- Broccoli, a popular primavera vegetable, is a nutrition star. It is among the top in vitamins A and C and in the B vitamin folate. It also is packed with disease-fighting plant compounds.
- Use frozen vegetables when fresh are out of season. Frozen veggies are just as rich in vitamins and minerals.

Packet Cooking

Though not a widely used method, packet cooking is surprisingly easy and delicious. Combine healthy foods and flavorings in a sealed packet, throw it in the oven or on the grill, and dinner is done.

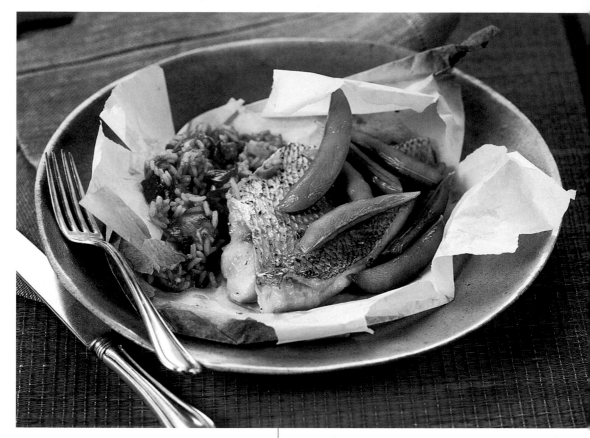

Red Snapper and Spanish Rice

1 packet Snapper & Snaps

1 cup Spanish Rice (1 baseball)

Calories 430, fat 5.5 g, saturated fat 1 g, cholesterol 65 mg, sodium 610 mg, carbohydrate 50 g, fiber 6 g, protein 44 g, calcium 140 mg.

SNAPPER & SNAPS IN A PACKET

Serves 4

   3 **cups sugar snap peas or snow peas**
   2 **tablespoons lemon juice**
   2 **teaspoons olive oil**
      Salt and black pepper to taste
   4 **red snapper filets, 6 ounces each**

1. Preheat oven to 400ºF, or prepare gas or charcoal grill.

2. In a bowl toss together peas, lemon juice, olive oil, salt, and pepper.

3. Coat four 15-inch lengths of parchment paper (or foil) with cooking spray. Place each filet on one half of the paper. Top with about ¾ cup of the pea mix. Fold the paper over the fish and peas and seal by folding over all edges.

4. Place the foil packets on a baking sheet in the oven or directly onto the grill and cook for 10 to 12 minutes.

SPANISH RICE

Serves 4

- 1 **medium onion, finely chopped**
- 1 **medium green bell pepper, finely chopped**
- 1 **celery rib, finely chopped**
- 2 **garlic cloves, minced**
- 4 **ounces mushrooms, sliced**
- 2/3 **cup long-grain white rice, uncooked**
- 1 **cup low sodium tomato juice**
- 1 **cup chicken broth, preferably reduced sodium**
- 1/2 **teaspoon salt**
- 1/4 **teaspoon black pepper**
- 1 **bay leaf**
- 4 **plum tomatoes, halved, seeded, and diced**

1. Lightly coat deep nonstick skillet with cooking spray. Sauté onion, green pepper, celery, and garlic until onion is almost soft, about 3 minutes. Stir in mushrooms and rice and sauté until rice turns golden, about 2 minutes.

2. Stir in tomato juice, broth, salt, black pepper, and bay leaf. Bring to boil over medium-high heat. Cover, reduce heat, and simmer, stirring occasionally, 15 minutes. Stir in tomatoes.

3. Cover and cook until rice is tender and liquid is absorbed, about 10 minutes longer. Fluff with fork to keep rice from sticking. Remove from heat and discard bay leaf.

4. Before serving divide into 4 equal portions and refrigerate extra.

Instead of Snapper

Flounder and sole: Packet cooking works particularly well for delicate fish that tends to fall apart during cooking. Season with just a squeeze of lemon, along with salt and pepper.

Salmon filet: Try Asian flavorings like hoisin sauce or sesame oil. Salmon steaks take longer to cook than filets.

Shrimp and scallops: These shellfish stay moist and succulent during cooking. Cook with minced garlic and a drizzle of olive oil.

Chicken breast: Combine strips of chicken breast with sliced red pepper and onion and a teaspoon of salsa for a new twist on Mexican fajitas.

Flank steak: Stays juicy and flavorful when sliced into strips and paired with thinly sliced onion. Season with a bit of teriyaki sauce.

Tofu: Cut into 1-inch cubes and combine with snow peas and mushrooms. Marinate first for extra flavor.

TIPS ON COOKING IN PACKETS

Cooking in a packet retains moisture and flavor and minimizes cleanup.

- Use parchment paper, foil (regular or heavy duty), or specially designed grill bags to hold the food.
- Add little or no liquid, since the packet retains all the moisture from the foods being cooked.
- Fold over edges well to keep cooking juices in.
- Cook in the oven at 400°F, or over indirect heat on the grill to avoid burning. 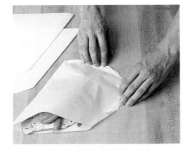 Cooking time varies with the type of fish, meat, or vegetables you are cooking. Root vegetables like carrots take longer than softer vegetables like peas or mushrooms.

Asian Noodles

We know lo mein and ramen best, but Asian foods are as rich with noodles as Italian cuisine. Mixed with fresh and flavorful ingredients, Asian noodles make great one-dish dinners any time of the year.

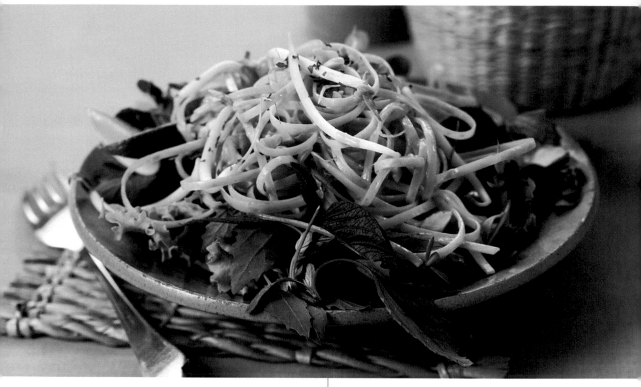

Noodles and Greens

1 cup Thai Noodle Salad (1 baseball)

2 cups mixed greens (2 baseballs)

Calories 430, fat 16 g, saturated fat 3.5 g, cholesterol 0 mg, sodium 250 mg, carbohydrate 64 g, fiber 6 g, protein 11 g, calcium 150 mg.

THAI NOODLE SALAD

Serves 4

    8 **ounces Asian rice noodles**
    1 **teaspoon peanut oil**
    2 **cloves garlic, minced**
    1 **medium onion, sliced thin**
    ¼ **cup vegetable broth**
    ¼ **cup sliced scallions**
  1½ **cups bean sprouts, thoroughly rinsed and drained**
    ⅓ **cup natural peanut butter**
    ¼ **cup light coconut milk**

    8 **cups mixed greens**
    ¼ **cup cilantro, chopped**
    2 **limes, juiced**
    2 **tablespoons chopped peanuts**

1. Prepare noodles according to directions on package. While noodles cook, heat peanut oil in a large nonstick skillet. Sauté garlic for about 30 seconds. Add onions and broth and cook until onions are tender, about 5 minutes. Drain noodles and add to oil mixture.

2. Add scallions and bean sprouts to noodles and toss gently until well-mixed.

3. Mix together peanut butter and coconut milk and add to noodle mix. Toss to coat. Before serving noodles divide into 4 equal portions and refrigerate extra.

4. Place 2 cups of lettuce on each plate, top with the noodles, and garnish with chopped cilantro, lime juice, and chopped peanuts.

Instead of Bean Sprouts

Asian vegetables are the secret delight of the produce section—delicious, healthy, and easy to cook. Try one or more of these varieties, cut into slivers, and sauté or microwave until color brightens:

Try	Features
Bok choy	Thick light green stems, dark green leaves, mild cabbage flavor
Chinese broccoli	Large leaves, yellow or white flowers
Chinese cabbage (Napa)	Light green leaves, lacy veins, delicate cabbage flavor
Pea shoots	New-growth stems and leaves, mild pea flavor
Watercress	Small leaves, sharp taste
Yard-long bean	Extremely long, resembles and tastes like green beans

ABOUT NUTS AND NUT BUTTERS

As you've no doubt guessed by now, we're nuts about nuts. A growing number of experts recommend nuts as part of a healthful diet, in part because the main form of fat in nuts—monounsaturated—has been linked to lower blood cholesterol levels. And they go nicely with many Asian side dishes. The catch: ounce for ounce, nuts have more than three times the calories of meat, so use them wisely. Here's what you get from some favorites:

Type	Calories per 2 tablespoons (2 thumbs)
Cashews	94
Peanuts	97
Almonds	104
Natural peanut butter	187
Cashew butter	188
Smooth peanut butter	190
Almond butter	203

TIPS FOR ASIAN SEASONINGS

Countries that share a continent don't necessarily share a cooking style, as we see in Asia. Each country uses its own unique combination of sauces and seasonings. Our recipe features the classic flavors of Thailand: coconut, peanut, cilantro, and lime. To travel through the other cuisines of Asia, consider the flavors of:

China: Soy sauce, five-spice powder, hoisin sauce, oyster sauce, garlic

Japan: Soy sauce, rice wine, sugar, fish stock, ginger

Korea: Soy sauce, sesame oil, garlic, chili peppers, fermented soy paste

Vietnam: Fish sauce, lemongrass, cilantro, garlic, shrimp paste

Indonesia: Tamarind, ginger, thick soy sauce, coconut, lemongrass

The Philippines: Coconut milk, garlic, ginger, vinegar, fermented shrimp paste

Continued from page 97

serious business. Rightly or wrongly, your performance against your goals defines success for you, motivates you, and, too often, lets you down. Goal-setting is so important, in fact, you'll discover that we revisit the subject a month from now. But until then it's time for some basics.

Take that initial weight-loss goal you set for yourself and think about it for a few minutes. Ask yourself three questions:

1. Is my goal a reasonable one, something I can achieve based on the progress I'm making so far?

2. How long is it likely to take to reach my goal?

3. What weight would I be satisfied with if I can't quite hit my ideal goal?

After you've given these weighty questions some thought, set out your goals for the coming months. We recommend having a goal in mind for the end of the 12-week program about two months from now. If that's not *your* ultimate goal, set another target on a longer time frame.

What's Your Healthy Weight?

One target worth keeping in mind is your healthy weight. Since height and weight are related, experts don't rely on pounds alone. Instead they use a formula called body mass index (BMI). On page 311 you'll find information on how to calculate your current BMI and the number of pounds you'll need to lose to reach a healthy BMI.

Because individual body types differ, the official BMI chart offers a recommended range, not a single magic number. Having your healthy weight in mind can often serve as a great motivator.

But keep your perspective. If you're overweight, losing just a few pounds will make you healthier. Studies show that people who drop 5 percent of their body weight significantly improve their blood pressure and cholesterol numbers, thereby reducing the strain on their hearts and arteries. They also lower their risk of diabetes. The closer you get to your recommended BMI, the healthier you'll be.

Think TRIM

As you think about workable goals for the coming two months and beyond, keep in mind the acronym TRIM. It stands for:

Time-bound: An effective goal should have a deadline—a time when you expect to reach it. Choose a date two months from now, when you will have completed the 12 weeks of the *ChangeOne* program. Select the day and mark it on the calendar.

Realistic: We've said it before, but it's worth repeating: if you set a goal you can't reach, there's no point in setting it. Choose a target that you're pretty sure you can hit. Odds are you won't go from a size 20 to a size 12 in the next few months. But you could get to a size 16, or even 14.

Inspiring: Your goal should be something that really matters to you—attainable, but ambitious enough to excite you. Maybe you don't really care all that much about pounds on the scale, for instance; what you're concerned about is getting into shape so that you can keep up with the kids on hikes and bike rides.

Measurable: A worthwhile goal has to be measurable. If it isn't, obviously, you'll never know when you've reached it. The first step is to make it as specific as possible. The next is to describe exactly how you plan to measure your progress. A few examples:

Instead of:	Make your goal to:
Lose as much weight as I can before summer begins	Drop 10 pounds over the next two months
Be better about my diet	Follow *ChangeOne* at least six days out of seven each week
Get back into shape	Jog for 45 minutes at least three times a week in preparation for a 10-K charity run
Try to be more active	Walk at least 30 minutes five days a week over the next two months
Eat fewer sweets	Treat myself to just one dessert a week over the coming month
Feel less embarrassed by the way I look	Lose 10 pounds and join a water aerobics class by Memorial Day

In addition to pounds on the scale, give yourself at least two other goals. Dropping several dress sizes, for example, or fitting into a pair of jeans you wore two summers ago.

It's Not All About the Scale

Why have another goal in addition to pounds on the scale? Because while weight is the measure that most people use, it's not necessarily the best one. Who really cares what the bathroom scale says? What most people really want is to look better. And the scale can lie.

For example, let's say you're doing a great job on your diet, dropping calories and burning fat. At the same time, you've gotten so gung-ho about exercise that you've started going to the gym. You're tightening up flabby muscles and even adding some strength. You look great! You feel terrific!

But when you step up on the scale, oops: your weight has barely budged. Why? As we've pointed out before, you're replacing fat with muscle, which actually weighs more than fat, volume for volume. You're changing your body composition for the better. The reflection in the mirror shows it. Maybe you've dropped a waist size or two as well. You feel stronger and fitter. But if you have no other gauge than pounds on the scale, you'll be disappointed.

Once you've settled on realistic and measurable goals, fill out the *ChangeOne* Contract on page 305. Why a contract? Because while it's one thing to decide on a set of goals, it's another to really commit to them. Make a deal with yourself in writing. The form even includes a place for you to sign. And while you're at it, have someone witness the contract. Telling people your goals can often serve as essential extra motivation.

If all that sounds silly, you may be surprised. There's something powerful about putting your John Hancock on any agreement, even one you make with yourself. Before you sign it, make sure the goals you've set for yourself pass the TRIM test. Check again to be sure they're goals you are willing and able to work toward over the next few months.

Changes Ahead: Dining Out

More and more of our meals are eaten away from home—in restaurants, delis, and fast-food places. The only problem with dining out is the food that many eateries serve these days: oversized portions that are loaded with fat and calories. This week, while you focus on dinner, make a list of a couple of restaurants you'd like to try. Next week we're going to invite you to go out to dinner to practice a few simple strategies to cut those portions down to size.

More Dinner Choices

Can't find something you like from among the six suggested dinners in this chapter? Check out pages 268–283 for more delicious *ChangeOne* dinners. Here's a sampler:

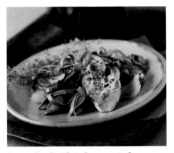

Sautéed Chicken with Caramelized Onions
page 269

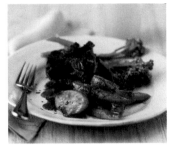

All-American Pot Roast with Braised Vegetables
page 272

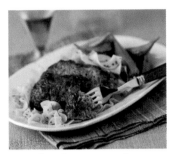

Heartland Meat Loaf
page 274

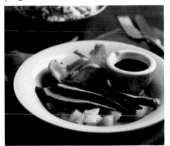

Sweet-and-Sour Glazed Pork with Pineapple
page 277

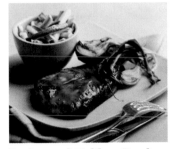

Barbecued Halibut Steaks
page 278

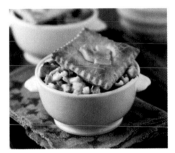

One-Crust Chicken Pot Pie
page 280

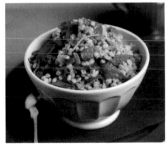

Barley Pilaf with Herbs
page 282

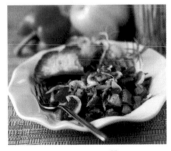

Summer Ratatouille
page 282

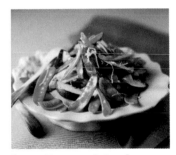

Snow Peas and Apple with Ginger
page 283

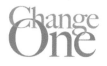

Week 5
Dining Out

Sure, you're watching what you eat. That's no reason to deny yourself the pleasure of eating out. Yes, the serving sizes surpass imagination, and in many restaurants the notion of cooking light means one stick of butter in the sauce instead of two. But if you approach dining out with common sense and a little bit of nerve, you can have a great meal while sticking with your plan.

This week dine out at least twice. Order exactly what you want, and don't take no for an answer!

Who knows? You might find it great fun getting the waiter and chef to deliver a more personalized meal to you. Remember, there's no need to fear a restaurant. You are the customer, paying to get what you want. So enjoy it, take your time, and savor the flavors—as *you* desire them.

A *ChangeOne* Evening Date

Dining out has become one of the great national pastimes. In 1970 the average American spent about one-quarter of the household food budget dining out. Today it's more like one-half. And why not? Never before have we had so many mouthwatering choices, from spicy Thai stir-fries and sizzling Mexican rice dishes to exotic Japanese sushi and good old American comfort food.

But there is a downside to dining out. Restaurant food typically contains 22 percent more fat than food consumed at home, experts say. And portion sizes? They've spiraled out of control at many eateries.

Portion creep happened gradually enough that most people didn't realize exactly how big those entrées had become until an organization called the Center for Science in the Public Interest (CSPI) began conducting clever sting operations a few years ago. The group rounded up meals from restaurants like the kind many of us dine in regularly. In one operation CSPI sampled almost two dozen Chinese

Dining Out Portions

These meal plans use both standard measurements and the *ChangeOne* portion-size guide. For this chapter we focused on dinner. It's the meal people typically eat out, and it often delivers the biggest portions. When you're going out for breakfast or lunch, you can review the portion sizes in those sections beforehand.

Type of food	Example	Amount	*ChangeOne* portion
One starch or one grain	Rice, pasta, noodles	$2/3$–1 cup	Tennis ball–baseball
	Roll	Medium	Tennis ball
One protein	Shrimp, scallops, crab	4 ounces	Baseball
	Chicken, turkey	3–4 ounces	Deck of cards
	Beef, veal	3 ounces	
	Salmon	3 ounces	
	Light-flesh fish	6 ounces	Checkbook
Vegetables		½ cup if with oil or butter; unlimited if steamed or raw	2 golf balls

restaurants. In another its investigators ordered from the menus of a variety of Italian restaurants, including several well-known nationwide chains.

What they found made headlines. Portion sizes and fat content at many of the nation's eateries have become so bloated that many meals border on health hazards. In some cases, CSPI found, a single entrée exceeded what many of us should eat in a whole day. At some Chinese restaurants, for instance, an order of kung pao chicken packed 1,400 calories. Love Italian food? A spaghetti and meatballs meal at some restaurants measured in at almost 1,000 calories.

One study found that in some cases, a single restaurant entrée exceeded what you should eat in a whole day.

Fettuccini Alfredo, or pasta in a cream sauce, soared to almost 1,800 calories in a single serving. Even half of one of these entrées puts you over your *ChangeOne* dinner target. Garlic bread to go with that? Eat a couple of pieces of the butter-soaked bread in many restaurants and you could tally up an additional 350 or more calories.

If you dine out a lot—and most of us have about four meals a week in restaurants or fast-food places—numbers like those can be discouraging. But even though the chef rules the kitchen, remember that you rule the table. You're the one footing the bill, after all. You choose what to eat and how much of it you want. You determine how quickly or slowly to enjoy a meal. You say when you've had enough. In some restaurants you can even give the chef specific directions for how you want your meal prepared.

Many of the strategies you'll use to take charge in restaurants are the same ones you've already been practicing: planning ahead, keeping an eye on portion sizes, and monitoring hunger and fullness signals. This week keep them in mind when you take yourself out to dinner. They'll help you sit down to a *ChangeOne* meal you'll enjoy without regrets.

Do Your Menu Homework

If you're considering a restaurant you've never tried before, stop by and look over the menu before you go in to make sure you'll be able to order the meal you want. Most establishments display their menus outside. Some even post them online. You won't be able to learn much about portion sizes, of course, but at least you'll know whether the menu includes some decent options. You could even pick the safest bets before you go in. That way you won't have to look at the menu and be tempted by steak smothered in hollandaise sauce or deep-fried cheese blintzes.

If you dine out frequently, keep your own personal list of diet-friendly restaurants in your area—places where you know you'll be able to get a great-tasting, low-calorie meal.

But there are some kinds of restaurants you should avoid altogether—unless you have an iron will. All-you-can-eat joints, buffet-style restaurants, even sprawling salad bars pose a hazard. Salad bars sound healthy enough, but many of them are stocked with calorie-rich dishes like creamy pasta salads. Better to order a simple garden salad with salad dressing on the side. Fried-chicken eateries and barbecue joints? Most of what's on the menu is so high in calories and fat that you'll bust your calorie budget before you satisfy your hunger. Fast-food restaurants? Unless you're willing to eat half that burger or chicken sandwich and wash it down with a diet soda, you're going to have a tough time finding a fast-food place that doesn't overdo the calories in its meal offerings.

And remember, you're shooting for at least two servings of vegetables. At the local burger joint you'll be lucky to get a piece of lettuce and thin slice of tomato.

But don't worry. There are still plenty of places where you can sit down to a good meal, as you'll discover paging through the suggested menus we review this week.

Check-In

What meal do you typically eat out? Breakfast? Lunch? Dinner? All of the above? If you dine out a lot, take a fresh look at the portion sizes in the first four weeks of *ChangeOne* so that when that plate of pasta or a burger lands in front of you, you'll know just how much to eat and how much to take home for later.

Many dieters find that keeping a visual equivalent in mind helps prevent portion creep. If you only treat yourself to a restaurant meal once or twice a month, definitely use the tips in this chapter to guide you when you open the menu. But enjoy yourself, too. Have that steak and eat it, too. If dinners out are an occasional treat, you don't have to worry. Still, pay attention to how full you feel. When you're satisfied, push your chair back and savor the feeling of being in control of what and how much you eat.

On the following pages we'll guide you through the good and not so good of some popular restaurant cuisines. But at the restaurant you'll need to be specific about your desires, or you'll end up with piles of high-calorie food on your plate. Take control from the start and don't let the restaurants dictate your dining experience. Beginning on page 122 you'll find some advice for getting exactly what you want—and nothing you don't want.

Italian Restaurants

Appetizer, pasta, main course, dessert—that's a standard meal in many Italian restaurants. Can you fit it into *ChangeOne*? Certainly, when you pay close attention to portions and include lots of vegetables. Check out our sample meals below.

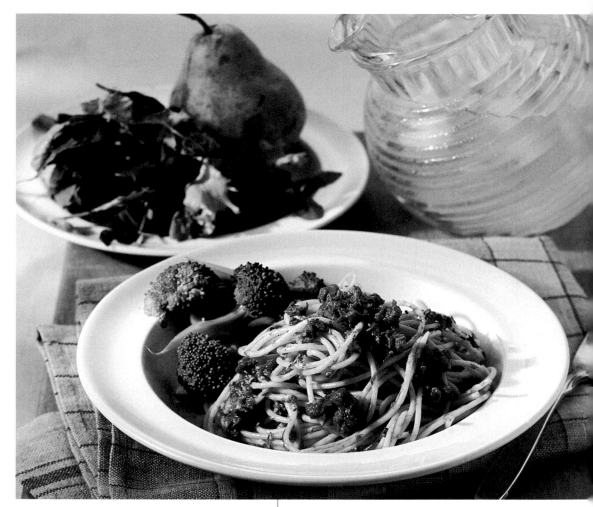

Menu 1

Green salad dressed with balsamic vinegar and a drizzle of olive oil

Spaghetti with red clam sauce (baseball)

Sautéed broccoli

Piece of fruit, or fruit salad (2 golf balls)

(Meal pictured above)

Approximate serving info (based on ChangeOne *sizes):* Calories 440, fat 11 g, saturated fat 1.5 g, cholesterol 15 mg, sodium 240 mg, carbohydrate 70 g, fiber 12 g, protein 20 g, calcium 200 mg.

Menu 2

Cup of minestrone soup (diner coffee cup)

Chicken breast cacciatore (deck of cards)

Plain pasta (tennis ball)

Spinach with garlic

Cup of fresh berries (2 golf balls)

Approximate serving info (based on ChangeOne *sizes):* Calories 440, fat 13 g, saturated fat 3 g, cholesterol 45 mg, sodium 1,140 mg, carbohydrate 56 g, fiber 12 g, protein 29 g, calcium 250 mg.

Choosing Your Meal

Soup

Italian soups are hearty, almost filling enough to be a meal if paired with a slice of crusty Italian bread and a green salad. Minestrone—a tomato-based soup with vegetables, beans, and pasta—is a great choice. Pasta fagioli features a fiber-rich combination of beans (fagioli) and pasta in a savory broth. Top either with a sprinkle of parmesan cheese for richer flavor.

Appetizers

Often listed as "antipasto" on the menu, appetizers run the gamut from fresh seafood salads to fried mozzarella, eggplant, and zucchini. To get the biggest bang for your buck, stick with the nonfried seafood or a virtually calorie-free fresh vegetable salad. If you're wondering how some of your current favorites stack up, here's a list of portions around 100 calories, ranked from best to worst in terms of calories and nutrition:

Appetizer	Serving size
Minestrone soup	1 cup (diner coffee cup)
Marinated shrimp	1/2 cup (2 golf balls)
Pasta e fagioli	2/3 cup (small coffee cup)
Fried calamari	1/3 cup (1/2 tennis ball)
Fried eggplant	1/2 cup
Mozzarella sticks	1 (1 thumb)

Main meals

Portions in many Italian restaurants are big enough to feed at least two. To keep your meal size in check, limit your pasta portion to about 2/3 cup (tennis ball). Here's a sampling of Italian dishes that all deliver about 250 to 300 calories:

Entrée	Serving size
Chicken cacciatore*	3 ounces chicken (deck of cards)
Veal marsala*	2 ounces veal
Veal scallopini*	2 ounces veal
Chicken or eggplant parmigiana*	3 ounces chicken or eggplant
Cheese lasagna	About 1 cup (baseball)
Ravioli and tomato sauce	About 1 cup
Baked ziti	3/4 cup (tennis ball)
Fettuccine Alfredo	3/4 cup
Spaghetti and meatballs	3/4 cup

Plus 2/3 cup cooked pasta

TIPS FOR ORDERING

Out with your spouse or children? Here's how to order for four, family style:

- One large salad, dressing on the side
- One appetizer
- Two pastas
- Two nonpasta main dishes
- Two vegetable sides

BEWARE

- **Pasta primavera:** Unless it's made the *ChangeOne* way (see page 98), this may be the biggest imposter of all; many restaurants make this dish with lots of cream.
- **Eggplant parmigiana:** Breaded and fried eggplant soaks up the oil.
- **Stuffed mushrooms:** Stuffing usually is a combo of cheese, fatty sausage, and cream.
- **Antipasto salad:** Mostly cheeses and salami slices.

Chinese Restaurants

Most of us can't go long without Chinese food. It's hard to resist dishes like crispy egg rolls, wonton soup, and tangy stir-fries. While some Chinese dishes can break your calorie bank, smart choices can be enjoyable additions to your weight-loss plan. Take the guesswork out of ordering with one of these menus.

Menu 1

Cup of wonton soup (diner coffee cup)

1 small egg roll (deck of cards)

Chicken chow mein (baseball)

Steamed mixed vegetables

Cup of pineapple chunks (baseball)

(Meal pictured below)

Approximate serving info (based on ChangeOne sizes): Calories 470, fat 19 g, saturated fat 4.5 g, cholesterol 130 mg, sodium 1,010 g, carbohydrates 52 g, fiber 8 g, protein 25 g, calcium 200 mg.

Menu 2

Cup of egg-drop soup (diner coffee cup)

Moo goo gai pan (tennis ball)

Brown rice (baseball)

Steamed broccoli

1 fortune cookie

4 orange wedges

Approximate serving info (based on ChangeOne sizes): Calories 420, fat 16 g, saturated fat 4.5 g, cholesterol 95 mg, sodium 1,590 g, carbohydrates 47 g, fiber 6 g, protein 26 g, calcium 150 mg.

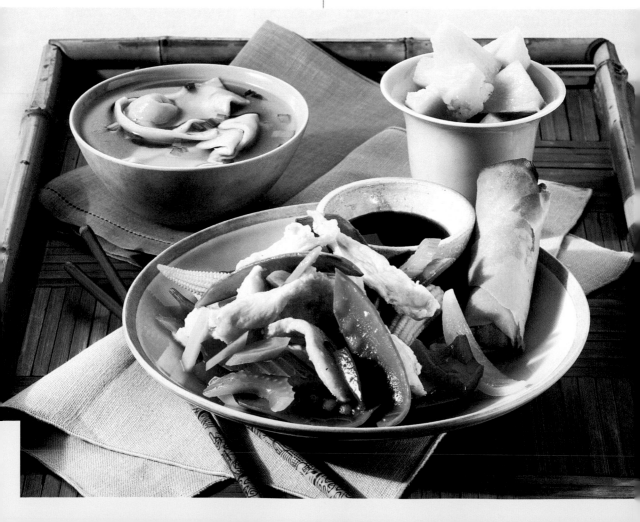

Choosing Your Meal

Soups

Chinese soup is a terrific starter. Your best bets are egg-drop soup or wonton soup. Hot-and-sour soup has about twice the calories of those. Likewise, velvet corn chowder and other hearty soups are more calorie-rich.

Appetizers

You *can* say "yes" to appetizers. Look for marinated vegetables or favorites that can be steamed rather than fried—wontons, dumplings, and spring rolls, for example. Here are some common choices in serving sizes that are around 100 calories, ranked from best to worst in terms of calories and nutrition:

Appetizer	Serving size
Marinated spinach salad	1 cup (baseball)
Dumplings, steamed	2 small or 1 medium
Spring roll, steamed	1 medium
Egg roll, all types	1 small
Spring roll, fried	1 small
Fried wonton	1 small

Main meals

Sharing entrées is half the fun at a Chinese restaurant. To avoid overdoing it, try to limit yourself to a couple of bites from each entrée and pick dishes with more veggies and fewer fried ingredients. We've ranked several favorites from lowest to highest calories, ranging from about 250 to 300 calories:

Entrée	Serving size
Moo goo gai pan	¾ cup (tennis ball)
Chicken chow mein	¾ cup
Sweet and sour pork	¾ cup
Chicken egg foo yung	¾ cup
Beef egg foo yung	¾ cup
Pork egg foo yung	¾ cup
General Tso chicken	⅔ cup (tennis ball)
Shrimp egg foo yung	⅔ cup
Chicken or beef fried rice	⅔ cup
Kung pao chicken or pork	½ cup (2 golf balls)
Moo shu pork	⅓ cup (half tennis ball)
Cashew chicken	⅓ cup

TIPS FOR ORDERING

- Order a one-pot soup. The portion is generous, with lots of soup broth to fill you up.
- Order a side of steamed vegetables to mix in with a saucy main course. The extra veggies add fiber and other nutrients to your meal and make your portion look more generous.
- Ask for dumplings steamed rather than pan-fried. They taste just as good and have fewer calories.

BEWARE

- **Tangerine or orange beef:** The citrus is hard to find— just fried peel with breaded, fried beef.
- **With walnuts:** Nuts are great, but not with the extra fats and calories they pick up when they're caramelized (sugared and sometimes fried), as is done in many Chinese restaurants.
- **Spicy eggplant:** This is one vegetable that soaks up lots of oil.

Surf and Turf

Steak houses and fish restaurants are an excellent dining-out choice. Many entrées are available grilled—a cooking method that lets fat drip away— and plainer side dishes help you control calories. But steaks that hang over the edge of the plate and fish filets that make side dishes look like garnishes hardly fit the *ChangeOne* strategy. Get your doggie bags ready!

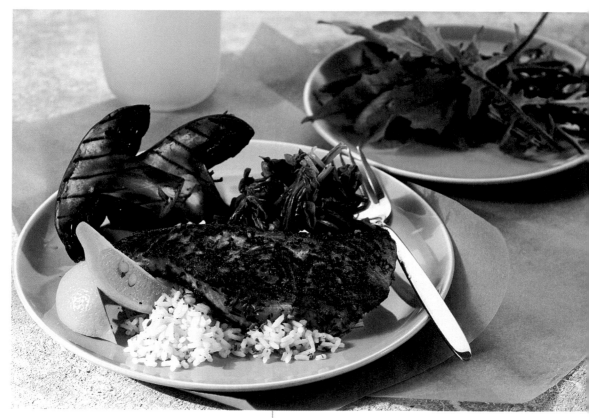

Menu 1

Grilled portobello mushroom

Green salad with fat-free dressing, or reduced-fat—adds about 30 calories

Grilled blackened salmon (deck of cards)

Sautéed spinach (2 golf balls)

White rice (tennis ball)

(Meal pictured above)

Approximate serving info (based on ChangeOne *sizes):* Calories 430, fat 16 g, saturated fat 3 g, cholesterol 55 mg, sodium 570 mg, carbohydrate 44 g, fiber 6 g, protein 28 g, calcium 150 mg.

Menu 2

Shrimp cocktail: 4 shrimp and 2 tablespoons cocktail sauce

Green salad dressed with balsamic vinegar and a drizzle of olive oil

Grilled beef tenderloin (deck of cards)

Green beans (2 golf balls)

Steamed asparagus with lemon

Small baked potato (tennis ball)

Approximate serving info (based on ChangeOne *sizes):* Calories 470, fat 9 g, saturated fat 3.5 g, cholesterol 115 mg, sodium 1,020 mg, carbohydrate 60 g, fiber 8 g, protein 37 g, calcium 100 mg.

Choosing Your Meal

Appetizers

Seafood appetizers are a popular offering in both surf and turf restaurants. As long as the seafood isn't fried or swimming in butter or olive oil, it's hard to go wrong with choices like shrimp cocktail, crab legs, or steamed mussels. Green salad is always an option—try topping it with shrimp and using cocktail sauce in place of dressing.

Main meals

In most cases you can be fairly confident in the cooking techniques of fish and steak restaurants. Grilling disposes of some fat as the food cooks, and wood or charcoal grilling imparts delicious smoky overtones. But stay alert: the standard 12-ounce tenderloin steak is a full four *ChangeOne* portions, and that's not counting the oversized baked potato with it. Keep in mind that just one tablespoon of melted butter has more than half the calories of the surf and turf entrées below. Here's a list of some popular main dishes, ranked from best to worst on the *ChangeOne* calorie range of about 250 to 300 calories:

Entrée	Serving size
Grilled sea bass	4 ounces (deck of cards)
King crab leg	1
Lobster tail	1
Blackened salmon	3 ounces (deck of cards)
Blue crab cakes	1½
Beef tenderloin	3 ounces
Rack of lamb	2 ounces (deck of cards)

Side dishes

At some restaurants side dishes come with the entrée. At others you can order them separately. Here are the portion sizes you should be aware of for popular selections like grains and potatoes:

Side	Serving size
Baked potato	½ large or 1 small (tennis ball)
Rice pilaf	⅔ cup (tennis ball)
Couscous	1 cup (baseball)
Spaghetti	⅔ cup (tennis ball)
Mashed potatoes	¾ cup
French fries	⅓ cup (½ tennis ball)
Garlic bread	1 slice

TIPS FOR ORDERING

These cooking methods are lean and healthy:

- **Blackened:** Rubbed with black pepper, paprika, and other spices and grilled.
- **Steamed:** Cooked without fat in a seafood steamer.
- **Reduction:** Sauce made by boiling down stock, wine, or balsamic vinegar.
- **Brochette:** Meat, fish, poultry, or vegetables on a skewer.

BEWARE

- **Béarnaise:** Sauce made with butter and egg yolks.
- **Beurre blanc:** Light-colored butter sauce.
- **Chateaubriand:** Large portion of beef tenderloin, usually for two.
- **Dijonaise:** Dijon mustard and cream sauce.

Diners and Coffee Shops

Americans love diners and coffee shops because they have something for everybody. The catch is that the number of choices can be overwhelming. And the huge portions at many diners give new meaning to the word "abundance." But there is good news: all of those choices make it easy to stick to your *ChangeOne* plan.

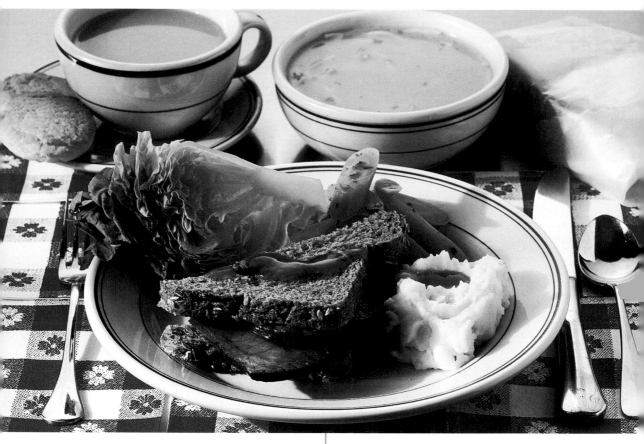

Menu 1

Small bowl of chicken noodle soup

Green salad with fat-free dressing, or reduced-fat—adds about 30 calories

Hot roast beef sandwich (take home half)

Mashed potatoes (½ tennis ball)

Cooked carrots (2 golf balls)

2 small butter cookies

(Meal pictured above)

Approximate serving info (based on ChangeOne *sizes)*: Calories 460, fat 16 g, saturated fat 5 g, cholesterol 50 mg, sodium 2,220 mg, carbohydrate 58 g, fiber 8 g, protein 23 g, calcium 150 mg.

Menu 2

Turkey breast (deck of cards)

Turkey gravy (dixie cup)

Cranberry sauce (2 thumbs)

Candied sweet potatoes (2 golf balls)

Green salad with fat-free dressing, or reduced-fat—adds about 30 calories

1 roll (tennis ball)

Approximate serving info (based on ChangeOne *sizes)*: Calories 440, fat 7 g, saturated fat 2 g, cholesterol 80 mg, sodium 1,050 mg, carbohydrate 63 g, fiber 7 g, protein 32 g, calcium 150 mg.

Choosing Your Meal

Soups

A typical diner offers two or three different soups each day, usually a broth with pasta or rice, a bean- or pea-based option, a chowder, or French onion soup. Lowest in calories are the broth-based soups like chicken noodle or beef barley. Bean or pea soups have more calories but also are more filling and satisfying. A bowl with bread and a salad is a meal. Highest in calories are soups made with cream, like chowder, or those with cheese.

Appetizers

Most diner appetizers are fried. Be sure to look at other sections of the menu, such as side dishes or breakfast, for surprisingly satisfying appetizers; or play it safe and order a side salad. The list below ranks popular choices by calories and overall nutrition, with calories ranging from about 35 to 65:

Appetizer	Serving size
Grilled vegetables	1 cup (baseball)
Tomato juice	1 cup
Barbecue chicken wing	1
Onion rings	2

Main meals

Here again, portion size is the issue. Also, lots of foods are fried and meals come in several courses. The three meals below are all right around the 450-calorie target for dinners:

Menu	Serving size
Chicken breast teriyaki	3 ounces (deck of cards)
White rice	1 cup (baseball)
Stir-fried broccoli	1 cup
Meat loaf	3 ounces (deck of cards)
Mashed potatoes	1/3 cup (1/2 tennis ball)
Green beans	1/2 cup (2 golf balls)
Dinner roll	1 (tennis ball)
Spinach omelet	2 eggs
Wheat toast	2 slices
Sliced tomatoes	

TIPS FOR ORDERING

Things to look for on the menu:

- **Grilled, broiled, roasted:** When done correctly, fat drips off.
- **Half portion:** Right around the *ChangeOne* recommended portion size.

BEWARE

- **Complete dinner:** Soup plus salad plus entrée plus sides plus dessert.
- **Dieter's plate:** Full-fat cottage cheese, fruit, and a burger patty; you could get fewer calories by ordering a regular burger.
- **Meal salads:** Enough to feed a family, with all the meat and cheese mixed in.
- **Potato skins:** When they're fried, not baked.

Mexican Restaurants

There's lots to love about Mexican fare—plenty of beans, fresh fish, grilled vegetables, and salsas. Many popular dishes could feed you and several relatives, however, and they're often drenched in cheese and sour cream. But choose wisely and you can have a delicious Mexican meal that fits nicely into your *ChangeOne* plans.

Menu 1

Cup of gazpacho

1 chicken fajita with:

>   Flour tortilla
>   Grilled chicken (deck of cards)
>   Grilled onions and peppers
>   Guacamole (thumb)
>   Unlimited lettuce, tomato, pico de gallo (fresh vegetable salsa)

(Meal pictured below)

Approximate serving info (based on ChangeOne *sizes):* Calories 430, fat 10 g, saturated fat 2 g, cholesterol 70 mg, sodium 1,310 mg, carbohydrate 47 g, fiber 6 g, protein 40 g, calcium 100 mg.

Menu 2

Shrimp or fish ceviche

2 steak soft tacos with:

>   2 corn tortillas
>   Grilled sirloin steak (deck of cards)
>   Grated cheese (palmful)
>   Unlimited lettuce, tomato, salsa

Approximate serving info (based on ChangeOne *sizes):* Calories 430, fat 16 g, saturated fat 6 g, cholesterol 155 mg, sodium 590 mg, carbohydrate 33 g, fiber 5 g, protein 40 g, calcium 250 mg.

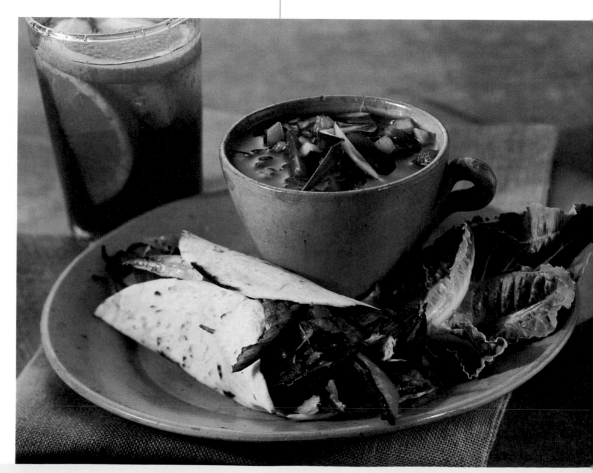

Choosing Your Meal

Soups

Two traditional Mexican soups deliver great taste without many calories. Gazpacho is a cold tomato soup brimming with diced green peppers and cucumber; with all those vegetables, it's wonderfully healthy. Tortilla soup starts with a base of chicken broth and gets its flavor from lime, cilantro, and pieces of chicken, with crumbled corn tortillas to round out the taste and texture.

Appetizers

Most Mexican appetizers are fried or dripping with cheese. If you must order quesadillas (grilled tortilla cheese sandwiches) or nachos (fried chips with an assortment of toppings), get one order for the whole table. Better yet, try ceviche, a fish or shrimp cocktail marinated in citrus and often accompanied by tomato and avocado.

Main meals

"Grande" is the best way to describe Mexican main courses. To avoid big portions, pick from the a la carte menu and get side orders of beans or rice if you want. One item with soup or a shared appetizer is about the right amount of food. Listed below are several favorites in the 250–300 calorie range when you eat the portion listed:

Entrée	Serving Size
Chicken fajita	Same as Menu 1
Steak soft taco	Same as Menu 2
Burrito	5 ounces (checkbook)
Hard-shell taco	2½ ounces
Beef and bean chimichanga	4 ounces (deck of cards)
Beef and cheese chimichanga	4 ounces
Tostada	6 ounces (checkbook)
Chicken taquito	5 ounces
Beef flauta	4 ounces
Cheese quesadilla	4 ounces

TIPS FOR ORDERING

- Ask the waiter to take away the tortilla chips. Better to not be tempted than to try to limit yourself to just a couple.
- Pick just one high-calorie topping—sour cream, grated cheese, or guacamole—and use it sparingly. Guacamole is best, healthwise.
- Make a meal of side orders—for example, black beans, rice, and grilled vegetables topped with salsa.

BEWARE

- **Fish taco:** The fish usually is breaded and fried. See if you can get it with the fish grilled.
- **Tostada or taco salad:** The fried tortilla bowl has more calories than the salad. Order it without the bowl.
- **Frijoles:** High-calorie beans if they've been fried; refried beans are cooked in lard and then mashed.

Take Control of the Table

Be the director of your dining experience right from the start, and you really can have it your way, all the way. Here are four guidelines that will put you in charge:

1. Ask and you shall receive

The wait staff should know how a dish is made, what the ingredients are, and how big the portion size is. So ask, already. Then have it your way. If the burrito looks good except for the fact that it's smothered in sour cream, ask the chef to hold the cream. If you'd like the grilled chicken breast without the skin, say so. If the vegetable side dishes are usually prepared with gobs of butter, request yours lightly sautéed in olive oil or steamed. Pizza tonight? The chef should be more than willing to make yours with half the normal cheese, or none, and an extra topping of vegetables.

2. Sign up for one course at a time

One of the pleasures of dining out is taking your time. Or at least it should be. Unfortunately, at too many restaurants waiters snatch up one course and rush in with the next before you've had time to put your fork down. There's a reason. Most restaurants want to turn tables around as quickly as they can to squeeze in as many seatings in an evening as possible. That's their business. Yours is to relax and take the time you need to eat only what you want—and no more. If you're worried about being rushed, order just one course at a time. Start with an appetizer. Once you're done, look back at the menu to consider what you'll have next. A useful rule of thumb: allot at least 20 minutes per course—the time your body needs to send satiety signals. Do you feel full? You're under no obligation to keep ordering.

3. Draw the line

Ask whether the kitchen can prepare half portions. Many restaurants are more than willing to do so. Some even offer half portions on the menu. If the dish you order turns out to be too big, ask the waiter right then and there to divide the portions and set half aside for you to take home. Don't wait until you've started to nibble. Don't depend on your willpower to eat only half of what's in front of you. If you know in advance that the entrées at a particular restaurant are outsized, ask for a half portion as the meal and request that the other half be brought at the end in a takeout container.

4. Rule the table

When you're dining out, you're in charge— not only of what you eat but of what's on the table. Lots of restaurants start you off with a basket of dinner rolls. If you're hungry when the rolls arrive, you'll automatically gobble up mediocre white-flour bread smeared with butter and loaded with calories without even giving it a second thought. Why waste the calories? Tell the waiter, "No bread, thanks." If you're famished when you sit down, order something more sensible to take the edge off your hunger before you do anything else—a side salad, a vegetable side dish, or a glass of spicy tomato juice, for instance. At the same time, ask for a glass of water. Heck, ask for a whole pitcher. Then you won't have to keep the busboy busy filling your glass. Remember to drink plenty of water with your meal. And don't forget who's boss. If something arrives at the table that you don't want, politely decline it. No one will mind.

Manage the Menu

Order wisely, and you can put together a meal that's long on flavor and short on calories. Here are five things to consider when you open the menu:

1. Be colorful

Meat and creamy sauces are usually beige, right? Where do most dishes get their brightest colors? From vegetables and fruit, of course. Choose the most colorful dishes on the menu, and chances are you'll order the healthiest, lowest-calorie selections. Spicy red salsas, deep purple beets, green

Help!

"I'm used to a glass of wine or beer with dinner. Can I enjoy a drink and still lose weight on ChangeOne?"

Sure. But before you raise your glass, remember one key word: moderation. Alcoholic beverages contain calories— about 120 calories in a glass of wine and 145 in a 12-ounce glass of beer. In fact, the average adult who drinks gets 10 percent of total calories from alcohol, surveys show.

But whether those calories "count" in the same way that food calories count is a subject of debate. Even though drinkers consume more calories than nondrinkers, they aren't more likely to be obese or overweight. What's more, volunteers in controlled studies who are given additional calories in the form of alcohol do not gain weight. If they replace some carbohydrates or fat in their diet with the equivalent number of calories in the form of alcohol, they may actually lose weight.

Why? Researchers suspect that alcohol may alter the way the body burns fat, causing it to "waste" calories.

But the new health benefits associated with some alcoholic beverages haven't been enough to convince health experts to advise nondrinkers to start imbibing. The reason: excessive drinking poses big health risks.

Still, if you enjoy a glass of wine or beer with dinner, go on enjoying it. But make sure you have just one. Drinking more than that can loosen your inhibitions and make it easier to break your resolve to stick to your diet.

salads, yellow corn, bright orange, and yellow sweet peppers turn your plate into a rainbow of colors. As long as vegetables arrive without added fat they're free on *ChangeOne*. Help yourself. And there's another reason for filling your plate with color. Many of the substances that provide fruits and vegetables with their colors are antioxidants—potent disease-fighters that have been shown to lower heart disease and cancer risk.

Help!

"Okay, so I know going out for fast-food isn't the smartest thing to do. But sometimes there's no other choice, especially if the kids have anything to say about it. Is there any way to order off a fast-food menu and still hold calories down?"

Sure, as long as you can resist the messages to add this and supersize that. Be a contrarian. Choose the smallest sizes. Ditch the secret sauce. Double up on lettuce and tomatoes. Order diet soda or water instead of sugary drinks. Here are 11 meal options to choose from:

- Chicken nuggets (four pieces), sauce (one package), garden salad with fat-free vinaigrette
- Grilled chicken flat bread sandwich (hold the sauce), garden salad with fat-free vinaigrette
- Junior hamburger, garden salad, fat-free French dressing
- Large chili, shredded cheddar cheese (two tablespoons), two saltine crackers
- Plain baked potato, Caesar side salad, fat-free French dressing
- Veggie burger, garden salad, fat-free dressing
- Grilled vegetable sandwich (hold the mayo), black bean soup
- Two beef soft tacos
- Chicken soft taco, pintos, and cheese
- Zesty chicken salad bowl (no dressing)
- Taco salad with salsa (no shell)

2. Order appetizers and sides

Another favorite dieting strategy: forgo the entrée section of the menu and order only from the appetizers and side dishes. With today's oversized restaurant portions, an appetizer or side often makes the perfect meal by itself. Skip things like the deep-fried mozzarella, of course, and make sure your choices include at least two servings of vegetables.

3. Dip into the sauce

Ordering salad dressing on the side and drizzling it on sparingly is one of the oldest diet tricks. Remember that you can order other sauces on the side, too, from gravy to guacamole. Give yourself no more than a tablespoon. And put your fork to good use. Instead of pouring on the sauce or salad dressing, dip the tips of your fork in the dressing and then spear a bite-sized portion. You'll make a little bit of a good thing go a long way.

4. Create your own smorgasbord

If you're dining out with friends who share your concern about overdoing it, agree to order and share entrées. If there are four of you, order two or three main dishes. You'll get a chance to sample a wider variety of items and keep portions down to size. Be careful, though: some people offered a lot to choose from end up eating a lot more. Decide in advance to sample only two or three forkfuls of each dish. With lots of dishes on the table, it's especially important to be aware of hunger and satiety signals. Sit back from time to time and think about whether you've had enough. If you have, put your fork down, raise a glass of water, and enjoy the conversation.

5. Be a discerning food critic

Remember the credo of smart dining: if it doesn't taste great, don't eat it. Sure you paid for it, and it's a shame to waste food. But to finish something you don't really like is the true crime. When you're dining out this week, be a tough critic. Pay attention to the first few bites. Decide whether it's good enough to finish, or whether you'd just as soon set aside calories for something else. If you dine out frequently, consider keeping a diner's diary, with mini reviews and notes on what you had. Use a star system to award top restaurants your own *ChangeOne* rating. You'll find yourself paying closer attention to the food you eat—and enjoying it more.

Changes Ahead: Weekends & Holidays

Restaurant meals are meant to be savored and enjoyed. So is the weekend. Whether it's a calm day at home or a wild outdoor excursion, so many of us use weekends for relaxation, family, and good food. Once you master the art of restaurant ordering, *ChangeOne* style, your next task will be to take on your weekend eating habits.

For some of us this will be a hard one. When we get together with friends and family, food seems to magically appear, in copious amounts. It's time to start thinking about the role food plays in your social and family life. Look back to last weekend and think through all you did and the role food played in things. Where were the temptations, the times when food was too available or the center of attention?

As you will see, we've been taught that food equals love—that mom pushing an extra slice of pie at you is her way of showing how much she cares for you. When you are ready to move on, we'll show you how to say no to all those food offerings, without guilt or sacrifice. Plus, you'll learn techniques for handling special occasions as well.

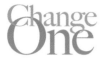

Week 6

Weekends
& Holidays

We almost called this chapter "Family & Friends." Why? Because on weekends and holidays, that's who you'll be spending your time with, and these people will have an incredible amount of influence over what you eat—and how much. In many cases they'll be instrumental in determining your long-term dieting success, either through their support or lack of it.

Weekends are also when the usual work-week routine is up for grabs. New temptations arise from every side: fancy dinners out, hot dogs and french fries at the ball game, Sunday brunches, and backyard barbecues.

This week dive into your weekend with gusto. We're proposing just this one change: focus less on food and more on active fun.

We'll show you that you don't have to hide from friends, family, or fun to stick to your new eating habits.

Get Together With Family and Friends

By now you know that the real secret to losing weight isn't as complicated as a lot of diet books would have you believe. Like a lot of the volunteers who tested *ChangeOne*, you may have found that making just two or three changes was all you needed in order to start slimming down.

The same principles that have guided you will serve you well when your routine suddenly switches gears on weekends and holidays. Sure, you'll need to be a little creative. But that's not such a bad thing. Learning to be flexible is important. Life, after all, has a way of throwing us a curve now and then. The more confident you feel about adapting your diet to new situations, the better your chances of success. Weekends and holidays are a great way to discover that you can control what you eat in almost any situation.

Why Not Take the Weekend Off?

If you've tried a deprivation-type diet in the past—the kind built around diet shakes or long lists of forbidden foods—you were probably tempted to take a vacation from dieting when weekends and holidays rolled around. But by making a distinction between days when you follow a diet and days when you're on "vacation" from it, you tell yourself that your diet is some kind of unnatural chore. It makes you eat one way to lose weight, but you really want to eat another, very different way in your everyday life. That's the recipe for a diet that will fail. Too many dieters lose weight, then go off their diets and return to the way they used to eat. Almost immediately the pounds begin to pile on again.

ChangeOne isn't about deprivation, as you know by now.

Check-In

Frustrated that you're not losing weight faster? There's no need to be if you're dropping a pound or two a week. That's a pace that will keep you on track not only to lose weight but keep it off. Wish you were losing that much? Look back at the Fast Track suggestions in the breakfast, lunch, snacks, and dinner sections. Choose two tips from any of those to put into effect this week. Fast Track turned out to be one of the most popular features of *ChangeOne* among our volunteers. Many followed the advice in all of them.

It's about good food and a rational way of eating that you can enjoy while you lose weight—and will continue to enjoy and benefit from long after you've lost the pounds. It is a diet you can live with every day.

That's the key. The more consistently you make smart eating choices, the more quickly they'll become second nature to you. That's why it's so important on weekends and holidays to find ways to use *ChangeOne* strategies even when your normal schedule is thrown up for grabs and you find yourself in situations where plates are piled high and beverages are flowing freely.

If you're celebrating something special—your birthday, an anniversary, a big wedding, whatever—live it up. But plan ahead. Strike a deal with yourself in advance. In return for getting the chance to indulge a little, agree to skip snacks during the day; set aside 45 minutes for a calorie-burning activity; or put together any combination that lets you, in effect, pay as you go. Keep track of what you eat during the day. Fill in a detailed food diary if you have time.

And remember, one indulgence doesn't mean you've failed. It doesn't even have to bring bad news on the scale. To gain a pound, you have to consume about 3,500 more calories than you burn. That's a lot of calories. Even the biggest holiday feast isn't likely to pack that many. The truth is, a big blowout isn't what typically spells trouble for dieters. The real danger is eating a little too much every day—or every weekend. If you do indulge yourself this weekend, just make a pact to follow the *ChangeOne* meal plans more closely during the coming week and you'll be fine.

When Food Is Love

One big reason weekends and holidays are difficult is that in all the world's cultures, food equals love. Food is a reward. Food is comfort. How do we celebrate Valentine's Day? With chocolate hearts. What do we do for someone's birthday? Bake a cake. How do we mark a wedding? With a feast. The simple act of offering someone food is a way to show love and affection. There's nothing wrong with that. We just need to keep a clear view of why we're eating.

This week and weekend notice the role that food plays for you with your family and friends. If the people who love you press you to eat more than you want or need, look for alternatives. If your mother says, "Eat, eat," to show she cares, say: "No thanks, mom. I'm full right now—but let me help you clear the dishes so we can have a chance to talk." If your friends' main device for getting together is dinner out, suggest alternatives that don't have to center around food: cards, bowling, dominos, or badminton, for instance, or a hike in a nearby park.

When you do find yourself at the table with friends and family, remember that you don't have to overeat to show you care. Food is only part of what makes sitting down with

Continued on page 134

Practicing the Art of Saying, 'No, Thanks'

"Have some more," your doting mother-in-law urges you. "You're going to waste away if that's all you eat."

"What?" Aunt Bev says. "You didn't like my casserole? You've always loved my casserole. Come now, just one more little serving. Dessert? But it's a special occasion. You can't say no!"

Of course you can say no—but sometimes only at the risk of hurting someone's feelings. Or so it may seem. But you don't have to let well-meaning urgings to eat cause you to overeat. You can always refuse. And by being diplomatic you won't hurt any feelings in the process. Here's how:

Be up-front. Casually mention to everyone in advance that you're on a diet and watching portion sizes. Make it clear that you don't want to offend anyone but that it's very important for you to keep an eye on how much you eat.

Compliment early and often. If you're oohing and aahing after the first bite, it won't seem as if you disliked the dish when you turn down seconds later.

Pace yourself. If you know Aunt Bev's feelings will be hurt when you don't sample her pecan pie, plan your meal accordingly. Help yourself to smaller portions of the main course so you have a little extra room—and some extra calories to spare—when dessert rolls around.

Say yes to a little. Sometimes it's easier to take a small portion than refuse everything and find yourself staring at an empty plate while everybody enjoys dessert. But be sure that you control the serving size, not Aunt Bev.

Use delaying tactics. You can avoid offending people by saying "Maybe later," or "I'm so full right now I wouldn't be able to enjoy it. Let me wait a little while." Once the plates are cleared away and the festivities move on to the next stage, no one will remember that you didn't have dessert.

Take it home. Another strategy to avoid eating more than you want is simple flattery. When the offer for seconds comes along, rave about how great everything was—and ask if you can take a serving home rather than have seconds now. And taking seconds home doesn't mean you *have* to eat them. If you don't intend to, make sure you dispose of the leftovers right away. We won't tell.

> "I'm so full right now I wouldn't be able to enjoy it."

Egg-Based Brunches

A leisurely Sunday brunch with family or friends is among life's great pleasures. And since you're combining two meals in one, you have a lot more calories in play. These two menus feature egg dishes as the centerpiece.

The Sunday Omelet

1 Vegetable-Cheddar Omelet

¾ cup oven-roasted potato wedges (lightly brushed with oil, seasoned, and baked at 375°F for 40 minutes)

1 cantaloupe wedge

Calories 420, fat 17 g, saturated fat 5 g, cholesterol 440 mg, sodium 430 mg, carbohydrate 43 g, fiber 6 g, protein 21 g, calcium 120 mg.

VEGETABLE-CHEDDAR OMELET

2 **eggs**
1 **teaspoon water**
2 **teaspoons chopped fresh herbs (dill, basil, parsley, etc.)**
⅛ **teaspoon salt**
⅛ **teaspoon fresh ground black pepper**
½ **cup (loose) thinly sliced fresh spinach**
1 **plum tomato, chopped**
2 **tablespoons shredded reduced-fat cheddar cheese**

1. Whisk the eggs, 1 teaspoon water, herbs, salt, and pepper in medium bowl. Toss spinach, tomato, and cheddar in small bowl and set aside.

2. Lightly coat nonstick omelet pan or small skillet with cooking spray and set over medium heat 1 minute. Pour egg mixture into pan and cook until eggs begin to set on the bottom. Lift up edge of eggs with heat-proof spatula, pushing cooked part toward center of pan and letting uncooked portion run underneath. Cook until eggs are almost set and bottom is lightly browned.

3. Spread spinach filling over half of omelet, leaving ½-inch border around the edge and reserving 1 tablespoon for garnish. Lift up omelet at edge nearest handle and fold in half. Cook 2 minutes. Slide omelet onto plate and garnish with reserved filling.

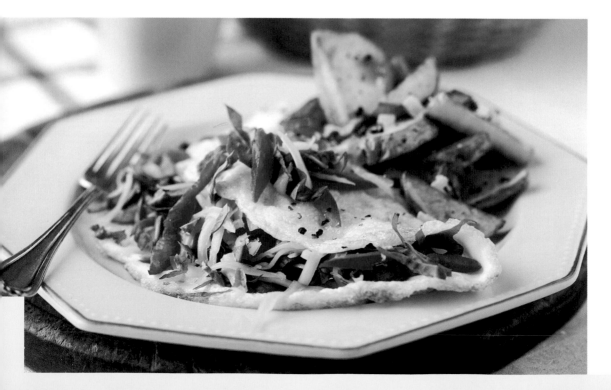

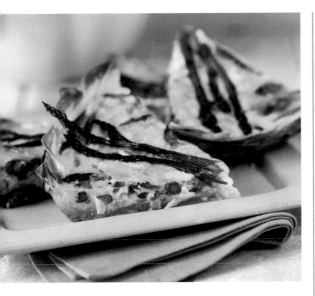

1. Preheat oven to 400°F. Coat a 9-inch pie plate with cooking spray and sprinkle with bread crumbs. Beginning in center, arrange potato slices in slightly overlapping circles out to the side. Lightly brush with olive oil and press down gently. Bake 10 minutes.

2. Set 8 to 12 asparagus spears aside. Cut remaining spears into 1-inch pieces.

3. Sprinkle crust with ¼ teaspoon salt and ¼ cup cheddar. Cover with asparagus pieces, then sprinkle with scallions and another ¼ cup cheese. Arrange whole asparagus spears on top.

4. Beat evaporated milk, eggs and whites, butter, mustard, pepper, and remaining salt in medium bowl. Pour into pie plate and sprinkle with remaining cheddar. Bake until knife inserted in center comes out clean, about 35 minutes.

Quiche and Fruit Bread

1 slice Zesty Cheddar-Asparagus Quiche

1 slice Peach Quick Bread (recipe on page 256)

6 ounces orange juice

Calories 350, fat 11 g, saturated fat 4 g, cholesterol 100 mg, sodium 490 mg, carbohydrate 48 g, fiber 3 g, protein 17 g, calcium 300 mg.

ZESTY CHEDDAR-ASPARAGUS QUICHE

Serves 6

- 1 **tablespoon plain dry bread crumbs**
- 8 **ounces small all-purpose potatoes, peeled and very thinly sliced**
- 2 **teaspoons olive oil**
- 1 **pound asparagus, trimmed**
- ½ **teaspoon salt**
- ¾ **cup shredded reduced-fat sharp cheddar cheese**
- 3 **scallions, sliced**
- 1 **can (12 ounces) evaporated fat-free milk**
- 2 **eggs and 2 extra egg whites**
- 2 **teaspoons butter, melted**
- 1 **teaspoon dry mustard**
- ¼ **teaspoon fresh ground black pepper**

ABOUT EGGS

Large eggs are the standard size for all *ChangeOne* recipes. But many cooks use extra-large eggs because they're more widely available. A large egg supplies 78 calories, an extra-large supplies 90, and a jumbo egg supplies 100. Most of the calories, fat, and cholesterol are in the egg yolk, which also contains beneficial compounds such as lutein, a pigment that aids eye health. According to research on eggs and blood cholesterol, most people are okay eating as many as seven whole eggs per week without increasing their cholesterol levels. To stretch your eggs, use additional whites. Egg whites are practically fat-free, and each one adds only 17 calories.

Seafood Brunches

Nothing says Sunday morning better than lox and bagels. But that's not the only seafood idea for brunch. Here's one classic—and one surprise.

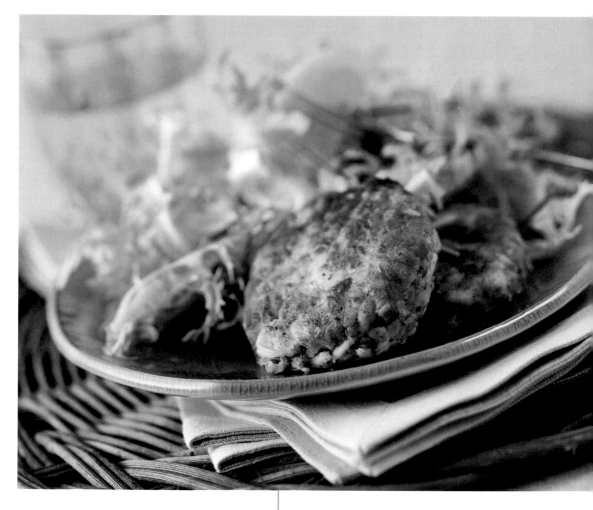

Crab Cakes

2 Chesapeake Crab Cakes

1 green salad with 2 tablespoons fat-free dressing, or reduced-fat—adds about 30 calories

1 small crusty roll (2 golf balls)

1 cup seasonal berries—raspberries, strawberries, blueberries, or black-berries, as available

Calories 440, fat 9 g, saturated fat 1.5 g, cholesterol 145 mg, sodium 1380 mg, carbohydrate 60 g, fiber 13 g, protein 32 g, calcium 250 mg.

CHESAPEAKE CRAB CAKES

Makes 8 cakes (serves 4)

$1/2$ **cup fresh bread crumbs**

1 **celery rib with leaves, finely chopped**

$1/3$ **cup finely chopped red pepper**

2 **tablespoons minced shallot**

1 **tablespoon finely chopped parsley**

2 **tablespoons coarse Dijon mustard**

2 **tablespoons low-fat mayonnaise**

1 **egg**

1 **teaspoon Old Bay seasoning**

1 **pound lump crabmeat**

$1/3$ **cup all-purpose flour**

2 **teaspoons vegetable oil**

1. Mix bread crumbs, celery, red pepper, shallot, parsley, mustard, mayonnaise, egg, and Old Bay seasoning in large bowl. Gently fold in crabmeat.

2. Preheat oven to 350ºF. Spread flour on waxed paper. Divide crab mixture into 8 even amounts, then form into patties with floured hands. Dredge in flour.

3. Lightly coat large nonstick oven-proof skillet with cooking spray and set over medium-high heat until hot but not smoking. Cook 4 crab cakes until brown, about 2 minutes on each side. Drizzle 1 teaspoon oil around crab cakes, gently shaking pan to spread oil after turning crab cakes over. Transfer to plate lined with paper towels. Repeat with remaining crab cakes and oil.

4. Lightly coat baking sheet with cooking spray, place crab cakes on sheet, and bake until very hot in center, 8 to 10 minutes.

Lox and Bagels

½ deli bagel, any flavor, topped with:

- **1 tablespoon reduced-fat cream cheese**
- **3 slices smoked salmon**
- **1 thick slice tomato**
- **1 slice red onion** (optional)
- **Capers** (optional)

1 cup fresh fruit salad (baseball)

1 mimosa (equal parts orange juice and champagne or sparkling water)

Coffee or tea

Calories 610, fat 7 g, saturated fat 3 g, cholesterol 17 mg, sodium 1,052 mg, carbohydrate 110 g, fiber 7 g, protein 17 g, calcium 120 mg.

HEALTH TIP

We lighten the calorie load on this classic breakfast by using reduced-fat cream cheese and only half a bagel. But you're not being short-changed: a deli or bagel-shop bagel weighs as much as five slices of bread.

TIPS ON BRUNCH MENUS

Try some or all of these ideas for your brunch menus:

Bread sampler:

- A basket of mini-muffins or crusty rolls

Salad variations:

- Spinach with reduced-fat dressing
- Sliced cucumbers tossed with rice vinegar, sesame oil, and a sprinkle of sugar
- Cubed tomatoes drizzled with balsamic vinegar and flavorful olive oil
- Baby lettuce and watercress

Cheese choices:

- Low-fat cottage cheese mixed with chopped cucumber, peppers, and radishes
- Part-skim ricotta flavored with vanilla extract, cinnamon, and sugar
- Assorted sliced reduced-fat cheeses

Fruit treats:

- Fresh fruit salad
- Tricolor melon ball salad (cantaloupe, watermelon, and honeydew)
- Sliced peaches drizzled with amaretto

Continued from page 129

friends and family a pleasure. We get together to talk and laugh, to catch up on the latest news, to reinforce the ties that bind by expressing our feelings for one another. If you're engaged in conversation, no one will notice that you've put your fork down and are sipping from your water glass. Food may nourish our bodies, but it's laughter and expressions of caring, after all, that nourish our souls.

Nurturing Yourself

Family and friends aren't the only people who urge food on us as a reward or show of affection. Some of us do it to ourselves. We eat to reward ourselves or to feel better when we're blue. Especially if you grew up being offered food to feel better, you may have internalized this reflex. Feel bad? Eat. The trouble, of course, is that you'll almost certainly overeat. When you do, you'll feel bad. And what do you do then? Well, eat some more.

Music, quiet, a phone call, a walk—all serve as small personal rewards.

How to escape? You may already have found part of the answer in becoming aware of genuine hunger cues and distinguishing them from environmental and emotional triggers to eat. But if you still have trouble resisting the urge to reward yourself with food, make a list of alternatives to eating. What else will make you feel better? If your day is full of stresses, reward yourself with five minutes of quiet time to relax and depressurize. (You'll find more stress-busting strategies in Week 9, "Stress Relief," which begins on page 180.) If you love music, take a few minutes out to play a favorite piece. If you really, really want something to eat, reward yourself with a stick of sugar-free gum, a suggestion we've made before because it *really* works. Make a habit of it, in fact. Over time, whenever the urge to treat yourself to food arises, you'll think of sugar-free gum.

Have a Plan in Place

Routines may change on weekends and holidays, but that doesn't mean everything has to be thrown up for grabs. Chances are you've already made at least a few plans for this weekend. Before it gets under way, think ahead. Write down a schedule for breakfast, lunch, and dinner, and fill in as many blanks as possible.

Think of it as a reverse food diary. Let's say your weekend plans include a trip to your mother's house to celebrate her 60th birthday with a big family potluck. Your schedule might look something like this:

Saturday

Breakfast: *ChangeOne* breakfast at home

Lunch: On the road

Dinner: Mom's house

Sunday

Breakfast: Mom's house

Lunch: Potluck at the park

Dinner: On the road

Once you've written up a schedule, identify the meals that are likely to pose the toughest challenges and brainstorm ways to prepare in advance to make them easier. In the example above, Saturday breakfast is a breeze, but grabbing lunch on the road could be treacherous, given the long strips

Smart Holiday Tricks

When the big winter holidays arrive, there's often no way to avoid being stuck in the house with lots of relatives, friends ... and food. Here are some ways to cope:

Be helpful anywhere but in the kitchen. This is a tough one, especially if you're at the in-laws. But it's easy to nibble when you're surrounded by food in various stages of preparation. Volunteer for other duties: cleaning up, setting the table, being bartender, running errands—anything that doesn't involve food.

Volunteer for any job that doesn't involve food.

Be the activity director. Take the lead in suggesting non-eating activities that the family can do together, from playing charades to building a snowman.

Grab a water bottle. When there are lots of high-calorie-beverages around, it helps to have an alternative ready. Keep a glass or bottle of water handy.

Keep "free" snacks and beverages on hand. Satisfy your munchies with very low-calorie treats like carrots, celery, sweet peppers, sliced jicama, and diet drinks. That way you won't have to rely on your willpower to steer clear of all those diet-busting rich foods.

Hang with the kids. If all the adults are circling the food table, spend time with the children. At most ages, kids are more likely than adults to be doing something active. Their energy and playfulness can help distract you from food.

Get lost. If the sight and smell of all that food becomes just too much for you, excuse yourself and get out of the house. Take a stroll or go for a drive.

Change One First Person

Bowling Over the Calories

After losing 18 pounds during her first five weeks on *ChangeOne*, Meredith Ross wasn't about to let a big weekend throw her off track—even two big weekends in a row, as she showed when she competed in state and national bowling tournaments.

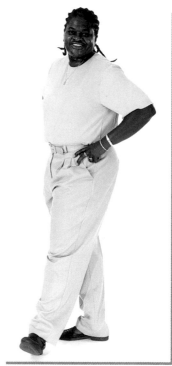

"I'm the sort of person who has breakfast, lunch and dinner the same time every day," says Ross, an information technology expert and top-notch amateur bowler. "When those tournaments come along, that schedule goes flying right out the window. Instead of having dinner at my usual seven o'clock, I'm sitting down with friends at one in the morning."

And as much as she loves bowling, Ross is the first to admit that bowling alley food isn't exactly inspiring. "We're talking hot dogs, hamburgers, french fries. Totally bad food."

So Ross set off on the two big weekends prepared with a big water bottle and a stash of granola bars. When she and her friends sat down to meals together, she'd pick and choose to find something that measured up to *ChangeOne*. Breakfast at the hotel was easy: oatmeal, juice, and a glass of milk. When dinner rolled around she skipped the fried foods and had soup and a salad. At lunch she asked the cook to put together a lettuce and tomato sandwich.

Her smart choices paid off. When she stepped up to the scale on the Monday following the two back-to-back weekends, Ross found that she had lost two more pounds.

"I was thrilled," Ross says. "I realized that, for me, the biggest change was learning what to eat. I've never been someone who ate a lot of food. But before I started *ChangeOne* I didn't know which foods to choose. Now I know. Vegetables. Whole grains. Grilled instead of fried. Even when my routine gets scrambled, I know now that I just have to remember those few rules and I can stay on my diet."

of fast-food restaurants between here and mom's. Family dinners are always a challenge—too much food, too many people urging you to eat. And a potluck on Sunday! Everyone will be bringing family favorites, and the table will be crowded with dishes.

Never fear. There are plenty of ways to plan ahead on a weekend like this. Here are seven ideas to get you started:

1. Do it yourself

The best way to control what you eat is to make it yourself—something we've mentioned a few times so far. If there's not much chance you'll find a decent meal when you're on the road, consider packing your own in advance. You'll save money, frustration, and time. If the weather's good and you can find a nice place to stop, you can turn a bag lunch into a picnic. When the weekend includes a potluck meal, contribute a *ChangeOne* dish. Fix two if you have the time. That way you'll have a choice of dishes you can rely on to be low in calories. Don't forget to bring along sugar-free beverages or sparkling water.

2. Celebrate special occasions with special food

At most big weekend and holiday gatherings, people bring big bowls of store-bought chips and dips along with lovingly prepared homemade delicacies, like Aunt Estella's chicken cacciatore or Grandma Peterson's rhubarb pie. Spend your calories wisely by skipping the run-of-the-mill munchies. Instead, choose from only the special foods that celebrate the occasion.

3. Practice your pace

The big holiday dinner is one time when everyone relaxes and enjoys a leisurely feast. It's a great chance to practice your best tortoise skills. For a long meal you may have to use every delaying tactic in the book. Drink a sip of water between each bite. Put your fork down frequently. Sit back in your chair and enjoy the conversation for a few minutes without eating anything.

4. Watch the alcohol

Wine, punch, beer, or other alcoholic beverages have a way of flowing freely at holiday meals. Don't let too much alcohol

Continued on page 142

Weekend Grilling

What better way to entertain than with your grill? But prepare yourself: meals you make for company on weekends tend to be larger than everyday meals. Plan to eat less at the other two meals that day.

Stand-Up Chicken

Crudité (raw vegetable) platter
(unlimited)

1 serving Beer-Can Chicken
(½ breast, or 1 drumstick and thigh)

1½ cups Grilled Summer Vegetables
(coffee mug)

½ cup German Potato Salad with
Dijon Vinaigrette (2 golf balls)

2 sesame breadsticks

1 piece Chocolate Snacking Cake
(recipe on page 284)

Calories 540, fat 8 g, saturated fat 2 g, cholesterol 85 mg, sodium 1,170 mg, carbohydrate 84 g, fiber 14 g, protein 37 g, calcium 150 mg.

GRILLED SUMMER VEGETABLES

Serves 4

2 small fennel bulbs, about 8 ounces each, cleaned

1 small eggplant, about 1 pound, cut lengthwise ½-inch thick slices

4 plum tomatoes, halved

3 large bell peppers, preferably 1 each green, red, and yellow, cut into ½-inch wide strips

1 medium red onion, cut into 8 wedges

½ teaspoon salt

½ teaspoon fresh ground black pepper

1 tablespoon orange juice

8 basil leaves, very thinly sliced

1 small garlic clove, very finely minced

1 teaspoon grated orange zest

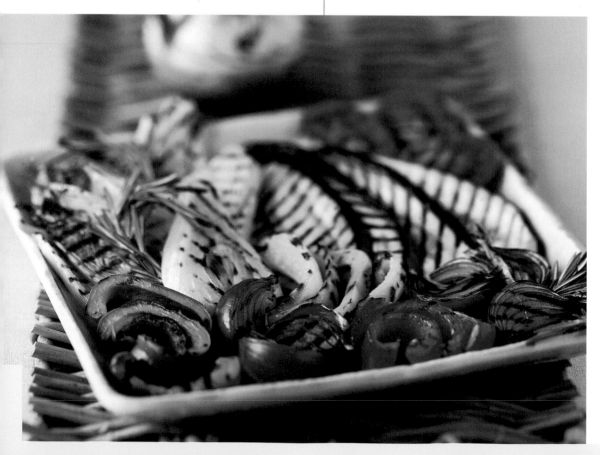

1. Preheat grill to high or start coals. Prepare fennel by cutting off fronds and setting aside. Peel bulbs and cut vertically into ½-inch slices. Coat fennel, eggplant, tomatoes, bell peppers, and onion with cooking spray, or a very light coating of olive oil, and sprinkle with salt and pepper.

2. Grill vegetables until tender and evenly browned, about 4 minutes on each side, turning once. Transfer to serving platter and sprinkle with orange juice.

3. Finely chop 1 tablespoon reserved fennel fronds and mix in small bowl with basil, garlic, and orange zest. Sprinkle over vegetables.

4. Before serving divide into 4 equal portions and refrigerate extra.

BEER-CAN CHICKEN

Serves 4

    1 chicken, 2½ to 3 pounds
    3-4 tablespoons dry spice rub, or make
         your own with equal parts paprika,
         onion powder, garlic powder, and
         salt and pepper to taste
    1 can beer

1. Prepare grill. If using a charcoal grill, place the coals around the outside edge of the grill. If using a gas grill, leave one burner off.

2. Rub chicken inside and out with dry rub. Loosen skin slightly and sprinkle a bit of dry rub between the skin and the flesh.

3. Open the beer can and pour out half. Place the beer can on the grill, in the center if using coal or over the unlit burner on a gas grill. "Sit" the chicken on top of the beer can; the can should fit inside the chicken cavity with its legs spread to form a tripod on the grill.

4. Close the grill lid and cook the chicken on medium heat until done, about 45 to 60 minutes. Carefully remove the chicken and can from the grill.

5. Cut chicken into 6 pieces—2 thighs, 2 drumsticks, 2 breast halves. One serving equals one thigh plus one drumstick, or ½ breast. Remove skin before eating.

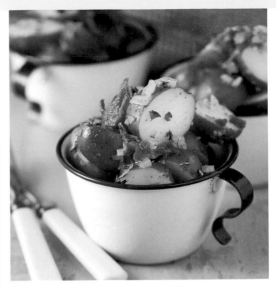

GERMAN POTATO SALAD WITH DIJON VINAIGRETTE

Serves 4

    1 pound small red-skinned potatoes,
       scrubbed and quartered
    ½ teaspoon salt
    3 slices turkey bacon
    1 small onion, chopped
    3 tablespoons cider vinegar
   1½ tablespoons sugar
    1 tablespoon country-style Dijon
       mustard
    ½ teaspoon olive oil
    ½ teaspoon pepper
    ¼ cup finely chopped sweet pickles
    ¼ cup finely chopped red bell pepper
    ¼ cup minced parsley

1. Bring potatoes, enough water to cover, and ¼ teaspoon salt to boil in large saucepan over high heat. Reduce heat to medium and cook until potatoes are tender, about 10 minutes. Drain and keep warm.

2. Cut bacon in half crosswise and cook in large nonstick deep skillet until crisp; transfer to paper towels to drain, and then crumble. Sauté onion in pan drippings until golden, about 7 minutes.

3. Shake vinegar, sugar, mustard, oil, black pepper, and remaining salt in a jar, and then whisk into skillet. Bring to a simmer and cook until fragrant, about 2 minutes. Add potatoes, half of bacon, pickles, and red pepper, and cook, stirring, until potatoes are coated and heated through, about 2 minutes. Sprinkle with parsley and remaining bacon.

Holiday Classics

Holidays and food go hand in hand, and most of us look forward to enjoying the same family favorites year after year. It's okay if you choose to leave *ChangeOne* behind for a holiday meal. But if you want to stay with the program through the holidays, check out our sample menu, and some new options on old reliables.

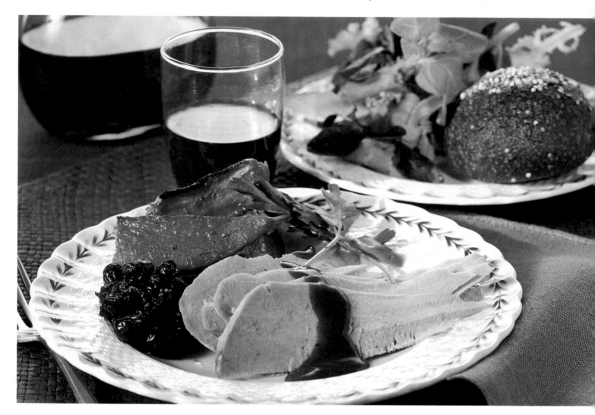

ABOUT FEEDING A CROWD

- Select at least two appetizers, one vegetable (like stuffed mushrooms or a crudité platter) and one holiday favorite (such as a low-fat cheese log).

- Offer a green salad as a low-calorie filler.

- Main meal choices should include one or two entrées, a starch side dish (pasta, rice, potatoes), rolls or bread, and one or two cooked vegetables.

- Prepare each recipe for about half the number of people at your dinner. For example, if you have 16 guests, prepare each dish to serve 8.

Turkey Dinner

3 ounces Apple-Stuffed Turkey Breast (deck of cards)

¼ cup gravy

2 tablespoons cranberry sauce

½ cup Orange-Glazed Carrots or Sweet Potatoes

1 green salad with 2 tablespoons fat-free dressing (2 salad dressing caps)

1 small crusty roll

Note the higher calorie count (below), so plan other meals of the day accordingly.

Calories 620, fat 7 g, saturated fat 2 g, cholesterol 105 mg, sodium 1,780 mg, carbohydrate 91 g, fiber 9 g, protein 45 g, calcium 200 mg.

APPLE-STUFFED TURKEY BREAST WITH ORANGE MARMALADE GLAZE

 1 **whole bone-in turkey breast (3 to 3 1/2 pounds)**
 1 1/2 **teaspoons salt**
 1 **teaspoon fresh ground black pepper**
 2 **celery ribs, cut into 1-inch pieces**
 2 **large apples, peeled and thinly sliced**
 1 **large onion, thinly sliced**
 5 **sprigs fresh thyme, plus 1 teaspoon chopped thyme**
 2 **teaspoons olive oil**
 2 **cups apple juice**
 1/2 **cup low-sugar orange marmalade**
 1/2 **cup dry white wine or apple juice**

1. Preheat oven to 350ºF. Rinse turkey, pat dry with paper towels, and rub skin all over with salt and pepper.

2. Combine celery, half of apples, half of onion, and 3 thyme sprigs and mound in center of roasting pan. Toss chopped thyme with remaining apples and onion in medium bowl. Stuff half of mixture under turkey skin; place remaining mixture in neck cavity.

3. Place turkey on top of mixture in roasting pan. Lightly brush turkey with olive oil and top with remaining thyme sprigs. Pour apple juice into pan. Roast 1 hour, discard thyme sprigs, and baste turkey with 1/4 cup marmalade. Continue roasting until turkey is golden brown and instant-read thermometer inserted in thickest part of turkey (not touching bone) reaches 170ºF, basting twice with remaining marmalade. Let stand 10 minutes to set juices. Transfer turkey to platter and slice. Discard skin.

4. Stir wine into apples and vegetables in pan (do not strain). Bring to boil over medium-high heat, scraping up browned bits from bottom of pan with wooden spoon, until liquid is reduced by half.

ORANGE-GLAZED CARROTS OR SWEET POTATOES

 2 **pounds carrots or sweet potatoes, peeled**
 1 **can (6 ounces) frozen orange juice concentrate, thawed**
 2 1/2 **teaspoons ground coriander**
 1 **teaspoon salt**
 3/4 **cup water**
 1 **tablespoon olive oil**
 1/3 **cup chopped fresh mint**

1. If using carrots, halve lengthwise and cut into 2-inch strips. If using sweet potatoes, cut into eighths lengthwise and cut those into 2-inch strips.

2. Combine carrots or sweet potatoes, orange juice concentrate, ground coriander, and salt in large skillet. Add water and bring to a boil over medium heat. Reduce to a simmer, cover, and cook until vegetables are crisp and tender, about 15 minutes.

3. Uncover, increase heat to high, and cook until vegetables are tender, about 7 minutes.

4. Add oil and cook, swirling pan until vegetables are glossy and sauce is creamy, about 1 minute. Stir in mint.

5. One serving equals 1/2 cup (2 golf balls).

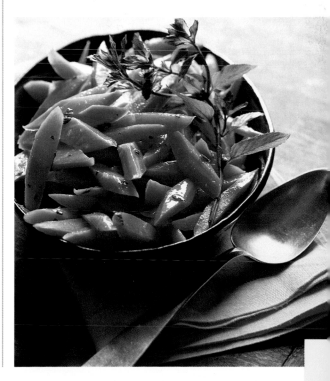

Continued from page 137
dissolve your best intentions to stick to your diet. Limit yourself to one glass with your meal. The rest of the time have sparkling water or sugar-free soft drinks. Love an icy cold beer on a hot summer weekend? Light beer should be an option, and the offerings in this category are getting better and better.

5. Get out and about

The extra leisure time on weekends offers a great opportunity to plan activities that involve burning more calories. Rally your relatives for hikes, bike rides, walking tours of the city, softball, croquet, a run on the beach, throwing a Frisbee, or just frolicking with the dog. Burn 500 extra calories this weekend and you can treat yourself to a big piece of Grandma Peterson's rhubarb pie without worrying about upsetting your calorie balance. Activities that the whole family can join in are also great ways to enjoy time together—and they don't center around food.

6. Take time for bedtime

Weekends are a wonderful opportunity to catch up on sleep you may have missed during the week. Lack of sleep can erode your willpower and determination. Obesity experts believe it can even cause you to put on pounds. Get to bed a little early one night this weekend. If that doesn't work, allow yourself to sleep a little later than usual one morning.

7. Fine-tune your expectations

If the coming week is a crowded schedule of holiday parties, be realistic about your goals. Instead of trying to continue losing weight, for instance, relax your goal to simply maintaining your current weight. When the holidays are done, you can start shedding pounds again. Setting standards that are impossible to meet mostly just leads to failure. Unless you have an upcoming modeling session for the cover of a fashion magazine, odds are you don't have to lose a certain amount of weight by a certain date. Remember, this is a weight-loss plan for your entire life. Don't put yourself under needless pressure right from the start. It's far better to take a little while longer to reach your goal than to put yourself under unnecessary stress.

Should You Enlist Family and Friends?

A bit of encouragement, a helping hand, even someone joining you on your walk around the neighborhood can be great morale boosters. So can a shoulder to lean on when things aren't going your way. Help from family and friends also can take the pressure off you and eliminate the unnecessary stresses in your life.

How important are the people around you when it comes to dieting success? At first, behavioral scientists assumed the answer would be "very." The more support dieters had, the assumption went, the better their odds of losing weight and keeping it off. But the results of studies looking at social support and weight loss have been mixed. Some people do better when they have a strong social network. Others do just fine on their own.

Knowing whether you tend to be a team player or a solo flier is the first step in finding the kind of support and encouragement you need to succeed. To find out, answer the questions in the Quiz on page 145.

Your Friends in Need

Social support comes in many forms, from the neighbor who joins you on your morning walk to the spouse who decides to do the *ChangeOne* program along with you. The first step in getting the help you need is deciding *what* you need. Check one or more of the following options:

❏ An activity partner
❏ Someone to talk to when I'm down or discouraged
❏ Someone who can answer specific diet questions
❏ Help in the kitchen
❏ Help around the house
❏ A lunch or dinner companion
Other: _____

Now make a list of possible candidates to fill the positions you've checked. Keep in mind that help and support sometimes come from unexpected places. A colleague at work may be more useful to you than a close family member. A neighbor you meet on one of your walks—someone who's also trying to slim down—may end up offering more help than a close friend.

If you're looking for emotional support, identify someone you're willing to confide in, even if that means admitting weakness or failure. If you're looking for practical help around the house, you probably already know whom to ask. So ask. Be specific about what you need and why you need it. If you're asking someone to do a real favor, think about what you can do for them in return.

Beware of Saboteurs

In a perfect world, family and friends would support you 100 percent. But we live in an imperfect world. Sometimes the people closest to you may be threatened by your efforts to change yourself.

Often it's especially the people closest to you, in fact, who have trouble with your decision to lose weight—a spouse or sibling, for example. If your spouse tends to be a little jealous, your decision to lose weight could be interpreted as a desire to be considered more attractive to other people. If your spouse could stand to lose a little weight, too—but isn't willing to try right now—he or she may resent your determination and success.

There are plenty of reasons that don't take a psychiatrist to figure out, of course. Following a diet requires changes in the kitchen and at the table.

And some family members may not want to be bothered by those changes. They may not like the extra time you spend planning lunches or dinners. They may feel uncomfortable finishing everything on their plate while you eat smaller portions.

Take a moment to think about the people closest to you. Among them, is there anyone who:

■ Continues to urge food on you even when you say you're not hungry?

■ Belittles your efforts to lose weight?

■ Throws obstacles in the way of your being more active?

■ Seems resentful or threatened by the fact that you've begun to lose weight?

■ Expresses anger or frustration when you leave food on your plate?

■ Undermines your efforts with negative messages? Perhaps they do that with comments like, "I don't know what makes you think you'll be able to lose weight this time," or, "Once the holidays roll around you're going to gain it all back

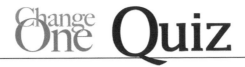

Team Player or Solo Flier?

Some people need the support and advice of people around them. Others do best on their own. To determine whether you're best suited be a soloist or a team player, answer the following 14 true-or-false questions. Your score will help you choose the best strategies to overcome obstacles and to keep your motivation high.

1. **I'm comfortable talking to other people about my weight.**
△ True
☐ False

2. **If things aren't going well for me, I typically turn to family or friends for advice.**
△ True
☐ False

3. **I'm embarrassed talking about my feelings with other people, even people close to me.**
☐ True
△ False

4. **Getting a little pat on the back now and then would help motivate me right now.**
△ True
☐ False

5. **When I set my mind to do something, I don't really need other people to push me.**
☐ True
△ False

6. **I have at least one person in my life with whom I can talk about almost any-thing.**
△ True
☐ False

7. **I tend to keep my personal feelings to myself.**
☐ True
△ False

8. **The people around me are part of the reason I've had trouble losing weight in the past.**
☐ True
△ False

9. **I've always tended to tackle problems on my own.**
☐ True
△ False

10. **I'm not really sure that the people around me have my best interests in mind.**
☐ True
△ False

11. **Just being able to talk things over with someone when I've got a problem can make things seem better.**
△ True
☐ False

12. **I'm very uneasy about letting people see my weaknesses.**
☐ True
△ False

13. **I've joined groups in the past, and they've really helped me.**
△ True
☐ False

14. **Frankly, I don't trust people to be honest with me or tell me what they're really thinking.**
☐ True
△ False

Turn to next page to tally your score.

Quiz Score

Tally up the number of colored shapes you checked—blue triangles or green boxes:

△ Blue _____

☐ Green _____

△ Blue answers indicate team players, people who benefit from the support of others. The more blue triangles you checked, the more likely you are to rely on a strong support network of friends and family. If you wish you had a little more help from the peanut gallery now and then, read on for tips on how to get the support you need.

☐ Green answers indicate the solo fliers—people who typically go it alone. The more green boxes you checked, the more likely you are to depend on yourself.

Most of us are a little bit team player and solo flier, of course. We turn to friends or family sometimes and depend on ourselves at other times. Don't be surprised if your score falls somewhere in the middle. Read on for advice on how to strengthen your social network, along with tips on how you can do a better job of helping yourself.

again anyway."

■ Constantly reminds you that you're on a diet and clucks over every bite you eat? That's not help, it's a constant irritation that could wear you down over time.

If so, you may be struggling against someone who's trying to sabotage the change you want to make. Often the hardest part in dealing with a saboteur is acknowledging that your personal relationships aren't perfect, and that someone close to you may be standing between you and improvement. It's easier to blame yourself or your lack of willpower. But it's crucially important to recognize when someone is making life harder, rather than easier. Otherwise they can undermine your chances of success.

Talk It Out

If you spot a problem like that this week and you think it comes mainly from a lack of communication, ask your problem person for a heart-to-heart talk. Explain why losing weight is so important to you—and why the sincere support and enthusiasm of people around you matters so much.

Point out things they do that make it hard for you or hurt your feelings.

And be specific about the kind of help you need from them. For instance:

- "I'd rather you didn't offer me seconds. When I say no, I feel as if I'm hurting your feelings. But it's very important to me right now to cut back on the amount I eat."

- "I'd really like to have you join me for a walk after dinner instead of watching television. Maybe we can make a list of the programs we really want to see and schedule around them."

- "It would help me a lot if we put snack food out of sight in the cupboard, rather than on the counter where I see it all

How To Be Your Own Best Friend

Can't find a support team? Doing just fine on your own? Whether you're a soloist or a team player, a few strategies can help you get through the inevitable rough patches. The key is to be your own best friend. Here are four ways to do that:

Banish negative thoughts. Most of us have heard the little voice that whispers, "You're never going to be able to make it," or, "You just don't have what it takes." Learn to recognize such negative thoughts and replace them with the kind of positive messages a good friend would offer. "Sure you can do it." "One slip-up is no big deal." "Keep up the good work."

Keep a journal. If that negative voice in your head just won't let up, try carrying a small notebook with you this week and jot down every negative thought that occurs to you. You may be surprised to find that the simple act of writing these thoughts down makes you see how irrational they are. If you can't dismiss them, take a moment to come up with a positive counter-message. "I'm trying to

improve myself." "I've stayed with a diet for five weeks, which isn't bad." "Hey, no one's perfect. I'm doing my best." By keeping a diary, you'll also become aware of the situations and circumstances that trigger negative thoughts. Avoid them if you can. If you can't, have your positive counter-messages ready.

Reward yourself for a good job. When you reach one of your goals—even if it's something as simple as sticking to *ChangeOne* through a long holiday weekend—give yourself a reward. For a little extra motivation, decide in advance what the reward will be: a new pair of walking shoes, a new piece of clothing, a spa or massage treatment, or tickets to a big game or must-see concert.

Learn to laugh at your foibles. Having a sense of humor can go a long way when you're trying to make a big change in your life. Take yourself too seriously and you'll slip into the kind of all-or-nothing thinking that makes people give up before they've even given themselves a chance to succeed.

> "Hey, no one's perfect. I'm doing my best."

the time. I have a tendency to eat when there's food out."

■ "It really hurts my feelings when you say I never stick with things. I'm really trying this time. Your encouragement means a lot to me."

■ "I appreciate that you want to help me lose weight, but continually reminding me I'm on a diet is driving me to distraction. For the most part, I want to handle this on my own. Let me ask for help when I need it. "

Ask your spouse or friend to talk about their feelings. Explore what you can do to make the situation easier. If a loved one feels threatened, make it clear that your love hasn't changed.

Be sure to have fun on weekends. It makes healthier eating so much easier.

In some cases, you may know that all the talking in the world isn't going to solve the problem. Then the best strategy is learning to recognize acts of sabotage and to find ways to defuse them. This week try to avoid tense situations that involve food. Spend less time in the kitchen, for instance, and more in other parts of the house. If leaving food on your plate is a hot button, serve yourself only as much as you want to eat.

No advice will fit every situation. Use your best judgment. And if you can't get the support you need from one source, you can often find it from another. You can always learn to lean on yourself for motivation and encouragement, too.

Enjoy Yourself

Enjoying yourself should come easy on weekends and holidays. But if you're constantly worried about being tempted by too much food, it's easy to forget that the point of weekends and holidays is to relax and have a good time. The meal suggestions on these pages offer plenty of great flavor and portions guaranteed to satisfy even a weekend appetite. So this weekend make sure to relax and enjoy yourself. Being physically active on weekends and holidays also adds enjoyment and gives you an opportunity to relax.

Why make a point of enjoying yourself when you're on a diet? Because the more you're able to find pleasure, with and without food, the easier you'll find it to stay with the program and turn healthy eating into a lifelong habit.

Changes Ahead:
Fixing Your Kitchen

Some of us love to cook; the rest of us don't. But cook we must, most every day. Next week we will focus on having a kitchen that is as friendly and simple as can be so that making *ChangeOne*-style meals is a cinch.

As you work through your weekend and holiday strategies this week, ponder your kitchen setup. Are you overstocked with snacks and unhealthy prepared foods? Or is your pantry so bare that making a healthy, fresh meal guarantees a trip to the store? Do you own a can of cooking spray? If yes, is the spray easier to get to than the butter in the refrigerator?

We think you'll be surprised at how much easier cooking healthy can be once you make a handful of small tweaks in the way you buy and store your food and supplies.

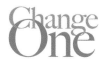

Week 7
Fixing Your Kitchen

"On days when warmth is the most important need of the human heart," the author E.B. White once wrote, "the kitchen is the place you can find it."

White's words still hold true. Even in today's world of takeout pizzas and microwave meals, the kitchen is still the warm heart of most households.

This week you'll transform the kitchen by tossing out the devilish foods on hand, replacing them with *ChangeOne* choices, and rearranging for easier, healthier cooking.

Why make changes in the kitchen? Because we don't ever want you to think of your kitchen as a place to be avoided. In *ChangeOne* we want the kitchen to remain a place of warmth, a place that encourages happiness and healthy eating at the same time.

Stocking Up Smartly

Making sure you have plenty of food in your pantry may sound like strange diet advice. After all, who wants a wealth of edible temptations around when you're trying to eat less, not more?

In fact, as many dieters discover, a bare cupboard can actually spell trouble. No matter how scant your provisions are, chances are there's a bag of chips from last week's party or a box of candy left over from Valentine's Day lurking somewhere. And if that's all there is to eat, guess what you're going to grab if you get hungry enough? Exactly.

By keeping plenty of healthy foods around you'll have plenty of choices, not just for snacks but for every meal of the day. And by organizing your kitchen smartly you can make sure the best choices are right in front of you when you swing into the kitchen or open the refrigerator door. What's more, a well-stocked, well-organized kitchen can save you time and spare you frustration. With the right selection of essentials on hand, you can put together a simple and delicious meal without having to make a run to the grocery store. Many home chefs are inspired to make interesting dishes simply by opening up the refrigerator, checking out what's there, and conjuring up tasty combinations. (You'll find three from-the-pantry recipes on pages 156, 159, and 162.)

Ask yourself, "Would I eat this?" Then, "Should I eat this?"

For a detailed analysis of your kitchen and tips on how to make it work better for you, take our "Inspection Time" Quiz on page 153.

The first step in designing a diet-friendly kitchen isn't shopping; it's clearing your shelves. So get the garbage sacks ready, along with a box for items you can give away to the local food bank. It's time to get rid of food you don't want—and don't need around to tempt you.

Start with the pantry. Ask yourself on each item, "Would I eat this?" If yes, then ask, "Should I eat this?" Keep in mind your family's tastes, of course. But don't be too generous. If you shouldn't eat it, chances are your loved ones shouldn't, either. Focus in particular on items that have sat around for more than six months.

Move to the refrigerator and freezer next. Clear out those funky old condiment jars, those squishy old peppers, those eight-day-old leftovers.

If it feels good to clear off the shelves, it should. And it'll feel even better when you fill up the space with foods that are healthier, fresher, and more interesting.

Go Shopping

Your next step is making a run to the grocery store to buy essentials. Exactly what those essentials are will depend on your taste, how often you prepare meals at home, and the kinds of foods your family likes. You'll find a master shopping list of kitchen essentials on page 157 to use as your guide. You don't need to stock them all, of course. The more choices you have on hand, though, the easier it will be for you to put together a *ChangeOne* meal or snack on the spur of the moment.

Before you head for the grocery store this week, keep in mind six essential strategies for smart shopping:

1. Have a snack before you go.
You'll get some exercise cruising the aisles and hauling bags, so go ahead and take the hunger edge off before you hit the store. An empty stomach can make you empty-headed. Nothing weakens willpower faster than being hungry. Chances are you've seen shoppers so hungry that they dip into a bag of chips or package of cookies even before they've reached the checkout line. Avoid trouble by shopping after you've eaten a meal. If you find yourself shopping for dinner on an empty stomach, have a *ChangeOne* snack before you start pushing your cart down the aisle.

2. Start with a list—and stay with it.
Your local grocery is full of temptations that can be hard to resist. Supermarkets are in the business of selling food, especially items with a big profit margin. The biggest money-makers are often the

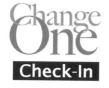

Check-In

Is someone making it harder rather than easier to eat right? If you realized last week that you have a saboteur working against you, consider taking an extra week to resolve the situation as best you can. Keep a record—write down every time someone says something or does something that seems designed to sabotage your efforts. At the end of each day look over your entries and brainstorm for ways to free yourself. Strategies include avoiding situations that involve food, countering negative messages with positive ones, or simply learning to ignore criticisms or unwanted enticements. Sometimes the best approach is to talk it out. At other times separating yourself from the source of trouble is a better solution. Use your judgment. Just remember that you're in charge of what you eat—no one else. Be considerate of other people's feelings, but stick to your resolution.

Change One Quiz

Inspection Time

How diet-friendly is your kitchen? There's only one way to find out. Put on your kitchen inspector's cap, grab a pencil and a pad of paper, and fill out the following checklist:

1. **What are the first three things you see when you open your refrigerator door?**

1. _____
2. _____
3. _____

2. **What are the first three things you see when you open the freezer?**

1. _____
2. _____
3. _____

3. **List the three handiest snacks in your kitchen:**

1. _____
2. _____
3. _____

4. **How many different kinds of fresh vegetables does your refrigerator crisper contain?**

❏ None
❏ One or two
❏ Three or more

5. **Is there a bowl of fresh fruit on the counter?**

❏ Yes
❏ No
❏ Usually, but not today

6. **Do you have the makings of a *ChangeOne* dinner in your cupboard and refrigerator?**

❏ Yes
❏ No
❏ Usually, but not today

7. **Where do you keep your grocery list?**

❏ Posted on the refrigerator door or in another prominent place
❏ Tucked away somewhere in the kitchen
❏ What list?

8. **Rate your collection of storage containers:**

❏ Plentiful and in a variety of different sizes
❏ Enough for a few leftovers
❏ What storage containers?

9. **How many "too-tempting-to-resist" foods are stored in your kitchen right now?**

❏ None
❏ One or two
❏ Three or more

10. **Which of the following is your kitchen lacking?**

❏ Measuring spoons
❏ Measuring cups
❏ Nonstick frying or sauté pan
❏ Set of sharp knives
❏ Vegetable steamer
❏ Microwave
❏ Rice cooker
❏ Set of small bowls and plates

Turn to next page to tally your score.

Quiz Score

Assessing your answers:

1, 2, 3. If the first items you see fit on the *ChangeOne* menu, your kitchen's in great shape. If not, your kitchen is working against you. Either get rid of the stuff you'd rather not be tempted by, or tuck it away where you have to work to get it.

4. Vegetables are free, so stock a tempting variety. That will make it easy to throw together a low-calorie meal without running to the store.

5. Put a bowl of fruit out where everyone in the family can see it. That way it will be the first place everyone goes when a snack attack strikes.

6. If you don't have the makings of a *ChangeOne* meal on your pantry shelf, you should. You'll be ready for anything, from a stormy night to a surprise visitor.

7. Invest in an erasable message board that you can mount on the refrigerator. It's a great way to keep a grocery list so that you won't be caught short when you want to cook a quick and simple meal.

8. Keep plenty of storage containers handy. Sure, they're great for leftovers. But you can also use them to divvy up giant food packages from the store into reasonably sized portions when you get home.

9. Why drive yourself crazy keeping foods you can't resist? Toss 'em. Or put them so far out of reach that you'll have to make a big effort to get them. One of our *ChangeOne* volunteers tucked his treat foods behind a couple of rows of wineglasses.

10. For a list of terrific time-saving, diet-friendly kitchen tools, check out page 302.

items that are prominently displayed at eye level or at the ends of aisles. Chances are you'll see row after row of snack foods, cookies, colas, donuts, and highly sweetened cereals. Steer your cart down almost any aisle and you'll be surrounded by brightly-colored packages specifically designed to lure their way into your cart. "All natural!" "Two for one!" "Giant family-size economy pack!" "Choose me!"

To avoid the hard sell, put together a shopping list in the quiet and comfort of your own kitchen. Build your list around recipes and meal plans. Use the guide to kitchen essentials on page 157, along with our lists of shopping strategies on pages 300–301.

Once you get to the market, stick to your list. Sure, if

fresh peaches or ripe tomatoes are in season, help yourself. Don't be afraid to tinker with your meal plan if you find something irresistible in the produce aisle or there's a good bargain at the fish counter. But don't reach for that jumbo size bag of cheesie-wheezies just because it's on sale this week. If it's not on your list—or your diet—it doesn't belong in your cart. If you don't find what you're looking for at the store, talk to the manager. Most grocery stores are happy to stock what customers want.

3. Steer your cart around the perimeter.

In most grocery stores, the healthiest choices are arranged around the perimeter of the store. That's where you'll find dairy products, the produce section, and the meat and fish counters. Processed foods, including those rows upon rows of brightly colored snack food packages, are usually in the center of the store. As a general rule, then, the more shopping you do around the perimeter, the less processed food you're likely to run across—and the more food you'll find that fits your *ChangeOne* diet.

4. Think small.

Giant food warehouse clubs have risen on the promise of saving money by buying in bulk. There's nothing wrong with saving a few dollars. But if you have a tough time stopping yourself once a jumbo bag of chips is open, take heed. If you're buying something to eat right away, buy a small package—preferably a single-serving size. If you buy jumbo sizes to save money, divide them into single-serving size, resealable plastic bags or containers right when you return from shopping.

5. Read the small print.

With few exceptions, all processed and packaged foods are required to carry detailed food labels that list ingredients and nutritional information. Learning to read a label will help you shop wisely. When your goal is to lose weight, the most important number on the label is calories per serving. Be

Continued on page 158

Managing Your Food

1. Use opaque storage containers for "treat" foods so you won't be tempted by the sight of the contents.
2. Put notes on food containers to remind yourself of what a sensible portion should be.
3. Decide in advance how much you plan to eat—before you open the container.
4. Attach a list of your favorite *ChangeOne* snacks to the refrigerator door as a reminder.
5. Put a date on leftovers—and a reminder on your calendar of when you plan to eat them.
6. Once a week tour your kitchen, making sure the healthiest foods occupy the most prominent positions.
7. Keep a list of essential items that are running low so that you won't be caught unprepared.

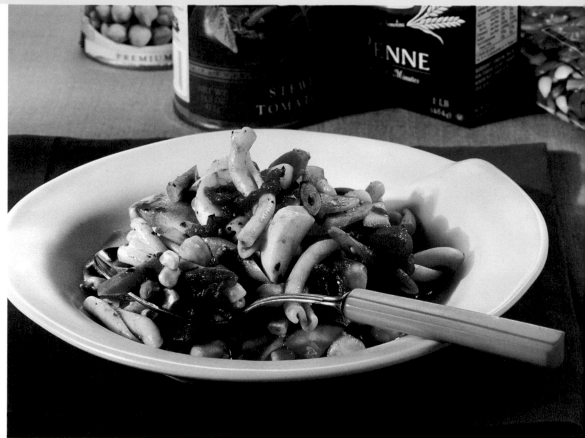

Stew from the Pantry

You can put everything but the kitchen sink into this quick and tasty stew.

2 cups Kitchen Sink Stew (2 baseballs)

1 slice Garlic Bread

Calories 420, fat 5 g, saturated fat 1 g, cholesterol 0 mg,
sodium 1,180 mg, carbohydrate 81 g, fiber 14 g,
protein 16 g, calcium 150 mg.

KITCHEN SINK STEW

Serves 4

1 **28-ounce can recipe-ready or plain stewed tomatoes**

1 **20-ounce can chickpeas (also called garbanzo beans) or other beans, drained and rinsed**

2 **cups frozen mixed vegetables**

1 **cup dry pasta (elbow macaroni or other small shells)**

1 **teaspoon dried Italian herb mix, or ½ teaspoon dried oregano plus ½ teaspoon dried basil (optional)**

2 **cups water, plus more as needed**

1. Combine all ingredients in a medium pot. Place on the stove on medium-high heat and bring to a boil. Reduce heat to low and simmer until pasta is cooked, about 20 to 30 minutes, depending on pasta size.

GARLIC BREAD

Serves 4

1. Slice Italian bread into 4 palm-sized slices, and store the rest.

2. Mince 2 cloves garlic and mix with 2 teaspoons olive oil.

3. Spread ¼ of mixture on each slice.

4. Top each bread slice with 1 teaspoon grated parmesan.

5. Broil until topping is warm, about 1 minute.

Kitchen Essentials

Use this guide to make sure your kitchen has all the items you'll need for healthy snacking and quick, easy-to-cook meals. Here we list some everyday staples, the basic provisions you should have on hand to be sure you can always put together a meal from a well-stocked pantry and refrigerator. For a guide to perishables—the fruits, vegetables, dairy products, and meats that you use in *ChangeOne* meals—look at the Shopping Strategies on pages 300–301.

In the pantry
- Baking powder
- Baking soda
- Cocoa powder, unsweetened
- Cornstarch
- Flours—whole wheat and all-purpose
- Sugars—white and brown
- Vanilla extract
- Vinegars—balsamic, red wine
- Oils—olive, canola, sesame
- Cooking spray
- Peanut butter*
- Broth—chicken or vegetable, canned*
- Soups—mushroom, minestrone, or vegetable, canned*
- Tomatoes, canned*
- Tomato sauce*
- Tuna, canned*
- Herbs, dried
- Italian spices, dried
- Mushrooms, dried

Condiments
- Salt and pepper
- Ketchup*
- Mayonnaise, reduced fat*
- Mustards*—Dijon, yellow
- Soy sauce
- Hot sauce
- Pickles and pickle relish*
- Capers*
- Olives*

Cereals, grains, and beans
- Cereal—ready-to-eat, whole grain
- Oatmeal (rolled oats)
- Couscous
- Legumes (kidney beans, chickpeas, black beans, etc.), canned or dried
- Pasta
- Rice—brown and white

Snacks
- Graham crackers
- Nuts, mixed
- Popcorn kernels
- Whole-grain snacks like crackers and pretzels

Fruits and vegetables
- Fruit canned in juice*
- Fruit, assorted fresh
- Raisins
- Garlic, fresh
- Onions
- Potatoes—baking or roasting, and sweet potatoes or yams
- Celery
- Bell peppers, green or red

In the refrigerator
- Butter
- Cheeses for grating, such as parmesan
- Eggs
- Milk—low-fat or nonfat
- Yogurt, plain—low-fat or nonfat

In the freezer
- Bagels—mini or small (2 ounces)
- Breads—whole wheat and pita
- Berries and other fruit, frozen
- Fruit sorbet or fruit/juice pops
- Beef or chicken bones for homemade stock
- Chicken breasts, individually portioned
- Ground turkey or lean ground beef
- Meatless burgers
- Pizza crust, frozen
- Prepared dinners— reduced-calorie, frozen
- Vegetables, frozen

Miscellaneous
- Carbonated water
- Vegetable juices
- Sugar-free soda
- Iced tea, unsweetened
- Evaporated skim milk, canned
- Herbs, fresh
- Tomato salsa
- Green chilies, canned
- Tortillas—corn and flour, small

These items may need to be refrigerated after you've opened them

Continued from page 155

sure to check how the label describes a serving size. The amount can vary widely even within the same category. Some cereal boxes list ¾ cup as a serving, for example, while others use 1 cup. Some foods may look as if they're low in calories until you discover that a serving size would fit into a thimble.

6. Keep treats at a distance.

Don't buy high-calorie items you have trouble resisting once they're under your roof. Do you really want them tempting you all the time? To ensure that treats remain treats, make them part of a special occasion. When the family wants ice cream, for example, go out for it. Don't make it too easy to splurge by keeping a half-gallon in the fridge. Kids clamoring for cookies? Take them down to the java hut or the bakery section of the store and buy a couple of good ones.

> **"Fudge-brownie ice cream— 50% off!" Uh-oh.**

Decide in advance how much you'll have. One small bite of everybody else's ice cream will let you sample a bunch of flavors and still keep you within the recommended serving size for dessert. A nibble or two on the kids' cookies will satisfy your sweet tooth and keep you on your diet.

Breaking the Chain

The single most important step for many of our *ChangeOne* volunteers was learning to shop for food smartly. If you prepare a lot of your meals at home, the decisions you make at the grocery store go a long way toward determining how well you eat.

To understand how important smart shopping is, visualize a chain. Scientists who study behavior talk about chains of behavior—individual decisions that connect like links on a chain. Let's say you give in to temptation one night and eat that whole pint of fudge-brownie ice cream in the fridge. At first that may seem like a single, impulsive act. But in reality it's the end of a long chain of choices.

Think back to the beginning. That pint of fudge-brownie ice cream didn't get into the freezer on its own, after all. The links in the chain might look something like this:

- You go shopping when you're hungry.
- Rushing out the door, you forget to bring your shopping list with you.
- At the store you see a sign that says "FUDGE-BROWNIE

Quick Black Beans and Rice

This side dish goes with just about anything; you can make it mild or spicy. Here we've given it a chicken companion.

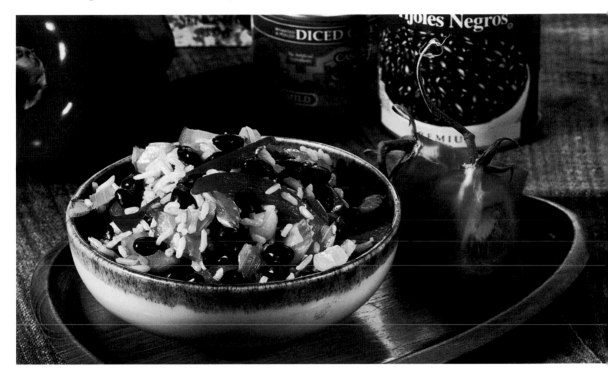

1¼ cup Quick Black Beans and Rice (2 tennis balls)

6 ounces Grilled Chicken Breast Filet (checkbook)

1 mixed green salad (unlimited) with 2 tablespoons (2 salad dressing caps) fat-free dressing, or reduced-fat— adds about 30 calories

Calories 440, fat 8 g, saturated fat 2 g, cholesterol 95 mg, sodium 870 mg, carbohydrate 45 g, fiber 10 g, protein 45 g, calcium 100 mg.

QUICK BLACK BEANS AND RICE

Serves 4
- **2 teaspoons olive oil**
- **1 red bell pepper, diced**
- **½ medium onion, diced**
- **1 stalk celery, diced**
- **1 clove garlic, minced**
- **1 16-ounce can black beans, drained**
  Optional seasonings: 1 tablespoon chopped chipotles in adobo, or
- **1 teaspoon chopped jalapeno pepper, or 1 tablespoon chopped green chilies, or 1 teaspoon hot sauce**
- **2 cups warm cooked brown rice**

1. In a large nonstick pan, heat olive oil. Saute pepper, onion, celery, and garlic until soft, about 5 minutes. Add black beans and optional seasoning, and heat until warmed.

2. Combine with brown rice.

GRILLED CHICKEN BREAST FILET

Serves 4

1. Place 4 chicken breast filets, about 6 ounces (checkbook) each, into a flat pan coated with cooking spray. Sprinkle with lemon juice, freshly grated black pepper, and 1 tablespoon (thumb) olive oil, or soak in your favorite marinade for 10 minutes.

2. Remove from pan and grill in oven (on broil) or on a grill until done, 7 to 10 minutes, depending on thickness.

ICE CREAM!—50% OFF!" Uh-oh.

■ You pop a pint in your cart.

■ You pop that same pint into the freezer, telling yourself you'll only have a little, and only on special occasions.

■ You're feeling low one night. You know you should get up and out for a walk to feel better, but ...

ChangeOne First Person

Lots of Little Packages

"I know I could probably find something a little fancier, or maybe a little healthier for me," Paul Rodriguez says. "But for me, convenience matters a lot. If something takes too long to put together, I'm not going to do it."

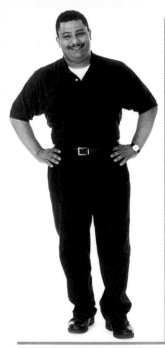

So after trying a variety of *ChangeOne* breakfasts during the first few weeks, Rodriguez finally settled on the ultimate convenience: individual-size breakfast cereal packages that he can buy 30 to a box at the local discount food warehouse. "I can have one at home or grab it and take it to work if I'm running late. I don't have to worry about pouring a certain amount into a bowl."

The same solution helped steer him away from the high-fat, high-calorie snacks he used to eat. Rodriguez now buys oatmeal bars— 100 calories each—in bulk at the same store. He packs one or two with him every day.

"Maybe later I'll want to branch out and be a little more creative. But right now it helps not to have to decide what I'm going to have for a snack. If I get hungry, I just reach for an oatmeal bar. It's been great."

After years of putting on pounds, Rodriguez was thrilled to see the weight beginning to slip way—15 pounds over the first seven weeks.

■ You're hungry. You open the refrigerator door, but because you haven't gone shopping lately there's not much there that you want.

■ You open the freezer door, and what's this? A pint of fudge-brownie ice cream leaps into your hands.

■ You know you should serve up just one small scoop and put the container back, but you're feeling lazy, so you open the lid and grab a spoon.

■ You know you should sit down at the counter and eat just a little, savoring every bite. But the TV is on and you wander into the living room. Instead of paying attention to the ice cream, you watch TV while you eat. The next thing you know the whole pint is gone.

How can you make sure this doesn't happen? Of course, you can break the chain at any one of its links. You can get the ice cream home, realize your mistake, and give it away. Or you can put the spoon down and not dig in. Sure you *can*, but if you're like most people, the best time to stop the chain is at the store. You don't have to resist eating something you didn't buy. That's something to remember the next time you're tempted by food you know could overwhelm your willpower and set your diet back.

Put Food in Its Place

Once you're back from your shopping spree, it's time to take a serious look at your kitchen. The strategy is simple. Put the healthiest choices in the most prominent spots on kitchen shelves and in the refrigerator. Put "treat" foods—the items you only want to reach now and then—out of sight, even out of reach.

Let's say you like to treat yourself to an oatmeal raisin cookie from time to time. Now imagine that those cookies are stored in a clear glass cookie jar on the counter. Every

Help!

"I have three teenage kids, and the kitchen is filled with foods they love—potato chips, soft drinks, ice cream, and all the rest. How can I diet-proof my kitchen against that kind of temptation?"

You can't—not entirely. But you can certainly make your kitchen more comfortable for yourself. If your teenagers are tall enough to reach high, ask them to keep their snack foods on the upper shelves. Assign them a low shelf for soft drinks and other sweetened beverages in the fridge. Insist on reserving the most accessible shelf in the refrigerator for foods that are on your menu. Ask the kids not to leave packages of junk food lying around, and tell them to put all food away in the designated places when they're done eating.

Don't stop there. Try to encourage the rest of the family to follow your example and eat food with fewer empty calories. Sure, it can sometimes seem like an uphill struggle. But many kids these days are surprisingly health-conscious. And since weight problems typically begin early in life, you'll be doing them a favor. Sit down with your kids and explain why losing weight really matters to you. If your children are still young, you can nudge their tastes in the right direction. One *ChangeOne* volunteer regularly offered his children healthy choices, and at ages four and six they now eat whole wheat crackers, broccoli, asparagus, grilled fish, and of course, lots of macaroni and cheese.

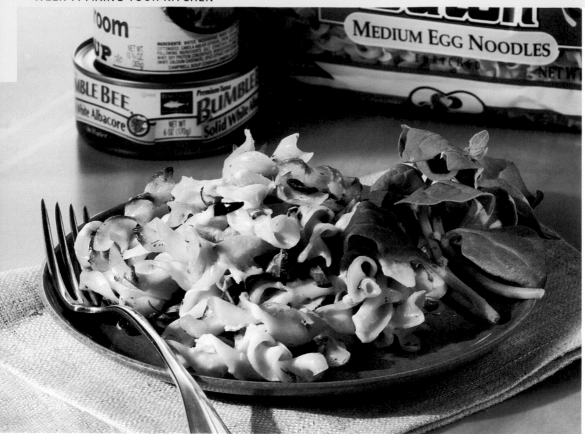

Casserole Dinner

Just add fresh or frozen vegetables to these pantry staples for an easy dinner.

1½ cups Homestyle Tuna Noodle
Casserole (2 tennis balls)

    Arugula salad (unlimited) with
1 teaspoon olive oil and
balsamic vinegar to taste.

Calories 420, fat 10 g, saturated fat 2 g, cholesterol 50 mg,
sodium 1,340 mg, carbohydrate 32 g, fiber 3 g, protein
47 g, calcium 200 mg.

1. Preheat oven to 375°F. Coat medium-size casserole dish with cooking spray.

2. Combine all ingredients. Place in casserole dish and bake until bubbly, about 30 minutes.

HOMESTYLE TUNA NOODLE CASSEROLE

Serves 4

- **2 6-ounce cans tuna packed in water**
- **1 can (14 ounces) fat-free cream of mushroom soup**
- **½ cup (4 ounces) canned evaporated skim milk**
- **½ cup sliced black olives**
- **1 4-ounce can chopped green chilies**
- **2 cups cooked noodles**

Instead of	Try
Tuna	Canned turkey
	Tofu
	Canned chicken
Mushroom soup	Fat-free cream of broccoli soup
	Fat-free cream of tomato soup
Egg noodles	Cooked pasta

time you swing into the kitchen for a snack, they're the first option you see. That means every time you enter the room you've got to rely on your willpower to resist turning a special treat into an everyday occurrence.

Why put yourself through that? Imagine, instead, that you keep a bowl of fruit on the counter and a few plastic containers with carrot and celery sticks front and center in the refrigerator. The cookies are safely stored away on the very top shelf of the pantry in a container with a lid that snaps shut—high enough that you need to get the stepladder out when you want them. Suddenly it's easy to grab something low in calories and rich in nutrition—an apple or a handful of carrot sticks. You will need to work to get at those cookies.

By the end of this week your kitchen will be a place where you can relax, not a place where you have to constantly feel like you're fighting temptations.

Changes Ahead: How Am I Doing?

In a typical conversation about weight loss, you talk about pounds. It's the easiest, clearest measurement of progress. But is it always the best measurement? No way.

Once you have your kitchen under control—and it might be wise to take extra time there given its importance and how many habits might need tweaking—we'll turn to the subject of progress.

If that sounds too simple to be important, it isn't. Self-assessment is tricky business. We tend to be very hard on ourselves. We forget the important markers—energy, attitude, overall appearance—and focus on unrealistic statistical measurements. So to prepare for this examination, think again about why you really want to lose weight. Think about how you judge your success or failure. And be prepared to look at yourself in a whole new mirror.

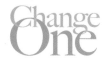

Week 8

How Am I Doing?

"How long does getting thin take?" Winnie the Pooh asks anxiously in A.A. Milne's classic children's book. You may be asking the same question just about now.

You probably have other questions, too. Why do you seem to lose weight some weeks and not others? Are you making reasonable progress toward your goal? What can you do to jumpstart your diet when weight loss stalls?

This week you'll assess how you're doing and find ways to get through trouble spots.

To get you started, take the "Seven Weeks of Progress" Quiz, which begins on the following page. You will use its questions throughout this chapter to focus on the best ways to overcome your unique weight-loss challenges.

Change One Quiz

Seven Weeks of Progress

Circle the appropriate number in the right-hand column to track your score.

1. **How do you feel about your weight-loss progress so far?**

Very satisfied	3
Satisfied	2
Disappointed	1

2. **How would you rate your energy level since you began *ChangeOne*?**

Improved	3
About the same	2
Slumped	1

3. **How would you rate your self-confidence while on this program?**

Improved	3
About the same	2
Worse	1

4. **How many days last week did you closely follow the *ChangeOne* menu for breakfast, lunch, dinner, and snacks?**

All or most	3
About half	2
Fewer than half	1

5. **How often are you able to stick to sensible portions when you dine out?**

All or most of the time	3
About half the time	2
Less than half the time	1

6. **Planning is crucial to dieting success; how well are you doing when it comes to planning where and what you'll eat?**

Very well	3
Good	2
So-so	1

7. **Feeling hungry can whittle away at anyone's willpower; how would you describe your experience on *ChangeOne* so far?**

Hunger isn't a problem for me	3
Now and then I get so hungry that I eat more than I should	2
Hunger is a problem for me a lot of the time	1

8. **How often do you experience strong cravings for specific foods (chocolate, ice cream, salty snacks, or candy, for instance)?**

Never	3
Now and then	2
Frequently	1

9. **What phrase best describes your family and close friends?**

Behind me 100 percent	3
Somewhat supportive	2
Not very helpful	1

10. **How would you rate your overall motivation right now?**

Excellent	3
Good	2
Shaky	1

11. **Stress can often get in the way when people are trying to change; how are you dealing with it?**

Very well	3
Well enough	2
Not very well	1

Continued on page 166

Continued from page 165

12. **Sometimes it seems there's food everywhere; how would you rate your ability to deal with temptations?**

I'm getting better at   3
eating only if I'm hungry

I give in to temptation   2
now and then, but not
as much as before

I still have a very   1
tough time saying no

13. **Where did you eat in your house during the past week?**

Kitchen and dining   3
room only

In front of TV or in   2
the bedroom

Both in front of TV   1
and in the bedroom

14. **How many days during the past week did you fit in at least 30 minutes worth of physical activity (walking, jogging, gym workouts, etc.)?**

All or most   3

About half   2

Fewer than half   1

Quiz Score

Scoring:
Add up the combined score of your answers and use the guide below to start evaluating your progress.

A score of 32 to 42: A big gold star for you. But put a check beside any questions that you scored as 1 and read the corresponding numbered tips in the following pages for advice on how to move ahead.

21 to 31: A little extra help could improve your chances of success. Mark the questions you scored as 1 and read the numbered tips that follow for advice.

14 to 20: Okay, you're having a tough time. Many people do when they first try to lose weight. Highlight the responses you scored as 1 and read the numbered tips in the section that follows for advice on these trouble spots.

Succeeding Your Way

No single approach works for everyone. Even diet experts have been surprised to discover how many ways there are to succeed—or fail—at dieting. Some people like to be told exactly what to eat and then follow a strict plan. Others take a few guiding ideas and handle the rest. Some people need a lot of support from family and friends. Others go it alone.

We've seen the same thing among the volunteers who tested the *ChangeOne* program. Some began to lose weight right with breakfast; others didn't hit their stride until they changed their approach to dinner. There were people who began to lose weight as soon as they changed the way they snacked. Others got the biggest bang for their buck paying attention to what they ate on the weekends. For some *ChangeOne* was a breeze. For others it wasn't always easy.

The quiz you just took should help clarify the challenges you've encountered on *ChangeOne*. To help you overcome these challenges, we'll review the quiz questions in detail in this chapter, offering tips and advice as we go to make sure you are getting all you can out of your efforts.

1 Disappointed in your results?
Reassess your goals; renew your commitment.

If you've lost eight pounds or more since you started *ChangeOne,* there's no reason to be disappointed. Experts say a healthy weight-loss plan should average one to three pounds a week. So eight weeks into *ChangeOne* you can expect to have lost anywhere from 8 to 24 pounds. Losing weight more quickly than that means losing muscle tissue along with fat, which could slow your metabolism and make it harder to maintain your weight loss down the road.

If you haven't started seeing the progress you'd like, there may be several reasons. If you've significantly increased the amount of exercise you're doing, you may be losing fat but adding muscle. Nothing wrong with that. In fact, it's the sure-fire way to look firmer and svelter. But because you're trading fat for muscle, you may not see as much difference on the scale. One sign that you're making progress: your waist size. If it's going down, you're changing for the better.

The most important thing now is not to get discouraged. Make a pact with yourself to use a little extra time and effort this coming month to reach your goal—and make sure the number is realistic. (We'll get into goal-setting in much more detail later in this chapter.)

2 Energy at a low ebb?
Have a snack—and get moving.

While people usually feel much better when losing weight, some people do experience periods of fatigue as well. When you take in fewer calories than you burn, you force your body to turn to the energy it has stored as fat. Falling short on calories can make you feel tired and even grumpy. There's another kind of fatigue: some people begin to get tired of dieting. But you don't have to let an energy drain get in the way of your weight loss.

If you're feeling deep fatigue every day, talk to your doctor. But if you simply have occasional slumps and less energy than you used to, try eating smaller meals and then snack more frequently during the day. Save the piece of fruit from breakfast to eat at midmorning, or hold off on the sliced vegetables you brought for lunch and have them as soon as you feel hungry in the afternoon. Eating more frequently can steady your blood sugar levels so you won't feel a slump when your energy supplies run low.

Eating more frequently can stabilize your energy levels, and being active can actually *increase* them.

Another way to combat fatigue is to fit extra physical activity into your daily schedule. It seems paradoxical to be more active when you have less energy, but research shows that physical activity can actually make people feel more energetic, rather than less. Activity provides a psychological boost that can banish the blues. Getting up and moving also increases your self-confidence. And regular exercise increases stamina, so you'll build reserves of energy for more activity.

3 Need a shot of self-confidence? Celebrate small victories.

It's easy to lose confidence if you're not reaching your goals and you're not quite sure why. There's always the temptation to blame yourself. You know how it goes: you tell yourself that you just don't have the staying power or the willpower to lose weight.

Banish those negative thoughts. You haven't failed just because the pounds are proving more stubborn to shed than you expected. For the moment, focus on your successes.

Here's a trick that worked for some of our volunteers. Let's say you've managed to lose five pounds so far, which may not sound like a lot. The next time you're at the grocery store, grab a five-pound package of flour, potatoes, whatever. Carry it around the store as you shop. Getting heavy? That's the amount of excess weight you used to carry all the time. Five pounds on the scale may not seem like much; but when you tote it around in your arms and think of it as the fat you've lost, you'll begin to realize the big accomplishment you've achieved already.

Remember, too, that pounds aren't the only measure of success. Make a list of other benefits you've gained by following *ChangeOne*. Maybe your clothes feel a little more comfortable. Maybe you're moving around more easily. Maybe you're simply eating a healthier diet. Whatever your successes are, celebrate them. And remember, if you can make one change, you can make two. If you can make two changes, you can do three. You get the idea.

4 Struggling with a particular meal?
Twice is nice: go back for seconds.

If you're pleased with your weight-loss progress so far but you aren't following the *ChangeOne* menu for all your meals, don't worry. Some people find they need to make only one or two small changes—giving up their fast-food habit or switching to sugar-free beverages, for example—to start losing weight.

Pounds not coming off fast enough? Go back to the meal that's giving you trouble and take another week to master it. Set aside enough time so that you can follow that chapter's meal plans to the letter, at least for one week. Try a few suggestions you didn't try the first time around. When you're always too rushed to have breakfast, get everything for the meal ready the night before. If eating too many snacks during the day is your downfall, distract yourself for a few minutes with something other than food— a short walk, an errand, or a chore around the house.

If you're not satisfied, take another week to master the meal that's giving you trouble.

5 Is dining out your downfall?
Zero in on portion control.

If your parents always praised you for being a member of the clean-plate club, you still may have trouble leaving food behind, especially when you've paid good money for it at a restaurant. With today's runaway portion sizes, dining out is a major challenge. Don't let the size of the serving plunked down in front of you determine how much you eat. Keep in mind the *ChangeOne* portion size visuals that we've been using—a baseball or a deck of cards, for example—to remind yourself what reasonable servings of food should look like. Ask the waiter to take away what you don't want and pack it for later. Pay attention to hunger and fullness cues, and eat slowly. For a refresher on navigating restaurants, look back to Week 5, "Dining Out," which begins on page 108.

6 Trouble planning ahead?
Make a list, check it twice.

Knowing where your next meal is coming from is critical to successful dieting. If you're having trouble planning ahead, try this: set aside 15 minutes the night before or first thing in the morning to make a list of what you'll need to do that day to stick with *ChangeOne*. Your list might include a quick shopping trip to buy what you'll need for dinner, a reminder of when and where you plan to get some exercise during the day, or a note to make a lunch reservation at a restaurant where you know you'll be able to order a sensible meal. Or look for a frozen meal that meets the *ChangeOne* guidelines. Keep several in the freezer. If you're having trouble finding time to pack a lunch, choose a meal that's quicker and easier to prepare: for instance, a macaroni salad you can make in advance and even divide up into single-serving containers.

7 Famished?
Eat more often.

It's fine to be hungry just before your next meal. But if you're getting so famished that you're tempted to give up the whole idea of dieting, it's time for a reassessment. For starters, this week fill out a Hunger Profile form (you'll find it on page 306) for a few days. Keeping tabs on your appetite will zero in on when you typically feel the hungriest during the day, and what you do about it. Next, begin helping yourself to a snack during those moments when you're feeling especially ravenous. Favor low-calorie, high-fiber snacks that will fill you up without putting you over your calorie target.

> You're more likely to stick to a diet that doesn't force you to go hungry.

If you're still hungry after lunch or dinner, help yourself to an additional serving of vegetables. Keep an eye on your weight. If you continue to lose weight, even if it's a little more slowly than before, that's fine. You're more likely to stick to a diet that doesn't force you to go hungry. If your weight remains steady, that's fine, too. Consider attacking the other side of the calorie equation: increase your activity level by adding 15 minutes of walking a day to what you already do. And keep in mind that many volunteers reported feeling hungry at the beginning of the program. But very quickly their appetites adjusted to *ChangeOne* portion sizes, and they began to feel perfectly satisfied as the weeks progressed—so hang in there.

8 Caving in to cravings?
Forge a new association.

Food cravings aren't hunger pangs. When you're genuinely hungry, you want food, any food. Food cravings are usually for something special—chocolate, potato chips, pizza, whatever. Sometimes food cravings are part of emotional eating. You want chocolate because it makes you feel better when you're feeling low. Food cravings can also be reactions to environmental triggers. You want ice cream after dinner or buttery popcorn when you get to the movie theater simply because all the cues remind you of these foods.

> Food cravings aren't hunger pangs. They are caused by emotional and environmental triggers.

The solution is to teach an old dog a new trick by creating a different, healthier association. Instead of having dessert after dinner this week, get up from the table and go for a stroll. Instead of buttery popcorn at the movies, bring along a *ChangeOne* snack. It won't take long before you associate movie-going with a granola bar or a piece of fruit instead of popcorn. For more on food triggers, emotional eating, and environmental cues, look back to Week 6, "Weekends and Holidays," which begins on page 126.

9 Need a helping hand or a friendly word?
Ask for it.

When the going gets tough, the tough often call on friends and family. If you're not getting the support you need, take this week to explore ways to enlist help or encouragement. The best way to get what you need is by asking for it. Be specific about the kind of help you need. Ask if there's anything you can do in return. Need to cast a wider net? Be creative. If you're looking for an exercise partner, for instance, post a flyer at work or on a neighborhood bulletin board. Wishing you had an eating partner? Consider starting a *ChangeOne* dinner club.

And keep in mind that even though the support of people around you can smooth the way, making a lasting change is ultimately up to you. Even without the active support of family and friends, you can make it on your own. Look back to "How To Be Your Own Best Friend" on page 147 if you need more encouragement.

10 Motivation in need of a tune-up?
Think back to the beginning.

Once the first flush of excitement is over, it can be tough to stay motivated on any diet. Now's the time to remind yourself why you wanted to lose weight in the first place. Write down your three top reasons for starting *ChangeOne*. Below that make a list of the benefits you've noticed so far. These may include the way you feel, the pounds you've managed to lose, the way your clothes fit, or the fact that you're getting more exercise than before. Assign each one a rating of one to three stars, depending on how important it is to you. Post your list somewhere where you'll see it every day (on the refrigerator door, for instance). By reminding yourself of the reasons you started *ChangeOne* and the benefits you've already gained, you'll add oomph to your motivation.

> **Remind yourself why you wanted to lose weight in the first place.**

11 Feeling frazzled?
Find a way to let off steam this week.

Being on a diet can be stressful. Add to that the other strains and stresses in your life, and the combination can seem overwhelming. If stress is threatening to derail your efforts to eat a healthier diet, it's time to take action. Next week we'll zero in on ways to deal with stress in much more detail.

For this week think of one change you can make in your life that will relieve some of the pressure. Ask someone to take on one of your responsibilities at home or the office.

Rearrange your schedule to find time to relax. Experiment with different ways to let off steam. Listen to your favorite music, sit quietly and concentrate on your breathing, take up yoga, or go for a walk or a workout. And if exercise is your answer, take heart in the fact that it eases stress *and* burns extra calories in the bargain.

12 Surrounded by temptations?
Take control of your surroundings.

If your willpower is being tested every time you turn around, take charge of your environment. As we suggested in Week 7, put treats out of sight and make sure that calorie-efficient choices like fruits and vegetables are the centerpiece of your kitchen. At work don't keep food around your desk or work area. If you find yourself in a situation where you can't remove the temptations, remove yourself—go for a walk, do an errand, or grab a *ChangeOne* snack. Remember, the less you have to rely on sheer willpower to avoid temptation, the more likely you are to reach your goals.

Give your willpower some help—don't make cheating easy.

13 Eating all over the house?
Practice the one-room, one-chair rule.

If you eat in practically every room of the house, you're creating associations with food everywhere you go. You'll have no escape from the urge to splurge. Set aside one room and one chair for eating at home. This week make a pact with yourself to go to the designated spot for every meal and snack you eat at home.

14 Sitting on the sidelines?
Get in on the action.

You don't have to start running marathons—all you have to do is find time to walk. This week find a way to add at least 15 minutes of walking during the main part of the day— before breakfast, over the lunch hour, doing errands, or an evening stroll; your eventual goal should be 30 minutes a day. And as we've mentioned above, physical activity can also help you feel more energetic and less stressed.

Goal-setting, Part II

Back in Week Four of the *ChangeOne* program, we asked you to sign a goal-setting contract with yourself. It's time to take another look at your contract—pull it out and give it a read. Were you fair on yourself? It's all too easy to have unrealistic expectations when you decide to lose weight—especially when it's the first time you've tried it in earnest. Even people who have dieted in the past tend to set goals that are tough to reach. And when they don't reach them, they give up.

By now you're an expert on what it takes to lose weight. You also know what you're willing and able to do. This is the perfect time to take a clear-eyed, no-nonsense look at what you want to accomplish. In addition, by revisiting your goals and committing yourself to them anew, you'll take a big step toward staying motivated. To get this reevaluation started, fill in the "How Do You Spell Success?" Quiz on the next page.

Don't Mistake Success for Failure

Almost anyone who sets out to lose weight on a diet can do it. The crazy thing about many dieters is that when they're doing well, they often don't realize it. *Seriously.* Many people who succeed end up thinking they've failed. That's because they get their minds wrapped around an unattainable goal and never see what they've achieved.

You may guess where we're going with the questions in "How Do You Spell Success?" Most people have several goals in mind when they decide to lose weight. A super ambitious goal is great if it jazzes you up at the start. But if it's too ambitious and you begin to think you'll never reach it, you can begin to feel frustrated, then disillusioned. You may actually succeed in losing a lot of weight and getting all the good stuff that goes with it, but if you didn't reach the mammoth goal, you may consider the diet a failure. Then you might give up, go back to your old patterns of eating, and gain back all the weight you lost.

To test the reality of the typical dieter's expectations, researchers at the weight-loss clinic of the University of Pennsylvania carried out a clever experiment. They asked a group of women at the start of a diet program to describe four different goals.

The categories will sound familiar. We borrowed them for the quiz you just completed. The researchers asked the

Change One Quiz

How Do You Spell Success?

Part I

1. How much did you weigh when you began the *ChangeOne* plan? _____

2. What is your dream weight? _____

3. Let's say you can't reach your dream weight; what's the most you can end up weighing and still be happy with the results? _____

4. If you can't reach that "happy" weight, what weight would you describe as acceptable? _____

5. Let's say that you lose weight, but still don't reach your "acceptable" weight; what ending weight would leave you feeling disappointed? _____

Part II

1. Look again at your "dream" weight; what is the number based on?

❑ The lowest my weight has been as an adult

❑ My ideal weight given my height

❑ What I weighed in high school or college

❑ The lowest weight I've been able to reach on a diet

❑ A healthy weight for me according to my doctor

❑ Other

_____

2. Numbers on a scale aren't the only way to measure the success of a diet. Besides weight, what other measures are important to you? On a scale of 1 to 5— not important to very important—rate the following items:

Smaller dress or pants size	1 2 3 4 5
How my clothes feel	1 2 3 4 5
How I feel (slimmer, more energetic, more attractive)	1 2 3 4 5
Specific health measures (blood pressure, for example)	1 2 3 4 5
Overall sense of health	1 2 3 4 5

3. If dress or pants size is an important measure of success for you, what goal do you have in mind?

Dress size: _____

Waist size: _____

4. What else do you hope to achieve by dieting? On a scale of 1 to 5—not important to very important—rate the following motivation:

Feeling more self-confident	1 2 3 4 5
Feeling sexier or more attractive	1 2 3 4 5
Being happier about myself and how I look	1 2 3 4 5
Feeling more in control	1 2 3 4 5
Not being embarrassed by my weight	1 2 3 4 5
Feeling fitter	1 2 3 4 5

Answers

Congratulations! You got every question correct. There are no wrong answers to the questions we just asked; they are too personal for that. But your answers do say a lot about your expectations. For insights on your comments and some thoughts about whether you are being fair to yourself, read on.

women in the program to specify:

- **Their dream weight:** The amount they would like to weigh if they could choose their ideal number.
- **Their happy weight:** A number on the scale that, even if it wasn't perfect, would make them happy.
- **Their acceptable weight:** The number that they would be willing to accept if they couldn't reach either their happy weight or dream weight.

Weight-Loss Goals: Myth vs. Reality

Myth 1: Your ideal weight is what you weighed when you were first married (or graduated from college, or before you had children).

If you're hoping to get back to what you weighed a few years ago, fine. There's a chance you really might get close to that weight again. But if we're talking 15 or 20 years ago, you might want to reconsider. Many people put on weight as they get older. And no matter how hard they try, they have a tough time being as active as they might have been in their early 20s. Don't live in the past. Set a weight-loss goal that's appropriate for the way you live now.

Myth 2: Your ideal weight is the number listed on a standard height-and-weight chart.

Yes, height and weight are often related. Taller people weigh more than shorter ones, all things being equal. But many other factors play a role in determining your weight. For example, your body type: big-boned and solid, small-boned and light, or in between. Your metabolism: whether you naturally burn brightly and move a lot, or take things more slowly. There are other factors as well, like the number of fat cells you have, or how much your parents and other relatives weigh. The numbers listed on a standard height-and-weight chart are just approximations. Don't let them determine if you've succeeded or failed.

Myth 3: Your ideal weight is the lowest weight you've been able to get to on past diets.

Okay, so you've lost that much before. But the fact that you're dieting again says you gained at least some, or perhaps all, of it back again. If you set a weight-loss goal that's too low to maintain, you'll get caught in yo-yo dieting— losing weight, gaining it back, and trying to lose it again. The best goal is one you can live with.

Myth 4: The less you weigh, the healthier you'll be.

Not true. In fact, many studies show that if you're overweight, losing just 5 percent to 10 percent of your current weight is all you have to do to get the bulk of the health benefits associated with weight loss: lower risks of heart disease, stroke, diabetes, and even some forms of cancer.

Myth 5: If you don't hit your dream weight, you'll never be happy.

You don't believe that, do you? A number is just a number. And if it's a number that leaves you frustrated and stuck in an endless cycle of losing and gaining weight, it's time to replace that number with a more reasonable one.

> Don't live in the past. Set a goal appropriate for now.

■ **Their disappointed weight:** A number that, even though it was less than what they currently weighed, would leave them feeling disappointed.

The women in the experiment had high hopes. They began the program weighing an average of 218 pounds. Their average "dream weight" goal was 149—a 69-pound loss. Short of that, the women said they'd be happy at an average of 155 pounds. If all else failed, they'd accept a final weight of 163 pounds. And they'd be disappointed if they ended the diet at a weight of 181, an average loss of 37 pounds.

How did they do? The women in the six-month program lost an average of 16 percent of their starting weight, or 35 pounds. Most experts would call that a strong success. The average weight loss at that point in a successful diet program is around 10 percent to 15 percent.

Though the researchers were thrilled, the women were not. On average they had fallen just short of the bottom target—their "disappointed weight"—which would have required them to lose 17 percent of their starting weight. Even the number they described as merely acceptable represented a 25-percent drop. Their dream weight required a 32-percent weight loss, more than double what experts deem a success.

Think about it. These women did great. They lost a significant amount of weight. But without a realistic goal to measure their progress, most of them were likely to consider the diet a failure. That's just crazy.

Divide Big Goals into Milestones

"Uh-oh," you're probably thinking just about now. "So this is where they tell me I can't lose as many pounds as I'd like."

Not for a second. All we want to do is urge you to make sure your first goals are realistic. Especially when you have a lot of weight you'd like to lose, it's helpful to think in terms of gradual milestones, rather than the ultimate weight you want to be. Once you reach your first milestone you can celebrate your success, take a deep breath, and head on to the next one. The milestone approach helps you gain confidence along the way. It also makes it easy to measure your progress step by step, rather than in a single leap. And that's really what *ChangeOne* is all about.

What's a reasonable first milestone? Many experts say you should first set your sights on losing about 10 percent of your starting weight. To calculate that, take your weight when you

Change One First Person

A Comfy Pair of Leggings

"I didn't really have a specific goal in mind when I started *ChangeOne*," Peg Hoh remembers. **"I certainly didn't have any fantasies of becoming a magazine model. I'd hit 50 and was chubbier than I wanted to be. For health reasons, mostly, I thought it was time to get into shape."**

An information technology manager, Hoh couldn't have been happier when she saw the numbers on the scale go down. By the eighth week on *ChangeOne* she'd lost 16 pounds. But about halfway through the program, something else began to matter to her a lot more than those numbers.

"One of the first changes I wanted to make was to become more active. I made up my mind to walk as often as possible when I got home from work. I bought myself a pair of stretch leggings to walk in. But I was so embarrassed by the way I looked in them, I wore a long sweatshirt so no one would see. It must have been a week or two later that I began to notice that they were fitting better. They just felt more comfortable. Even my husband said he could really see the difference."

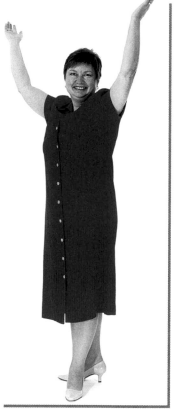

By then Hoh was walking several miles after work most days. She'd also begun eating breakfast, something she hadn't done before. "Those two changes really made the difference for me. Eating breakfast helped me take control of food, rather than having food control me during the day. Walking has really helped me deal with stress. Walking is like meditation for me. I love it."

Something else she loves is how comfortable her new leggings have become. "For me, now it's not so much a weight thing. Maybe I'll get down to my ideal weight, maybe I won't. But I know just by the way my clothes feel that I look better. And when I'm out there walking, I know that I feel better. That's enough reason to stay motivated."

started *ChangeOne* and knock the last number off. If you weighed 222, for instance, 10 percent is about 22 pounds.

Once you reach your first milestone, allow yourself a few weeks to savor the new, slimmer you and to consolidate the changes you've made. Take the time to enjoy all of the other benefits you're likely to experience, from the way you look in the mirror to the way your clothes fit. Then, when you're ready, set the next milestone for weight loss. For many people weight loss slows as they shed pounds. That's perfectly natural. To avoid becoming discouraged, we recommend setting subsequent milestones at about 5 percent of your starting weight—11 pounds if you started out at 222, for instance.

A Contract with Yourself

Okay, now let's take another look at the *ChangeOne* Contract we asked you to sign at the end of Week Four. Now that you have more experience under your belt—which has moved up a notch or two, we hope—take a look back at your contract. How are you doing? Do the goals you set back then still seem reasonable? Are they the goals that matter most to you?

Write up a revised contract if your earlier goals aren't working for you. This is a contract with yourself, after all. You're doing what you're doing—eating better, being more active, and losing weight—for your own sake, nobody else's. You decide the goals that mean the most and work the best for you. By putting them in writing, you'll be able to keep them in mind—and gauge your progress along the way.

Changes Ahead: Stress Relief

Our lives are filled with stress, and that's not always a bad thing. Stress comes in many forms and intensity levels, and much of it is normal and healthy. The trouble comes when we're unable to balance our daily stresses with time to recuperate and relax. Next week we will be looking at how stress can affect the way you eat and sabotage your weight-loss efforts. To prepare for the coming week think about the ways you deal with stress. Do you turn to food when the going gets tough? Does your day allow for time to relax and enjoy? Are excessive responsibilities and the interests of family getting in the way of caring for yourself?

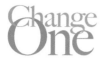

Week 9

Stress Relief

All we're asking you to do this week is relax. That's right, relax. Take a moment or two to shake off the stresses and strains of daily life.

Sound easy? If only it were so. Life can be so hectic these days that taking even a minute off from the pressures of work and family seems impossible. While achieving a stress-free life is unlikely, you can definitely loosen the hold that tension and anxiety often have on you.

That's important, especially when you're trying to lose weight. A rocky period at work or friction at home has knocked many dieters off their program. Stress can rob you of the energy you need to stay focused and motivated. If the pressure gets fierce enough, you may be tempted to say, "Forget it, I just can't do it," and give up your best intentions to stick to a healthier diet.

This week you'll identify sources of stress in your life and try out techniques to manage or even eliminate them.

Take the Pressure Off

Like a lot of people, you may find yourself reaching for food when demands get to be too much. That's hardly surprising. Just the act of eating can make you feel better when your nerves are frayed or you're feeling down. Recent studies have shown that eating—especially eating something high in carbohydrates—can lower your level of stress hormones and make you feel less frazzled.

In fact, you may feel better after eating because that's exactly what your body was signaling you to do: eat something. Stress itself can trigger hunger, scientists are learning. Here's how it works. Say you're on your way to a very important meeting. You're already running a little late when traffic comes to a sudden halt ahead of you. Instinctively, your body readies itself to do something to deal with the problem. Your brain signals your adrenal glands to churn out a variety of hormones, including the stress hormone cortisol. One of cortisol's jobs is to trigger the release of glucose and fatty acids, in case your muscles need energy.

Back in our hunter-gatherer days, this system made sense. Stress didn't take the form of traffic jams; instead, it was usually a real physical threat—a charging animal perhaps. A "fight-or-flight" stress response evolved to prepare us within seconds to do battle or run away. These days the challenges we face aren't as straightforward as that. Sure, you might be tempted to stop the car, get out, and run the rest of the way to your very important meeting. If you did, you'd burn off the energy your body had made available. But chances are you sit there and smolder until traffic begins to move again. Afterwards, the result of your surge in cortisol is an

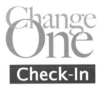

Check-In

At about this point in *ChangeOne*, you're probably having an easier time with some of the changes you've undertaken than with others. No surprise there. Last week you may even have targeted the part that's giving you the toughest time. That's great. But if you get so frustrated that you begin to wonder if it's worth the trouble, ease off. Focus on changes that feel more doable right now. If fitting in activity every day just isn't in the cards, don't worry. Concentrate instead on reining in portions. If paying attention to hunger cues has made a big difference for you, put your energy there and don't worry that you're missing breakfast now and then. Go with your strengths. Target the changes that offer the biggest payoff and concentrate on turning them into easy habits. Go easy on yourself.

increase in appetite—your body's way of guaranteeing that you'll replace the energy it released in the form of glucose and fatty acids.

A flood of these hormones wouldn't pose much of a problem if it happened only now and then. But a steady tide of tense situations can keep cortisol levels high all day, making you feel hungry almost all the time. As if that's not bad enough, cortisol also triggers enzymes that activate fat cells, priming them to store energy as fat. The most susceptible fat cells are those around your middle, which are particularly sensitive to the effects of cortisol.

You see the problem. Stress makes you hungry. Eating makes you feel better. Stress promotes fat. And you put on weight instead of taking it off. Watching your efforts to lose weight fail can then create even more pressure and tension.

Now is the time to make sure you don't get caught in the spiral of stress and eating.

If stress is getting the better of you, remember that everyone's life has its hassles, small and large. One major difference between people who succeed and those who don't, psychologists say, is how they deal with everyday tribulations.

To see how well you handle stress, take a few minutes to fill out the test on the next page. Your answers will help you analyze how you cope with the challenges of daily life.

Help!

"I feel jittery and short-tempered much of the day. I thought it might be too much caffeine—but I have only a couple of cups of coffee in the morning, that's it. What's going on?"

Watch the caffeine you're getting from sources other than coffee. Caffeine is a stimulant, and in some people it can aggravate stress. Besides coffee, there's also caffeine in teas, colas, chocolate, and some pain relievers. The best way to know if too much caffeine is a problem is to ease back on the amount you consume, but don't go cold-turkey. Caffeine withdrawal can cause headaches and may make you feel even more jittery and short-fused. A better way is to begin mixing regular coffee with decaffeinated coffee. Over a few weeks, gradually add more decaf and less of the high-octane brew. Then, if you decide to give up coffee altogether, you'll have an easier time.

Step One: Solve Problems That *Can* Be Solved

The most direct way to deal with stress is to eliminate the situations that wear you down. Yes, that's easier said than done, but the more irritations and annoyances you can unload, the easier it is to tackle the big issues. You may find there are plenty of petty aggravations you can fix quickly once you start paying attention to them. Every time you feel yourself getting hot, stop and see if you can find a solution. If

Change One Quiz

Stress Test

Read each statement below and check those that apply to you right now:

○ A lot of things in my life seem to be out of control right now.

△ I have several good friends I can call if I need to talk something through.

○ When I'm feeling frazzled, I often have the urge to eat.

△ I'm feeling pretty good about my life right now.

○ I often feel overwhelmed with the thought of everything that has to get done during the day.

△ I feel better once I've made a list of what I have to do.

○ Trying to lose weight has definitely added to the pressures I feel.

○ It's really been frustrating for me to try to find time to be more active.

△ Taking control of my diet has made me feel better about myself.

○ Sometimes I resent all the responsibilities I have.

△ I'm pretty good at taking problems in stride.

○ Lately I notice myself losing my temper when even little things go wrong.

△ Even when things get a little crazy, I still feel as if I'm in control of what's going on in my life.

○ If someone puts me on hold while we're talking and then doesn't come back on the line soon, it really makes me mad—mad enough to hang up sometimes.

○ I don't have much patience for people who make mistakes.

△ Even though my life is pretty crowded, I'm good at keeping my priorities straight.

△ I don't worry much about things I can't control.

○ When I'm under a lot of pressure, I sometimes find myself running in three different directions at once.

○ I frequently wake up in the night feeling anxious about my life.

△ No matter how hectic the day has been, it's easy for me to relax and unwind once I get home.

○ I wish I had more control over what happens in my life.

△ Exercise is a good way for me to let off steam.

○ Social situations often make me nervous.

△ Frankly, I don't tend to sweat the little things—I figure they'll take care of themselves.

Quiz Score

What your score means:

How many of each color did you check? If you tallied more blue triangles than red circles, your responses indicate that you've got the pressures of everyday life well in hand. But if the red outnumber the blue it could spell trouble—stress is hurting your life. If the numbers are about equal—and even if the blue slightly outnumber the red—be aware that a bad day could send you into the red zone. Whatever your score, there are plenty of effective ways to keep cool, calm, and collected. Just read on.

you find yourself shrieking because you can never seem to find the car keys or your glasses, for instance, establish a place where you put the keys, glasses, cell phone, or whatever, each time you put them down. Post a reminder on the door, if you have to, until you get into the habit.

If getting dinner together makes your blood pressure rise because half the time you don't have what you need on hand, take time on Sunday to stock the pantry for the week. Make double batches of storable dishes to cut your cooking time significantly.

Not all problems are that simple to eliminate, of course. Let's say your boss gives you more work than you can manage. On top of that, you haven't been given the authority you need to do the job. That's a classic high-stress dilemma. What to do about it? The direct solution is to talk to the boss and explain the problem. Frame the talk not as a complaint ("You're overworking me") but as a search for solutions ("It would help me a lot if we could decide on priorities, and if I had your support for making a few key decisions").

Or say your problems are at home—tension in your marriage, for instance, or trouble with one of the children. Talking it through with the person closest to you might help you get to the source of the pressure and relieve it. Yes, it can be hard to ask for help—but it gets easier when you first ask yourself, "What am I getting out of letting things go on the way they are?" You might explain to your spouse or kids why reducing tension in the household is so important to you now: you're trying to make changes that will make your life better. If the problems are more complicated than the family can handle alone, consider enlisting the help of a counselor.

Only you can know which problems you can confront directly and which you may have to learn to live with. Certainly, there are going to be irritations—and worse—that you can't eliminate, at least at the moment. But you can accept them without being overwhelmed by them—and without letting them derail your diet.

If You Can't Stand the Heat ...

For people who compulsively reach for food when tensions reach the boiling point, the simplest solution is the ultimate in common sense: get away from food. If there are problems at home, don't deal with them in the kitchen. Go to another room of the house to hash them out, and don't take food with you. Under tons of pressure at work? Keep snacks out of easy reach. This week remember our rule: don't eat to relax. Try one of these techniques first. Then wait 5 or 10 minutes to see if you're still hungry. If so, dig in.

Step Two: Accept the Things You Can't Change

There are people who can shrug off almost any setback. Others get frazzled when even the smallest things don't go right. In either case, the demands may be the same. The difference is in the individual responses. Psychologists don't understand all the reasons why people react so differently to stress. Having a sense of humor seems to help many people. Being able to distract yourself is an added plus. Just having something you really enjoy doing offers a time-out from the pressures of life. Playing a musical instrument, reading a good book, helping out at a local soup kitchen—all of these can take your mind off problems and give you a much-needed vacation from fretting.

Naturally, you can't completely change your personality. But experts say you can change the way you react to hassles and frustrations. On the following pages we offer seven ways to cool down when your temper flares or the problems in your life feel overwhelming. This week try out several of them. If one doesn't seem to work for you, move on to another. Your goal: to have at least two stress-busting techniques you can turn to when the pressure builds and your nerves begin to feel frazzled. Knowing how to relax and let off steam will help you stay focused and motivated.

1. Run Away

One of the most effective ways to defuse stress is to run away from it—or at least walk briskly. In a 1998 study that asked 38 men and 35 women to keep diaries of activity, mood, and stress, volunteers reported that they felt less anxious on days when they were physically active than on days when they didn't exercise. Even when stressful events occurred, people in the study said they felt less troubled on their physically active days.

Why? Exercise acts as an antidote to life's pressures in several ways. First, it is a simple distraction from problems. Second, it may change the chemistry of stress, blunting the effects of hormones like cortisol. Exercise has also been shown to ease the symptoms of moderate depression. That in turn may help people deal better with daily hassles and aggravations. And then there's the fact that exercise burns calories, an added bonus for dieters. Physical activity makes it easier not only to lose weight but to keep calories in balance once you go off your diet, and that's enough to make anyone feel good.

Virtually any kind of physical activity seems to relieve the effects of stress, although some researchers think that activities that involve repetitive movements—walking, running, cycling, or swimming, for instance—may offer the best defense. Many people consider swimming to be one of the most relaxing exercises, a soothing way to literally go with the flow. Repeating a physical movement over and over again somehow seems to ease mind and body.

Think about some ways to make your workout even more relaxing. If you're a walker, be aware of the way your arms swing from front to back and the rhythm of your gait. Repeat a soothing word or phrase each time you exhale.

An Ancient Cure for Frayed Nerves

Looking for a simple way to relax, refresh your energy, become more limber, and strengthen muscles at the same time? Yoga may be just the ticket. Exercise scientists have long known that yoga offers a great way to stretch, increase strength, and improve balance. Now psychologists are discovering it can also ease a troubled mind.

When researchers at the University of Wurzburg in Germany tested 12 women before, during, and after a 60-minute yoga class, they found that the women's heart rates dropped dramatically during the routines. The women also reported feeling less irritable than they did before the class.

Another recent study showed that yoga may well be one of the best stress-easers around. At Oxford University, a psychologist divided 71 men and women into three groups. One group practiced simple relaxation techniques like deep breathing. The second visualized themselves feeling less tense. The third did a half-hour yoga routine. The relaxers and the visualizers felt sluggish afterwards. The people in the yoga group reported feeling more energetic and emotionally content after their class.

How to get started? On pages 243–246 you'll find a simple stretching routine that includes several modified yoga positions. Give it a try this week.

If you enjoy the routine, you may want to sign up for a yoga class. Many fitness centers or yoga studios offer them. You'll also find helpful guides in yoga videos or instruction books.

Yoga is among the best stress-busters around.

If you work out on an exercise cycle or stair machine at a fitness club, you might find yourself parked in front of a bank of television sets. Watching TV can prevent you from getting into the soothing rhythm of your workout. Scientists have found that watching television makes people more jittery, not less. So ignore what's on the screen. Concentrate instead on your breathing and the repetitive movement of your arms and legs. If the gym plays music that gets on your nerves, bring a personal stereo with earphones and your own favorite music, or use noise-blocking earplugs and enjoy a quiet interlude.

You'll find plenty of aggravations you can fix if you take the time to recognize them.

2. Do One Thing at a Time

Chances are you've heard of Type A behavior—the hard-driven, competitive, take-no-prisoners personality profile once thought to be linked not only to high levels of stress but to greater risk of heart disease. The original term for Type A behavior was the "Hurry Syndrome," because Type A's tend to do everything faster than more relaxed personality types. Type A's feel so rushed, in fact, that they often try to do three things at once. They're the ones you see eating lunch, talking on their cell phones, and driving—all at the same time.

If you find yourself falling into this behavior, make an effort this week to focus on the task at hand. Instead of balancing your checkbook while you're talking on the phone, give the phone call your attention, then return to the checkbook. If you're constantly being interrupted with phone calls while you're trying to work on something, let the answering machine take messages. Call people back when the time is right for you.

In short, do one thing at a time, and you may feel your stress meter begin to tick down.

3. Put Out the Fire

Anger can be stressful, especially the "hot-headed" kind that lashes out and doesn't solve the problem that ignited it. But never expressing your anger can be harmful as well. If you feel your temper about to flare, stop, take a deep breath, and ask yourself three quick questions suggested by Redford Williams, a Duke University researcher who

Change One First Person

Taking Control, One Week at a Time

Dianne Barnum was no stranger to dieting or diet books. "I've read lots of them, and tried lots of programs," says Barnum, who lives in Brookfield, Connecticut. Fifty pounds heavier than she wanted to be, she'd never found a plan that worked for her. When the chance to try *ChangeOne* came along, she was among the first to sign up.

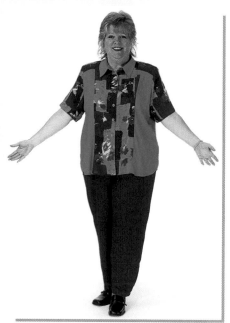

"Frankly, I wanted a lot from a diet. I wanted a program that was based on solid advice and the kind of foods I like. But I also wanted it to be doable. No counting calories all the time. No adding up food points. I didn't want to have to spend all my time writing things down. I wanted to be able to go on living my life—going out to restaurants with my husband, socializing—and make sensible eating part of it. But I also really wanted to start shedding pounds."

She did. She dropped 17 pounds through Week 9, and by the end of the first 12 weeks she was down 22 pounds. But she didn't stop there; after five months on *ChangeOne* she'd lost 40 pounds. "The most important thing I learned was how to take control. It's easy to blame other people or the things around you when you're overweight. But the simple truth is, you're the one who decides what you're going to put in your mouth, no one else. Once I realized that, all I needed was knowledge about smart choices and sensible serving sizes."

On course to lose the 50 pounds she set as her goal, Barnum continues to look for one change a week to keep her on track. "It may be something as simple as finding a new recipe I haven't tried. Or experimenting with a new food. I'll vary my exercise program just to keep it interesting. Whatever it is, every week I try to make one more change. And what a difference that's made in the way I look and feel. I look at myself in the mirror now and see a different person. And I love it."

pioneered work in anger control:

Is this really important to me? If the answer is no, leave what sparked your anger behind. If the answer is yes, then ask yourself:

Am I justified in being angry in this situation? Argue the pros and cons, as if you had to make your case in court. If your answer is, "No, I don't really have much to gripe about," you're likely to feel your anger and stress begin to melt away. Of course the answer may be, "Yes, that guy nearly ran me off the road, and he's so busy talking on his cell phone he didn't even notice it!" If so, then ask yourself just one more question:

Is there anything I can really do about it? Honking like crazy isn't going to change anything. It's only likely to make you angrier. So in the case of our driver, the best response is to let it go, take a deep breath, and keep out of the guy's way.

But if your answer to the last question is another "yes," then you're in luck. You have the chance to make a real change for the better. Let's say you're angry because one of the kids keeps leaving junk food lying around in the kitchen when you've specifically asked him or her to put it away. Lay down the law. Explain why you don't want junk food lying around. Get mad if you have to, but then let your anger go. If you have trouble doing that, ask yourself the first question again, but with a little twist: "What do I get out of staying angry?" Chances are the answer is "not much," except unpleasant aggravation.

> "What do I get out of staying angry?" Chances are, not much.

If all else fails, try imagining this is your last day alive and write down how you'd be dealing with the situation if you knew, assuming that you still have to go to work and do normal things. You're likely to find out that you have better things to do than stay angry and tense.

4. Call a Friend

Sure, it sounds a little sappy. But talking to someone else—even just calling someone to say a quick hello—does more than take your mind off your troubles. Swedish researchers recently reported that people with a strong sense of social connection to other people were almost one-third less likely to die after they'd had a heart attack than those who were socially isolated. Part of the reason, the researchers believe, may be the stress-easing effect of close relationships. If you don't have a circle of friends you feel like you can turn to, consider beginning to build one by volunteering for a local charity, joining a club or a church group, or signing up for an exercise class.

5. Talk to Yourself

Sometimes we're our own worst enemies. Instead of easing our pressures, we add to them by thinking in terms of absolutes, using words like "never," "should," or "always." "I should never have done that." "Things always go wrong for me." "I'll never be able to lose weight at this rate." If that sounds like you, be alert to moments when you're being unreasonably hard on yourself and try to lighten up. Counter the negative messages with a steady dose of positive ones.

> **Most of us have a hard time letting our minds go quiet and our bodies relax.**

Don't be embarrassed to say them out loud if you're alone. "Whoa. Easy there. Give it a rest." Replace the harsh absolute with a more reasonable and forgiving thought: "So it's going to take awhile to lose the weight. So what? No one's pushing me but myself. I'm doing fine." Take the broad view. Things don't always go wrong for you, after all.

The truth is, things occasionally go wrong for everyone. And when they do, everyone has the same challenge: to sort things out and get on with life.

6. Laugh It Off

Laughter actually can be strong medicine, researchers say. The act of laughing eases muscle tension, relieves stress, and has even been shown to lower the risk of stress-related illnesses such as heart disease.

In a study published in 2001, the Center for Preventive Cardiology at the University of Maryland Medical Center tested 300 volunteers for their propensity to laugh at everyday events. Those with a ready laugh were less likely to have heart problems than those who rarely broke a smile, the scientists found. Even among people with elevated blood pressure or cholesterol, the ability to laugh offered protection against heart attacks.

Now it's not always easy to laugh when things go wrong. But if you need a good chortle, try renting a favorite movie comedy, watching your favorite sitcom, or keeping a humorous book handy. Cartoon collections—"Doonesbury," say, or "The "Far Side"—offer plenty of laughs. If you frequently fume in rush-hour traffic, try renting or buying an audio book, preferably a funny one.

7. Practice Relaxation

Another proven way to ease stress is what Harvard University cardiologist Herbert Benson calls the relaxation response. According to Benson's studies, the method taps an innate mechanism that can be used to counteract the human "fight-or-flight" response that triggers stress. His research shows that the relaxation technique can lower blood pressure and ease muscle tension. Benson suggests setting aside 20 minutes and following these six simple steps:

- Find a quiet place where you won't be disturbed. Sit in a comfortable position, one that allows you to relax your body. Close your eyes.

- Starting with your feet and moving up, relax your muscles. End with the muscles of your face. Take a moment to experience the feeling of being completely relaxed.

- With your eyes still closed, breathe in and out through your nose, concentrating on each breath.

- As you exhale, begin to silently repeat a short phrase or single word, such as "peace," "calmness," or "easy does it." Choose a word that helps you focus your mind and banish distracting thoughts.

- Continue repeating your soothing word or phrase and concentrating on breathing. The experts usually recommend doing this exercise for 10 to 15 minutes. Don't set an alarm, though, or you'll constantly be thinking about it. Have a watch or clock handy and open your eyes now and then to check the time. And don't be discouraged from doing the relaxation routine if you don't have a full 15 minutes. Even a few minutes will help.

Silently repeating a word like "peace" or "calm" can help you achieve it.

- Sit quietly for a few more minutes, first with your eyes closed and then with them open. Savor the way your body and mind feel.

Sound easy? In fact, most of us have a hard time letting our minds go quiet and our bodies relax. You may need to practice relaxing a few times before you master the art. But with some practice you'll find that you can slip quickly into relaxation and away from stress.

Making the Change

Choose at least three of the strategies in this chapter and try them this week. You probably already have an intuitive sense of which ones are best suited to your temperament. But don't be afraid to try at least one that sounds a little far out. You may be surprised at how effective it can be.

Whatever you choose, don't put added pressure on yourself by thinking you have to squeeze yet one more change into an already crowded schedule. Most of these stress-busting techniques take no time at all. Even those that do, like practicing the relaxation response or exercising, are well worth the extra time. By taking a few minutes to relax, you may find that you're more focused and productive when you get back to work. Certainly, you'll feel calmer. And that's a change that will help you stay in charge of your diet and your life.

Changes Ahead: Staying Active for Success

When someone says they don't have the time to do something, what they often mean is they choose to spend their time doing something else. It's all a matter of priorities.

So when you say you don't have the time to exercise more, what priority of yours is higher than exercise? It's a question worth pondering this week as you work on destressing your life.

We realize that we've already asked you this week to invest time in relaxation, and that meant setting aside some other task. Next week we're going to ask you for even more time. But as you'll learn, you can grab exercise time in small pieces throughout the day, and with surprisingly little sacrifice. So as you proceed through this week, think of how you spend your time, and whether the TV rerun or that fourth phone call of the night is as high a priority as good health and maintaining weight loss.

Comfort Foods for Relieving Stress

"Comfort food," we've come to call it: simple, satisfying, home-cooked meals that conjure up relaxed family dinners in a cozy kitchen. Each of us has certain dishes we find comforting, often recipes we associate with childhood. Sitting down to one of them can be a great way to kick back and recover from a difficult day. Here are six suggested *ChangeOne* comfort-food meals guaranteed to transport you to easier times:

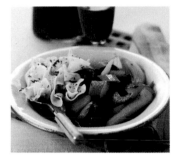

Beef Stew
page 92

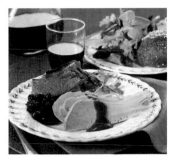

Apple-Stuffed Turkey Breast
page 141

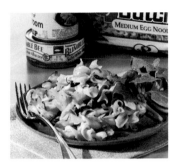

Homestyle Tuna Noodle Casserole
page 162

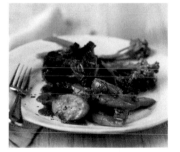

All-American Pot Roast with Braised Vegetables
page 272

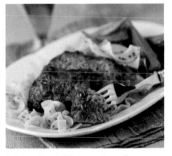

Heartland Meat Loaf
page 274

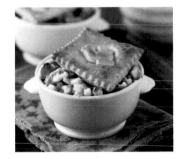

One-Crust Chicken Pot Pie
page 280

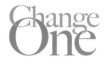

Week 10

Staying Active for Success

Let's face it: most of us have it easy these days. By some estimates we burn about half as many calories as people did a century ago just going about their everyday lives. That shortfall, many experts think, is a major reason so many of us struggle with our weight.

From the first week of this program we've been pushing exercise on you in subtle and not-so-subtle ways. This week we're getting serious about it.

Each day, find a few moments to squeeze in a short walk, a relaxing stretch, some extra activity. Start developing a new habit: moving around, whenever you can!

Becoming more active isn't essential to shedding pounds. But it sure helps. And it becomes even more important when you're trying to keep the pounds off. An active lifestyle, research shows, is the single most important key to long-term dieting success.

Rebel Against Inactivity

Over the past 20 years health experts have confirmed a simple but profound fact: we were built to be active. Physical activity helps keep arteries clear, hearts strong, and immune systems revved up. The more active we are, the evidence shows, the lower our risk of having high blood pressure, high cholesterol, diabetes, osteoporosis, depression, and even some forms of cancer.

For dieters, getting up and moving is especially important. Consider that it takes a 500-calorie-a-day drop to lose one pound of body fat in a week. One way to shed that pound is to eat 500 fewer calories than you need. Another is to burn an extra 500 calories a day doing serious exercise. For a 200-pound man, for example, that's about 40 minutes a day of steady jogging at five miles per hour, seven days a week.

Some people favor exercise. Others eat less. But most successful dieters find it's a whole lot easier to split the difference: to eat roughly 250 calories less a day and to burn an extra 250. That way your diet doesn't have to be quite so spartan. And you don't have to spend every free moment working up a serious sweat on a stair machine at the gym. In fact, as you'll see, you don't even have to become a formal exerciser.

But burning calories is only one reason to include physical activity in your *ChangeOne* program.

We were built to be active. Exercise makes us less susceptible to most every major disease.

Improve your long-term odds of success

By adding physical activity to a diet program, especially 10 weeks into it, you definitely enhance your chances of continuing success. Dieting may be the best way to lose weight initially, but exercise turns out to be the best way to ensure that you keep it off.

In a landmark 1996 study, researchers at Baylor College of Medicine compared three weight-loss approaches: diet only, exercise only, and a combination of exercise and diet. At the end of the first year the combination group had lost the most weight, followed by the diet-only group, with the exercise-only group trailing the pack.

But during the second year, a dramatic turnaround occurred. The diet-only group regained all of the weight they'd lost, and then some. The combination group regained some of the weight, but still remained slimmer than when they started the program. The exercise-only group fared best of all, regaining only a few pounds. The reason, experts surmised, was that people get weary of pure dieting and eventually give it up. Being physically active, on the other hand, becomes a pleasure, something people are willing to make a part of their lives.

Tame hunger

In a study published in 2002, Stanford University researchers compared volunteers in a diet-only program with a program that combined diet and exercise. After a year people in the combination group reported feeling less hungry than those in the diet-only program. The combination group also found it easier to make smart food choices and avoid temptations. There's one very simple reason for that: when you expend more energy through exercise, you can eat more without gaining weight. Also, research shows that exercise itself can dampen appetite.

Maintain the burn

One of the drawbacks to eating less is that your body compensates by burning fewer calories. That's why people often find it difficult to continue to shed pounds as they lose weight. The best way to make your body burn enough calories even as you lose weight is through physical activity.

Preserve muscle

Another drawback to dieting is that your body may find the energy it needs by burning not only fat but also muscle cells. That's a problem for three reasons. First, muscle gives

Don't Slow Down

You may have heard that certain kinds of aerobic exercise are better than others at burning off fat. Don't believe it.

It's true that leisurely exercise of roughly 40 minutes or longer will prompt your body to start tapping into fat cells for energy. But fitness experts say that increasing workout intensity will better serve your weight-loss goals over the long haul.

There are several problems with taking it too slow: most people don't exercise long enough to begin burning into their fat stores; by going at a slower pace, they burn fewer calories; and since everyone's squeezed for time these days, longer, slower workouts just don't make a lot of sense.

The best reason to exercise vigorously is that you'll burn more calories while you're working out, and the high intensity means that you'll continue to burn some calories after you stop. Remember, you want to create a calorie deficit, and the more energy you expend during (and after) exercise, the bigger that deficit will be. Work out as hard as you comfortably can.

you a shapelier physique. If one of your goals is to look better in the mirror, you'll want to keep muscle—maybe even add some. Second, well-toned muscles help you keep your balance and stay strong enough to work and play with ease—in a word, they keep you agile. Third, when you lose muscle tissue your metabolism slows down, because muscle tissue requires a lot of energy to maintain. The more muscle you have, the more calories you burn, even when you're doing nothing at all.

Lose fat faster

Add exercise to your diet program and you'll speed your fat-burning rate. Scientists at Queen's University in Canada recently compared the effects of diet versus exercise by tracking the progress of 30 men. Over three months volunteers in both the diet and exercise groups lost more than 16 pounds. But those who exercised lost almost two pounds more body fat than the dieters did. And it's fat, after all, that you want to lose.

Look and feel better

A recent study from the University of Maryland offers further evidence of the many benefits of combining a weight-loss program with exercise. Researchers asked 24 overweight, inactive women to begin walking three times a week; at the same time the women also scaled back their calorie intake. The diet advice was simple: the women were asked to cut 250 to 350 calories a day from what they were eating while following nutrition guidelines very much like those of *ChangeOne*.

After six months the volunteers had lost 8 percent of their body weight. For a 180-pound woman, that's a loss of 14 pounds. Nice, but get this: their total body *fat* had fallen by 15 percent. That means each woman had shaved off an average of 27 pounds of fat, replacing about half of it with muscle. Further, the women's aerobic capacity—a measure of their lungs' ability to take in oxygen—jumped 8 percent. In short, thanks to the diet and exercise combo, the women were fitter, slimmer, stronger, and had more stamina.

Check-In

It's been six weeks since you first drew up a *ChangeOne* Contract, and two weeks since we asked you to take it out again and assess your progress. With two more weeks of changes under your belt now, we're going to have you take one more look at it. Make sure the goals you set still make sense and are workable. Do you still consider your expectations realistic? If not, adjust them. Again, this is a long-term contract with yourself. Push hard to stay motivated, but not so hard that you get frustrated and give up.

Making the Change

Most people who disavow exercise discover that they actually enjoy it once they get into the swing of things. So keep an open mind. Here are some ideas to get you started:

Convince yourself it's worth a try. Beyond weight loss, experts say, there are some 50 proven benefits to exercise, from a healthier heart to a rosier outlook on life. Think about the benefits you're looking for and make a list of the five that matter most to you.

Picture yourself on the move. Top-flight athletes often visualize themselves performing their moves in order to fine-tune their performance. The same technique can help spur you to action. Picture yourself happily riding a bike, doing water aerobics, or hiking on a local trail. Imagine all the pleasant things you'll experience, from beautiful scenery to a surging sense of self-confidence.

Tell all. Announce your activity plans to friends and family. Knowing they know will further encourage (or shame) you to follow through.

Leap the hurdles. Look for clever ways to get over the inevitable obstacles. If you're pressed for time, try laying out your exercise clothes the night before. If you have a business trip coming up, choose hotels with exercise facilities or running trails nearby. Preoccupied with family matters? Find activities you all can do together, like hiking, badminton, volleyball, or bicycling.

Turn Downtime Into a Moving Experience

Of course, you never have free time, right? Don't be so sure. No matter how busy things seem, chances are you have plenty of opportunities to be more active. Get started this week by completing the Personal Time Analyzer form on page 309. Make a couple of copies. On at least two days this week—preferably a weekday

Help!

"I'm just not an exercise person. Never have been, never will be. Isn't it possible to lose weight and keep it off without working up a sweat?"

Sure, it's possible. But maybe you're reacting to the myth that exercise has to involve gyms, pumping iron, spandex, aerobics bunnies, and public displays of sweating. As you'll see in this chapter, you can get plenty of activity without the spandex and dumbbells. Your day provides plenty of opportunities for walking, stair climbing, and other everyday activities.

And those short bursts can have a long-lasting effect. In a study at the Cooper Institute in Dallas, scientists recruited 235 men and women. Half agreed to do a standard gym workout several times a week. The other half incorporated physical activity into their everyday lives. Both groups burned about the same number of extra calories and lost the same amount of body fat, on average. But the everyday-activity folks turned out to have one big advantage over the gym-goers: they were more likely to continue their on-the-fly workouts long after the study ended.

and a weekend day—fill out a time analysis. Write down what you do and how much time you spend doing it, hour by hour. Mark whether you're sitting still or up and moving. Active pastimes include walking, vacuuming, raking leaves, climbing stairs, riding a bike—any activity that requires enough effort to make you slightly winded. Inactive pastimes involve sitting, stretching out on the sofa, or standing around.

Once you've filled out the form, identify at least two chances in the day when you can get up and get going. Your goal should be to turn at least 30 minutes of inactive time into activity every day by the end of the week.

We're sticking with 30 minutes even though government health experts recently upped their recommendation to an hour. Sure, if you want to do more you'll get better results, but studies show that you'll reap the weight-loss benefits you want by doing at least 30 minutes worth of moderately strenuous activities—think brisk walking—most days of the week. Start with 10 to 15 minutes a day for the first half of the week, then add another 10 to 15 minutes. You don't have to do 30 continuous minutes. You can divide up the time any way you want: three 10-minute walks, for instance, or 10 minutes spent climbing stairs coming and going from work and a 20-minute walk in the morning.

Some opportunities may be obvious. If you commute by bus, train, or subway, get off one or two stops early and hoof it the rest of the way. If you ride an elevator or escalator coming and going from the office, take the stairs instead. If you usually park yourself in front of the television after dinner, choose a half-hour show you can live without and go for a walk instead. If you must watch the show, at the very least

You Choose

Here are some everyday activities and the amount of calories burned after 30 minutes. The figures are based on a 180-pound woman's expenditure:

Activity	Calories burned
Watch a baseball game	66
Play baseball	**354**
Shop online	66
Walk around the mall	**141**
Drive to the car wash	66
Wash your own car	**129**
Watch ballroom dancing	66
Go ballroom dancing	**129**
Ride a lawn mower	66
Push a lawn mower	**258**
Play a video game	66
Play Frisbee	**129**
Use a leaf-blower	75
Use a rake	**171**
Sunbathe	66
Go swimming	**300**

Change One First Person

Having a Lot More Fun

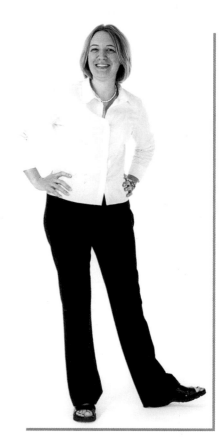

Two weeks before she started *ChangeOne*, Lynn Schmelder joined a gym, hoping to get back into shape for the summer. And for a couple of weeks she was really into it, grabbing time over her lunch hour to work out on one of the cardio machines. It didn't last long.

"I just got bored with doing the same thing over and over. I began to have to force myself to go. And then pretty soon I wasn't going. That's happened to me before—I've joined a gym, all excited, and then stopped going after the initial excitement wore off."

With a nudge from us at *ChangeOne*, Schmelder decided to give exercise one more try. But this time she was determined to ward off boredom by going for variety. Lots of it.

"I started doing aerobics, and I found that I really loved it. I like being with other people in a class. I like learning new moves. The instructors are great. So right now I'm going three to four times a week. I do regular aerobics, step aerobics, and kick-boxing.

"What a difference! Before, I had to drag myself to the gym. Now I can't wait to get there."

Staying active has also made a difference on the scale. When she started *ChangeOne*, Schmelder weighed 159 pounds; she's now down to 148. "My clothes fit better. I have so much more energy. And I'm having a lot more fun."

And she's also come to realize that, for her at least, the only way to stay active is to find things she really enjoys doing. "If you have to force yourself to do it, you won't keep it up. Willpower only goes so far. The key is to find things that are fun and interesting, things you really enjoy for their own sake. Then nothing can stop you."

do a few simple exercises during the commercial breaks.

With a little ingenuity you'll find other ways to turn downtime into active time. If you love to read, consider getting that latest thriller on tape and listen while you make a circuit on foot around the neighborhood. And being a devoted sports fan doesn't mean you have to become a couch potato during games; get a portable radio and walk while you listen to the play-by-play. If your work day is filled with meetings, suggest to your clients or colleagues a walk-and-talk session. Frequent travelers should make it a point to take a brisk stroll around the terminal while waiting for a flight; a long airport wait could turn into a respectable workout.

Other ways to fit an activity in every day this week:

Plan ahead: Decide where and when you'll have time for extra activity, and mark it on your calendar. Treat exercise as you would an appointment. Find an open time slot on your calendar and reserve a workout. If you use a computer, set it to remind you of your appointment. At the end of each day tally up how much extra activity you fit in. If you fell short of your goal, brainstorm ways to get a little more exercise the following day.

Have a fallback: Let's say Plan No. 1 is to walk for 15 minutes after lunch. That's great, unless someone at the office is celebrating a birthday and you end up being part of the festivities. Then it's time for Plan No. 2: walking for 30 minutes after dinner, when you usually would do your second 15-minute walk. Make sure your plans include both weekdays and weekend over the next seven days.

Make it useful: If you have trouble doing exercise just for the sake of exercise, look for ways to make it useful. Find bona fide reasons to go for a walk, for example. Instead of having the newspaper delivered, walk to the newspaper box or a nearby store. If you typically drive to a market that's within walking distance, save on gasoline and lace up those walking shoes. If there are chores around the house or yard that need doing, make a list and get cracking. The bottom

Help!

"The last time I tried exercising, I ended up being so sore the next morning that I could barely get out of bed. Is there anything I can do to prevent that?"

A little bit of soreness is normal. But if you're uncomfortably sore, it means you overdid it. This time around, don't try to go from 0 to 60 in 10 seconds. Ease into an exercise program a little at a time. Beginning on page 236 you'll find an eight-week fitness program designed to get you into shape slowly but surely. Another tip that may help: try doing a few stretching exercises before and after you walk or do other physical activities. You'll find a quick and simple stretching routine on pages 243–245.

Walking: Your Best Bet

Walking is the exercise of choice for most dieters. No wonder. You don't need a gym membership. You can do it virtually everywhere —around the block or around the mall, for example. It's gentle on joints, and you can burn a surprising number of calories. On flat terrain, a half-hour walk can chew through 100 to 150 calories, depending on your weight. Hike up some hills and you can erase 200 to 250 calories. Here's how to prepare:

Find Shoes That Fit

The only equipment you really need is a decent pair of walking shoes. Finding them is a cinch. What matters most is comfort. If it feels good on your feet when you try it on, odds are it also provides enough support. When shopping for shoes:

■ Wear the socks you plan to exercise in. That way you'll be sure to get the best fit.

■ Try on both shoes. Most people's feet aren't exactly the same size. Choose a pair that fits your larger foot.

■ Allow a little extra room. Feet swell when you walk, so buy shoes with about a thumb's width between your longest toe and the end of the shoe. Make sure the heel doesn't slip, though, or you could end up with painful blisters.

Check Your Form

Sure, walking comes naturally, and it's smart to stay close to the technique you've always known. But these tips will help you stay comfortable and get the most out of your walk:

■ Stand up straight. Imagine a string pulling you up from the top of your head. Let that string pull you up as straight as possible. Relax your shoulders.

■ Look ahead. Keep your neck straight and your head held high to avoid unnecessary strain to the neck and shoulders. If you have to look down to see where you're going, lower your eyes, not your head.

■ Move those arms. Bend your elbows and let your arms swing naturally at your sides. You'll prevent swelling, tingling, or numbness—and you'll burn up to 15 percent more calories by keeping your arms moving.

■ Don't carry that weight. Some people try to get in extra exercise by toting a couple of light dumbbells along for the journey, but fitness-walking experts say that's risky; the weights can pull you off balance and strain muscles in your back or legs.

> All you need is a decent pair of shoes and a good path for the journey.

Stay Safe

Walking is one of the safest activities you can do. Still, it's wise to take a few precautions:

■ If you're walking at night, wear a piece of reflective clothing.

■ If the path is dimly lit, bring a good flashlight.

■ When the weather's warm, be sure to drink a tall glass of water before you set out and another when you return.

If your path is rugged or bumpy, protect your ankles, particularly if you have a history of twists or sprains. Consider wearing a comfortable elastic bandage for support, and keep your eyes focused on the path.

line is to find a way to stay active, wherever and whenever you can. To help you reach this goal, we've included a Daily Activity Log on page 308, which will help you chart your time, efforts, and progress.

If you still need motivation—and who doesn't—take a look at some more compelling benefits to regular activity.

To burn more calories: The minute you get off the sofa or out of your office chair and start walking, you more than double the number of calories you're burning. A 180-pound woman burns about 2.2 calories a minute sitting in a meeting or parked in front of the TV. The same woman strolling around the neighborhood at a leisurely pace of two miles an hour burns 3.6 calories a minute. If she increases her pace to three miles an hour, she'll hit 4.7 calories a minute. At a brisk pace of four miles an hour—a mile every 15 minutes—she'll burn 7.2 calories a minute. Fifteen minutes at that pace will burn nearly 110 extra calories.

To boost your metabolism: Aerobic exercise—activity that leaves you feeling slightly winded—increases your calorie-burning rate while you're doing it. But if you want to boost your metabolism permanently, add strengthening exercises to your routine. As you know, muscle tissue is metabolically more active than fat tissue, which means it uses more calories just to maintain itself. Dieters who add muscle by doing strengthening exercises help keep their metabolism running high.

To look great in the mirror: A combination of aerobic and strengthening exercises is your best bet. Most dieters focus on the pounds on the scale, which is fine, to an extent. But the majority of us really want to look better. And once you begin to shed fat, the reflection in the mirror will look a whole lot better if you begin to tighten up slack muscles and burn body fat.

To become more fit: You'll need to crank the intensity level up a bit. Our 30 minutes a day of moderate exercise is good for overall health, but it is not enough for high-level fitness. One method scientists use to measure exercise intensity is counting heart beats. The harder you're working, the faster your heart beats. To increase your fitness level, most experts recommend exercising for at least 20 minutes at 60 percent to 80 percent of your maximum heart rate (to learn your targets, see the chart on the next page). To track your heart rate during exercise, stop for a minute and find your pulse, either on the inside of your wrist near the base of your thumb, or on your neck just to the side of your throat. Count how many times your heart beats in 15 seconds, and then multiply that by four. Or consider purchasing a heart-rate monitor; they're easy to use, and you can find them at most sporting goods stores.

Have Some Fun

If you're already active, devote this week to being a little *more* active. Try a workout that you haven't done before. Take a hike in a place you haven't visited. Set up the volleyball net that's been collecting dust in the garage. Pull the bike out and put some oil on the chain.

If physical activity hasn't been a big part of your life, give it a serious try this week. Don't push yourself too hard at the beginning. Try to make it a pleasure by finding pleasant places to walk, putting on headphones with your favorite music, or inviting a friend to join you. Just getting up from that easy chair and moving around will get your heart beating a little faster, your muscles working, and your calorie-burning engine churning.

Targeting Your Heart Rate

As you age, your maximum heart rate decreases. That in turn reduces the intensity at which you should exercise. To learn your target rates, check your age group below:

Age	Maximum heart rate	60% max	70% max	80% max
20	200/minute	120/minute	140/minute	160/minute
25	195	117	137	156
30	190	114	133	152
35	185	111	130	148
40	180	108	126	144
45	175	105	123	140
50	170	102	119	136
55	165	99	116	132
60	160	96	112	128
65	155	93	108	124
70	150	90	105	120

Changes Ahead:
Keeping on Track

We're near the end of the 12-week program, and by now you should have the key *ChangeOne* skills pretty well in hand. Time to start looking to the future and how to maintain your weight-loss successes for the months and years ahead. Next week we'll help you build a self-monitoring system. In preparation, think through all the ways you monitor your health and weight. Is it through the fit of your clothing? The mirror? The scale? Your moods? Armed with these personal tools, you'll create a warning system to remind you when you might be straying from your desired weight.

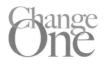

Week **11**

Keeping on Track

By now you're hitting your stride. You're dropping pounds, and the success feels great.

Still, as almost any successful dieter will tell you, it's essential to monitor your progress. The pressures that surround us to eat, eat, eat, don't go away. Portion sizes have a way of creeping up. Plans to go for a walk or hit the gym can fall by the wayside. And the pounds have a way of sneaking back.

This week you'll devise your own "first-alert" program to sound an alarm if you begin to get off track.

We're not suggesting that you measure every bowl of cereal or pasta serving for the rest of your life. But staying alert to how you're feeling, what you're doing, and how much you're eating will have a huge payoff in terms of weight, health, and self-confidence.

Schedule a Regular Checkup

With the end of the 12-week program just around the corner, it's time to take a moment to appreciate how far you've come. If you're like some of our *ChangeOne* volunteers, you may have already reached your target weight. Now it's time to make the transition from a diet that contains fewer calories than you need to one that balances your calorie intake with the number that you expend.

If you began *ChangeOne* hoping to lose a significant amount of weight, you may still have some pounds to go. There's nothing wrong with that. Slow and steady is the best kind of progress to make.

Wherever you are on the path to your desired weight, start planning now for the future. Almost any diet program will help you lose weight during the first few months. That's the easy part. If you've dieted before, you know that the real trick is maintaining weight loss—which requires turning the healthy changes you've already made into lifelong habits.

Sadly, that's where most diet plans falter. We've already mentioned one pitfall: call it the on-off trap. People go on a diet to lose weight and go off it once they've shed the pounds. And unfortunately, that means going right back to the way they ate before. You know how the story ends. Before long the numbers on the scale are right back where they started.

> **Most any diet will help you lose weight; the trick is maintaining the weight loss.**

There's another pitfall, and one that's probably more common. As people near their desired weight, they begin to ease up a little. They stop paying as much attention to portion sizes. They splurge a little more often on rich desserts. They grab an extra snack. Nothing dramatic. But if they're not watching, all those little nibbles can add up to a pound here and a pound there. Before they know it, they've gained back a chunk of the weight they lost.

Regaining a few pounds shouldn't be a big deal. You already know what it takes to lose those pounds, right? But losing ground spells real trouble, for several reasons. If you begin to gain weight back again, it's natural to assume that the diet isn't working and to abandon it completely. Worse, it's easy to begin to blame yourself and replay all kinds of negative messages in your head: "I'm a failure." "I'll never be able to lose the weight and keep it off." "I'm destined to be fat." Losing weight only to gain it back can also make you reluctant to try again. And when you do, you might feel discouraged from the start.

If your weight is holding steady, get on with your life. Forget about dieting for awhile.

Thanks to the careful work you've already put in, this is far less likely to happen to you than it is for people on faddish diets. You've learned that eating should be a pleasure, not something that you have to fear. You've seen that you can lose weight and keep it off while eating regular food that you actually like to eat. You've also discovered on *ChangeOne* that you can eat sensible portions without feeling hungry. Along the way, you've seen which changes have made the biggest difference for you.

Now all it takes to ensure that weight creep doesn't happen is to keep a watchful eye not only on your weight but also on how your clothes fit, how you feel, how much you exercise, and what's on the menu.

The *ChangeOne* First-Alert Program

Starting this week, take a few minutes once a week to do a quick self checkup. Record your weight. Estimate about how much physical activity you were able to get. Rate your overall mood. And jot down any issues or problems you may be dealing with. That's it. To make your weekly checkups even easier, we've included a *ChangeOne* Progress Log on page 310, which will allow you to track four weeks of checkups. At the end of those four weeks, chart how your weight has changed on the simple graph at the bottom of the form.

We're not suggesting you fill out weight-monitoring forms for the rest of your life. But we do recommend logging your progress for the next two months. If your weight is holding steady and you're comfortable with how things are going, tuck the form away in a drawer and get on with your life. Celebrate your success. Forget about dieting for awhile.

But don't forget to pay attention. Weigh yourself once a week. Keep track of how your clothes feel or where you notch your belt. Be alert to your moods. If you notice a change for the worse—if your favorite trousers start feeling a wee bit snug or you're going through a rocky period at home—grab a copy of the progress report and start filling it in weekly again.

Remember, most people's weight goes up or down a little, week by week. You probably already know how much yours normally varies. If the scale creeps up more than five pounds from your desired weight, it's time to take action. Don't panic—you haven't failed. And don't give up. You already know exactly what it takes to lose weight. You've done it before, and you can do it again.

ChangeOne First Person

A New Mindset

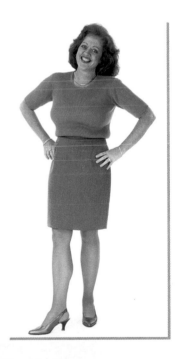

"Before I started *ChangeOne*, I really thought I'd have to see big improvement on the scale—I mean four or five pounds a week—to stay motivated. My mindset has definitely changed," says Mary Saltsman, an administrative assistant from Stormville, New York.

"The first few weeks were the toughest, maybe because I had such unrealistic expectations. But now I'm seeing the pounds come off, one pound a week, and that's just fine with me."

Saltsman lost 18 pounds during the 12 weeks, and she has maintained the weight loss since. Along the way Saltsman has made a few important changes. With teenage kids at home, she can't entirely steer clear of fast-food restaurants. "But even the kids are beginning to change some eating habits. Chicken nuggets have definitely taken a back seat to salads with my daughter, for instance. At regular restaurants, I now typically have a hearty soup and a salad when I dine out. More than anything else, I realize when I'm full now. I know enough to stop."

Tally Your Activity

Keeping track of exercise isn't as easy as watching pounds on the scale. True, if you go to a gym, it's no big deal to log each trip and what you did on a calendar. But if your exercise consists of doing everyday physical activities—taking the stairs, walking from the far end of the parking lot, doing a circuit around the block during commercial breaks—keeping track can be trickier.

One approach is to fill out an activity log, tallying up the time you spend every day. (Remember, we've included one for you on page 308.) Your goal should be to add at least 30 minutes of moderately intense activity daily.

Another strategy, which many people come to love, is using a step-counter, also called a pedometer. Step-counters are devices about the size of a pager that can be attached to your belt or waistband. By way of a mechanical pendulum that moves back and forth with each step you take, the device automatically records your every step.

A step-counter is easy to use, invaluable for tracking activity— and inexpensive.

The simplest devices, the ones that just count steps, are the best buys. Pedometers that compute the distance you've covered aren't very accurate; models that claim to tell you how many calories you've burned are even more unreliable, since they can't distinguish between a leisurely stroll and a heart-thumping run. A basic step-counter will run between $25 and $50 and can be found at most sporting goods stores.

For the first few days wear the counter but go about your usual day. At the end of each day, jot down how many steps you took. This number will serve as your baseline. Then set your first goal to increase the amount of walking you do. Without doing anything but going about your daily business, you're likely to take about 3,000 steps. Doing roughly 15 minutes worth of walking, stair climbing, and other everyday activities will add about 2,000 steps. The optimum goal for weight maintenance is around 12,000 to 15,000 steps a day.

Okay, so you're not there yet—don't worry. Scale up your weekly goals gradually. Start by shooting for 7,000 steps one week, for example, and the next week increase your goal to 9,000 steps. Like many people, you may find that using a step-counter will give you a little push when you need it. From time to time each day check to see how many steps you've taken. If you're barely up to 2,000 steps when lunch-time rolls around, consider a brisk walk after you eat. If you're done with dinner and are still short on steps, turn off the television and take a hike.

If you decide to use a step-counter, include the average number of steps you take on your four-week progress log. That way you can track your increasing activity at a glance.

Monitor Your Moods

While you're keeping tabs on your weight, how your clothes fit, and how much exercise you get, also be alert to how you feel—happy, sad, enthusiastic, busy, bored, gung-ho, whatever. You'll find a place on the progress log to record what your overall moods were like during the previous week.

Staying in touch with the way you feel is important for several reasons you probably already recognize. For a lot of people, stress, boredom, loneliness, or feeling blue are triggers for eating. If you're among those emotional eaters, keeping tabs on your mental state will help you begin to see patterns. You may see that the times your weight tends to creep back up again are times when you're bored.

The solution could be as simple as making a list of three things to do when you're feeling that way that don't involve eating. Let's say that stress at work is your downfall; every time you start checking the "stressed out" box on your progress report you can almost be sure your weight will start to climb. Simply recognizing that pattern can help you change it—by finding healthier ways to deal with stress than eating, for instance, or by increasing your exercise time.

Remember the First-Alert Plan

Like many people, you may discover that paying attention to your moods allows you to notice early warning signs of trouble. You realize that you're beginning to feel worn down by stress before you become completely frazzled. You notice the first signs of feeling blue.

That awareness can help you remedy the situation before you find yourself in a deep slump. Get together with friends. Schedule something you really love. Set aside extra time for exercise, which is a proven mood-booster. Turn your attention back to healthy eating as a way to avoid overeating when you're feeling discouraged or down.

The truth is, everyone feels down now and then. Sometimes there's a perfectly good reason for it. Money problems, relationship difficulties, a bad day at work. But some people find their moods dragged down again and again when there's no good reason except a feeling of low self-esteem. Given the emphasis our society places on being thin, it's not surprising that many people who struggle with their weight end up having a negative image of their bodies. The problem is compounded by a tendency on the part of many people to think that being overweight is the result of a lack of willpower. It's not that at all. It's the result of a complicated mix of factors, from genes and family eating patterns to body type and psychology.

Forget the "perfect" body myth; focus on a healthy, smart weight that fits you.

So here's another reason for monitoring your moods: if your mental state tends to turn sour because of low self-esteem, take time to remind yourself of how far you've come in making healthful changes. Remember that not all of us are magazine cover models. Healthy bodies vary tremendously in terms of size and shape. Don't get into the trap of wanting the "perfect" body. Concentrate instead on achieving a healthy, reasonable weight for who you are.

Of course, that's easier said than done. Sometimes feelings of low self-esteem reach all the way back to childhood, making them very hard to change on your own. Feeling sad or hopeless can be no more than just a passing emotion for some people, but for others it can be a symptom of clinical depression. If you find yourself struggling without success against feelings of sadness, hopelessness, or low self-esteem, talk to your doctor. There is a proven link between depression and weight gain. And treating depression, studies show, can have the additional effect of helping people get down to a normal weight.

Taking Action

If you notice your weight beginning to climb—or your clothes or belt beginning to feel tight—search for the reason. You may know exactly why you're gaining weight. Stress at work, perhaps, or long stretch of holiday party-going. Maybe you've just stopped being as strict as you were before about

Back to Wearing Clothes She Loves

"I've never had much luck dieting. But this time around, something just clicked for me," Tina Settembrino says. At the end of the 12-week program, Settembrino, a production associate who lives in Wappingers Falls, New York, is down two dress sizes.

"People stop me all the time and say, 'Wow, you really look good.' I feel good, too, healthier and more confident. I've tried to make a point of being aware of that, so it helps keep me motivated."

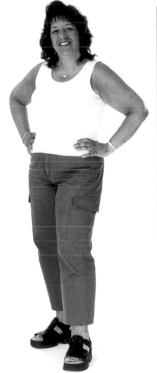

Another big incentive to stick with the program: being able to wear the clothes she wants to wear. "Before, I did most of my shopping at a local store that specializes in business clothes for larger women. We're talking baggy outfits," Settembrino says with a laugh. "But now that I'm slimming down, I'm back to shopping at the mall, buying clingier clothes. It's great."

Keeping an eye on how her new wardrobe fits helps keep her on track. "If I feel as if I'm slipping a little, if my clothes feel a little tighter or I think my portion sizes are beginning to creep up, I start right at the beginning, with breakfast. I go through each meal of the day, taking another look at what I'm eating and how much I'm eating. It's a great way for me to take control again without feeling overwhelmed."

keeping portions under control. The notes you've jotted down should tell you a lot. To do more in-depth trouble-shooting, fill in the diagnostic checklist below.

Once you've zeroed in on the specific problem, take action. Don't try to address all your issues at once. That's what *ChangeOne* is all about, after all: focusing on one change at a time.

Having trouble with a specific meal? Check back to the first four weeks of *ChangeOne* for advice on how to take control of breakfast, lunch, dinner, or snacks. Eating when you're not really hungry?

Make a conscious effort to stop and ask yourself whether you're actually responding to an emotional or environmental cue. If you're not truly hungry, distract yourself by doing something else—take a walk, do a chore, brush your teeth, or grab a stick of sugar-free gum. Feeling just plain over-whelmed? Your best bet may be that tried-and-true jump-start for any weight-loss plan: the food diary. Keep one for a week. Even if you make no other change, chances are you'll see progress on the scale.

Diagnostic Checklist

When the first-alert warning bell rings, use this checklist to identify the sources of trouble. ☺ A smile means you're doing just fine. ☺ A neutral expression means you're holding your own. ☹ A frown—well, you know what that means. After you're done, look over the categories that scored a frown. These are the areas to focus your troubleshooting efforts.

	☺	☺	☹	FOR HELP:
Breakfast				Page 22
Lunch				Page 38
Snacks				Page 58
Dinner				Page 82
Dining out				Page 108
Stress				Page 180
Resisting pressures to eat				Page 129
Environmental triggers				Page 62
Emotional eating				Page 66
Self-esteem				Page 212
Stopping when I'm satisfied				Page 84
Motivation				Page 172

Keeping track is so important that we urge you to set aside a particular time each week to conduct your *ChangeOne* checkup. Many prefer to do theirs on Sunday evenings. Use whatever day and time works best for you. Just try to stick to it. Put a reminder on your calendar. Post your weekly checkup form on the refrigerator or beside your desk—wherever it's easy to find. If you have a tendency to misplace pieces of paper, record your weight and activity level in a couple of places—a notebook or your computer, for instance. That way you'll have a backup. And if all is going well, then you'll have several reminders to tell yourself, "Congratulations! Be proud!" By learning the *ChangeOne* way to lose weight, you have changed yourself in untold wonderful ways.

If you notice the pounds coming back, diagnose the cause and find a remedy.

Changes Ahead: *ChangeOne* ... for Life!

With your own early-warning program in place, you can begin to relax a little and enjoy yourself without worrying that your waistline will suffer. Next week, in fact, is devoted to making sure that eating remains the pleasure it's meant to be. We're going to invite you to shake things up a little—to try something new in the kitchen or at your favorite restaurant. Treat yourself to something special. Have a blast; you deserve it. Over these past 11 weeks you've made some important changes. You've worked hard. Next week is your time to celebrate those changes and to look ahead at how to make them last a lifetime.

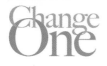

Change
One

Week 12

ChangeOne
...for Life!

It's celebration time. Put down the book for a moment, take a deep breath, and let out a victory yell.

You've reached Week 12, the end of the formal *ChangeOne* program. Over the past three months you've done something remarkable. You've redirected your life. You've changed the way you eat. More important than that, you've proved to yourself that you are in control. You've learned that small steps in the right direction can add up to a giant leap forward.

So in this final week, have fun. We want you to be playful with food. At least twice, try a new combination or flavor you've never had before.

Why? Because the enemy of weight loss is boredom. Eat the same way all the time, under tight restrictions, and you'll soon rebel. And if *ChangeOne* is about anything, it's about a love and respect for good food.

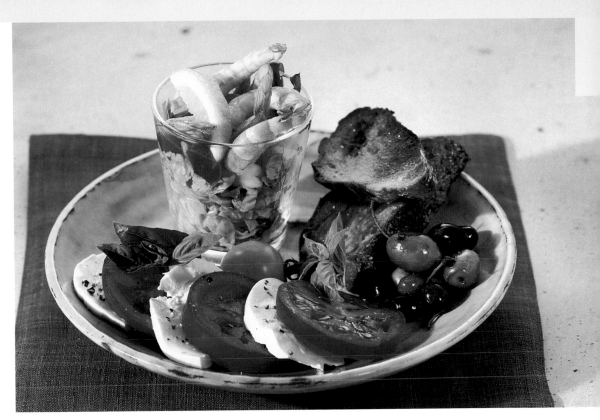

An Appetizer Dinner

Appetizers let you enjoy a diversity of flavors, textures, and cuisines. Plus, it's a playful and social way to eat. Here's just one approach.

MEDITERRANEAN TREATS

1   4-ounce shrimp cocktail
    (4-6 shrimp, plus cocktail sauce)

1   ounce fresh mozzarella (coaster)
    atop tomato salad with slivered
    basil and balsamic vinegar

10 herbed olives

1   slice crusty bread

Calories 430, fat 13 g, saturated fat 4 g, cholesterol
190 mg, sodium 1,350 mg, carbohydrate 46 g, fiber 5 g,
protein 33 g, calcium 250 mg.

VARIATIONS

For balance and calorie control, pick one
item from some or all of the following:

■ **Protein foods:** Ceviche, ½ cup;
  Thai satay (grilled chicken or beef
  strips), 2 skewers; smoked salmon,
  2 ounces; prosciutto, 3 thin slices;
  steamed mussels, 1 cup (out of shell).

■ **Vegetables:** Unlimited, as long as
  they are not prepared with added fat.
  As an option you can top them with
  1½ ounces fresh mozzarella, 1 ounce
  cheese slivers, or 1 tablespoon peanut
  butter, but keep the add-ons to reasonable portions.

■ **Nibbles:** 10 olives, handful of nuts.

■ **Bread:** 1 slice, your choice of flavor,
  or try a medium-sized hard roll.

Reward Yourself

Give yourself a big pat on the back, but don't stop there. Reward yourself with something special. Make it a complete extravagance, if you want—a weekend getaway or a night on the town. Or choose something that reinforces your changes, your results, and the new you: running shoes, a new bike, a gift certificate for yoga classes, or an enticing cookbook.

Why make a big deal about rewarding yourself? Because too often we tend to be aware of when we've fallen short and take our progress for granted. Even people who have lost weight and made healthy changes in the way they live may think they've failed—unless they celebrate their successes.

Why pat yourself on the back? Too often we emphasize our failures over our successes.

Acknowledging a job well done also serves as a way to mark those milestones we talked about before—the small steps you take that add up to a giant leap forward. Unless you celebrate them, you may not even be aware of how far you've come. And when we say celebrate your victories, we mean all of them. Some of your successes are easy to recognize. Eating a healthier breakfast, for instance. Or taming runaway snacks. But other positive changes may be more subtle, though more important: discovering that you can decide on a plan of action and stick to it; gaining self-confidence; banishing a negative voice that used to echo in your head; learning that you can slip for a day or two and get yourself back on track.

Small steps? Sure. But each one of them makes an important difference. This week take a little time out to think about the obvious and not so obvious ways you've changed over the last 12 weeks. Give yourself kudos for every positive step you've taken.

Aren't the people around us supposed to give us a big pat on the back when we've done something wonderful? Sure they are. And maybe you're lucky enough to have someone who does give you accolades for what you've accomplished. Still, it's important to give yourself a job-well-done, too. As helpful as other people can be, changing for the better is up to you and you alone. You have to be your own best friend. By giving yourself rewards, you also reinforce positive self-messages—a powerful antidote against those discouraging words that can sometimes repeat in your ears.

Trust Your Instincts

Yes, you'll celebrate your success this week. But—and no surprise here—we've included a lesson for the long haul. Relax. It's a lesson you'll love.

First, a question: what's the toughest challenge dieters face when it comes to keeping the weight off? When we asked our *ChangeOne* volunteers at the beginning of the program, many of them listed things like "snacks," "hunger," and "a sweet tooth." Most people starting a diet figure the hardest part will be resisting temptation. In fact, as we mentioned at the start, the biggest pitfall dieters face over the long haul is something much more basic: boredom.

People often give up on a diet because it gets tiresome. They grow weary of tracking calories or consulting long lists of foods they should or shouldn't eat. They rebel against the rules that most diets include.

We've made sure *ChangeOne* doesn't include a lot of strict rules, banned foods, complex theories, and other guidelines that tie you up. A healthy diet, after all, is about eating sensible servings of tasty and (mostly) nutritious food. You can eat just about anything, but if your choice is rich in calories, you'll have to watch portions. It's that simple.

But even with the varied *ChangeOne* menu, you could be feeling a little restless. So this week you'll shake things up. Fix something you haven't eaten before. Get creative in the kitchen and concoct a dish of your own. Treat yourself to a fancy meal at a restaurant you've been anxious to try. Forget the *ChangeOne* meal plans for a whole day. Heck, take the whole week off, if you want. Imagine that you're taking the training wheels off and going for a solo spin after 12 weeks of learning how to keep your balance. This week let the *ChangeOne* principles guide you as you venture out on your own.

To get started, turn the page for a party of festive ideas; then go to page 222 for more eating adventures.

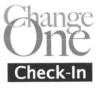

Check-In

Think back to where you were when you started *ChangeOne*. Write a list of the positive changes you've made since then. Put a star beside the changes that have had the biggest impact on how you look and feel. And then, as we suggested back in Week 11, put the list away, out of sight and out of mind. But remember where you put it. If in the coming months you find yourself falling off track, look back at it. You'll find listed there the changes that work best for you. Zero in on them and chances are you'll be able to take control of your weight again.

Taco Party

Tacos migrated from Mexico to become one of the most popular dishes in the United States. But why eat fatty restaurant tacos? It's more fun to make tacos at home. Set out a self-serve buffet of tortillas, chopped vegetables, low-fat cheese, and grilled or sautéed meats or beans, as shown. A serving is two tacos, based on our taco-building approach.

How to build a taco:

1. Put corn or small flour tortilla on plate.

2. Top with ¼ cup (golf ball) of either lean ground beef, ground turkey, shredded turkey, meatless crumbles, or fat-free refried beans.

3. Add 2 tablespoons (2 thumbs) shredded reduced-fat jack or cheddar cheese, guacamole, and/or sliced olives (total of 2 tablespoons).

4. Cover with vegetables and sauce— chopped tomatoes, shredded lettuce, diced red and green peppers, minced red onion, diced or sliced jalapeno peppers, chopped green chilies, salsa.

5. Fold over and eat.

For corn tortilla and ground beef: Calories 430, fat 22 g, saturated fat 10 g, cholesterol 80 mg, sodium 670 mg, carbohydrate 33 g, fiber 5 g, protein 27 g, calcium 300 mg.

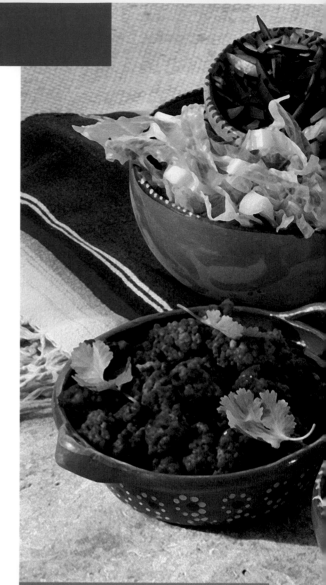

TIPS ON CHEESE

Mexican queso fresco is a soft white cheese with a mild flavor, similar to Monterey jack cheese. Check the label to make sure yours is made from pasteurized milk, which limits the chances of bacterial contamination. Other popular taco cheeses include pepper jack and cheddar. Look for grated reduced-fat varieties to save a few calories, or shred your own using a grater with fine holes. Chill the cheese well before grating to help prevent it from falling apart.

ABOUT REFRIED BEANS

Traditional Mexican refried beans, frijoles refritos, are made by sautéeng diced onion and sometimes garlic in lard, then adding and mashing pinto or other types of beans. Make your own lower-fat, lower-calorie version by cooking onion in a nonstick skillet with a teaspoon or so of olive oil and a splash of chicken or vegetable broth until the onion is soft. Add a can of pinto beans plus a teaspoon of ground cumin and mash the beans as they cook in the skillet. Or you might find fat-free canned refried beans in the specialty foods section of your grocery store.

TIPS ON TORTILLAS

- Corn tortillas have fewer calories than flour tortillas because they aren't made with added fat. And corn tortillas can deliver another bonus: when they're made with lime, a calcium compound, they dish up a decent amount of this important mineral.

- Colored corn tortillas are made from corn kernels that grow in a rainbow of colors, most commonly blue and red. They are just as nutritious as regular corn tortillas. Some say that blue corn tortillas have a stronger corn flavor. In any case, they add to the festivity of a taco party.

- Crisp tortillas usually are fried, and that gives them about double the calorie count of a soft tortilla.

HEALTH TIP

Keep your total portion of cheese, chopped olives, and guacamole to no more than 4 tablespoons. While they add great flavor and texture to tacos, all are high in fat and calories.

Try Something New

How you'll shake things up this week is up to you. If you've been sitting down to cereal every morning, see how a yogurt parfait grabs you. If you've been packing a sandwich, take yourself out for lunch this week. If you've been following the *ChangeOne* dinner meal plans scrupulously, pull a couple of cookbooks down from your kitchen shelf and try out a few new recipes. Do a *ChangeOne* makeover of an old family standard. Throw a big dinner party. Take the family out for a lavish meal. Splurge on a dessert you haven't had for a while. Visit the local farmer's market or produce stand and take home something you've never tasted before.

Giving yourself a little freedom doesn't mean putting your progress at risk. Last week you set up a first-alert system that will warn you if you get off track. Trust it. And trust your instincts to guide you. Gaining the confidence to make healthy choices is one of the measures of lasting success.

Colorful fruits and vegetables add pleasure to your plate. Clockwise from top: kale, spaghetti squash, bok choy, broccolini, long beans—wrapped around, (from top to bottom) chayote, two passion fruit, and kohlrabi—mango, two starfruit, plantain, prickly pear, and kabocha squash.

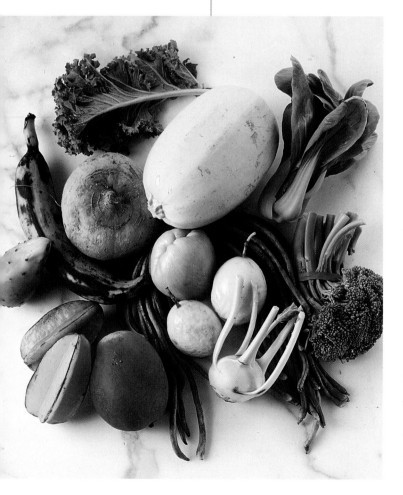

Not sure how to add excitement to the menu this week? Here are a few suggestions:

Make your own salad bar
For a family dinner one night this week put together a salad bar and invite the crew to create their own salads. Include at least two vegetables that aren't usually on the menu—jicama, beets, radicchio, edamame, or artichoke hearts, for instance. Warm up a loaf of whole wheat or whole grain bread. For dessert serve up a selection of colorful sorbets topped with berries.

Throw a taco party
As you've seen, tacos are a terrific way to serve up lots of vegetables—tomatoes, lettuce, grilled sweet peppers, and onions. Put all the ingredients

out on the counter and let everyone make their own. Mix things up by using black beans instead of refried beans, help yourself to as much salsa as you want, don't forget to dab on some guacamole, and go easy on—or skip—the sour cream. Look back to pages 220-221 for more ideas.

Slim down an old family friend

Choose a favorite casserole, pasta, or other dish and give it a boost by adding a serving of vegetables. Broccoli is terrific in tuna casserole. Garbanzo beans (also called chickpeas) make a great addition to spaghetti with tomato sauce. Green peppers can liven up, and lighten up, a bowl of chili. If fish sticks are a family favorite, serve them with a special salsa for added zest. If you'd like, use a calorie-counter to tally up the precise calories in your makeover meal.

Order a feast of appetizers and sides

Choose a restaurant with a wide range of appetizers and vegetable sides, and have a feast. Share the dishes with your dinner companions and you can order practically every small dish on the menu without having to worry about portion sizes. Start with only as many dishes as there are people at the table. If you're still hungry, order more. Steer clear of fried foods, of course, and include plenty of vegetables.

Throw a big dinner party. Take the family out for a lavish meal. Splurge on a dessert.

Go fish

Chances are your local fish market features at least a few kinds of fish you haven't tried. Be adventurous and cook up something new for you—orange roughy, giant prawns, or mahi mahi, for instance. Choose a recipe that involves baking or grilling, not frying. There are many low-calorie ways to give fish a burst of exotic flavor. Many markets now offer spices that create the "blackened" flavor of traditional Cajun cooking, for instance. Spicy salsas or a scattering of capers are also terrific on fish.

Bake bread

As a special treat, take the time this weekend to bake your own loaf of bread. If you don't have a bread machine, consider investing in one. They simplify bread-making. Pop the ingredients in, head out on a couple of errands, and by the time you're back, the house will be filled with the aroma of

Tantalizing Tuna

Most tuna salads are dripping in mayonnaise. But why settle for such a high-fat, ordinary tasting treatment? In this alternative version, lemon juice, plain yogurt, and Dijon mustard add moisture and tanginess.

VARIATIONS

- For Italian tuna salad, replace the yogurt and mayo with fat-free Italian dressing.

- For Indian tuna salad, add 1 teaspoon curry powder and 2 tablespoons raisins.

- For Tex-Mex tuna salad, replace the relish and mustard with 2 tablespoons salsa.

TUNA SALAD SANDWICH

Serves 2

- 1 **can white or light tuna in water, drained**
- 1 **tablespoon lemon juice**
- 1 **tablespoon plain yogurt or yogurt cheese (see page 29)**
- 1 **tablespoon reduced fat mayonnaise**
- 1 **tablespoon pickle relish**
- 1 **teaspoon Dijon mustard**
- 1 **tablespoon minced onion**
- 4 **slices wheat bread**
  Lettuce and tomato

1. Place tuna in small bowl and combine with lemon juice. Add yogurt, mayo, pickle relish, mustard, and onions; combine well.

2. Line 2 bread slices with lettuce and tomato. Top each with half of tuna mixture. Top with remaining slices of bread.

Calories 260, fat 5 g, saturated fat 1 g, cholesterol 30 mg, sodium 760 mg, carbohydrate 31 g, fiber 3 g, protein 22 g, calcium 80 mg.

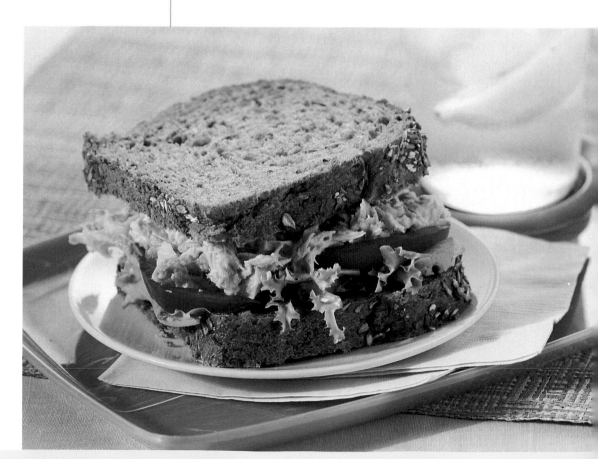

fresh baked bread. Choose recipes that include whole wheat flour and, even better, whole grains like oats.

Have a pizza extravaganza

Most markets sell do-it-yourself pizza crusts that make preparing a home-made pizza fast and easy. Get a group together for a pizza party. Include at least two vegetable toppings. Use shredded cheese rather than slices and you'll get more coverage with less cheese. Try smoked mozzarella instead of plain for more flavor.

Make a new acquaintance

It's easy to get into a rut, especially when you go shopping. This week look a little more closely at things you've been skipping in the produce section and take home a vegetable you haven't tried before. Many markets carry once-exotic leafy greens like arugula, watercress, radicchio, and chard. Never tried jicama? Roasted fennel? A fresh artichoke? Then you're missing out on some of the world's great taste treats. This week add a new vegetable to your repertoire.

Create your own signature pasta

No other dish is as versatile as Italian pasta. Pasta itself comes in a wide range of shapes and colors, from familiar fettuccine to fun shapes like wagon wheels, bow-ties, shells, corkscrews, tubes, and ears. And the ingredients that show up in pasta are virtually limitless—from shrimp or chicken to savory olives, artichokes, basil, diced ripe tomatoes, fava beans, tuna, capers, mushrooms, cauliflower, broccoli, parmesan cheese … you get the idea. Put on your chef's hat this week and create your own pasta masterpiece.

Travel the world

America's melting pot has created a rich variety of ethnic cuisines unmatched almost anywhere in the world, from Italian and French to Indian and Moroccan restaurants. This

Pasta Shapes and Sauces

Yes, everyone knows spaghetti goes with tomato-based sauce, but what about the rest of those noodles? In general, the lighter and more delicate the pasta, the lighter its sauce should be. Thicker or textured pastas go best with heavier and chunkier sauces. Here's a pairing of pasta shapes and sauces:

- Angel hair (thin spaghetti): light sauces.
- Conchiglie (shells): cheese-flavored sauces, and also good in soups.
- Farfalle (bowties): chunky sauces.
- Fettuccine (ribbon): creamy sauces, tomato-based sauces.
- Fusilli (twisted spaghetti), ravioli (stuffed pillows), rotelle (spirals): chunky, tomato-based sauces.
- Macaroni (elbows), ziti and penne (hollow tubes): meat sauces.
- Tortellini (small stuffed dumplings): tomato-based sauces.

week sample a cuisine you haven't tried before, or at least one you don't eat very often. If you're an avid home cook, try preparing something from a cuisine you've never explored before. Check your library or local bookstore for a cookbook that specializes in a particular ethnic cuisine. Chances are you'll discover a world of new ingredients and tastes.

Find a New Move

While you're shaking things up this week in the food department, do the same with exercise. The goal is simple: find something fun to do this week that you haven't done before, something that involves being active. Take the plunge at the local pool. Go for a hike in a nearby park. Take the kids canoeing. Go power-walking at the local mall. If you haven't given the *ChangeOne* workout on pages 236–237 a try, do it this week—but only if it sounds like fun.

And don't hide behind the excuse that you don't like being active. Don't tell us that you don't like strolling in a beautiful park, playing catch with the kids, walking past the shop windows downtown, or riding a bike around the neighborhood. Those are the kinds of activities that make life worth living.

Strike a Balance

ChangeOne is based on the simple principle that to lose weight, you have to take in fewer calories than you burn. To maintain your weight, you have to balance calories in and calories out.

That notion of striking a balance is a powerful one and worth keeping in mind as you move forward. As far as diet goes, there are many ways to build that healthy balance. One is to watch every bite you eat. Another, more relaxed way is to be aware of what you eat throughout the day, bal-

The Food Diary Revisited

We've touted the virtues of keeping a food diary more than once. It's a great way to see exactly what you eat and to spot patterns that may be scuttling your efforts to lose weight, such as skipping breakfast or going overboard on snacks. From time to time while you're dieting, filling out a food diary for a day or two is also an effective way to make sure you're still on track.

As you strike out on your own this week, consider keeping a food diary for at least a couple of days. Don't let the diary get in the way of being adventurous. Use the form on page 307 to record what you eat—that's all. When the week is done, you can look back at the form to see how you did setting out on your own. Check on how the number of low-calorie dishes compared to the number of higher-calorie treats. Do a quick accounting of the average servings of vegetables. Use what you learn from the food diary to fine-tune your food choices over the coming weeks. If you noticed yourself falling short on foods from the produce aisle, for instance, make a point of including a salad at dinner or a piece of fruit with lunch.

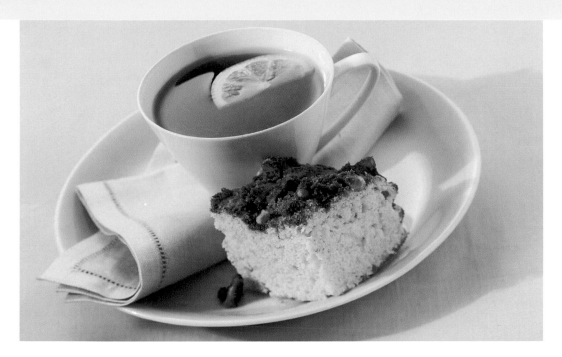

Cake for Breakfast

Classic streusel coffee cake is a high-calorie indulgence. This lightened version uses less than half the butter and substitutes buttermilk for the sour cream.

STREUSEL-TOP COFFEE CAKE

Serves 16

- ¼ **cup packed light brown sugar**
- 2 **tablespoons chopped walnuts**
- 1 **teaspoon cinnamon**
- 2 **cups plus 2 tablespoons flour**
- 4 **tablespoons unsalted butter, melted**
- ⅔ **cup granulated sugar**
- 1 **tablespoon baking powder**
- ¾ **teaspoon salt**
- 1 **egg**
- 1 **cup low fat buttermilk**
- 1 **teaspoon grated lemon peel**

1. Preheat oven to 400°F. Spray a 9-inch square baking pan with cooking spray.

2. In small bowl combine brown sugar, walnuts, cinnamon, and 2 tablespoons flour. Add 1 tablespoon of the melted butter to the walnut mixture and stir until crumbly.

3. In large bowl stir together the remaining 2 cups flour, the granulated sugar, baking powder, and salt until combined. Make a well in the center. Add the egg, buttermilk, lemon peel, and remaining butter. Stir until just combined.

4. Scrape batter into the prepared pan. Sprinkle with walnut topping. Bake for 40 minutes or until a toothpick inserted in the center comes out clean.

5. Allow cake to cool. Cut into 16 squares. A serving equals 1 square. Wrap leftovers in foil and freeze for up to 1 month.

Calories 150, fat 4 g, saturated fat 1 g, cholesterol 5 mg, sodium 200 mg, carbohydrate 25 g, fiber 1 g, protein 2 g, calcium 80 mg.

VARIATIONS

Choose one of the following:

- Add some chopped mixed fruit.
- Add ¼ cup of mini-chocolate chips.
- Split the batter in half, mix ¼ cup cocoa powder into half the batter. Drop batter into prepared pan, alternating spoonfuls of plain and chocolate batter. Swirl with a knife to create a marble pattern.

ancing a little indulgence here with a little restraint there. If you treat yourself to a sumptuous brunch with friends, for instance, go light on supper and try to fit in extra exercise. If there's a big birthday dinner planned in the evening, go easy on snacks and have a simple lunch.

As you've probably learned by now, one day of overdoing it on food doesn't mean the end of your diet. Cut back on portion sizes for the next day or two and you'll be able to regain your balance. Even a week of overdoing it won't bring your diet crashing down. Naturally, people worry about the big holidays at the end of the year, when every occasion seems to center around food. The reality is you can enjoy yourself over the holidays without much danger of putting on a lot of weight.

It used to be held as a gospel truth that people typically gain about five pounds during the holidays. Not true, according to recent research from the National Institutes of Health, which tracked 200 men and women from late September through early March using weight and other health measurements. The average weight gain was about one pound. And it turns out that extra pound may have had less to do with eating than with exercise. People who said they weren't physically active during the roughly six months of the study typically gained about 1.5 pounds; those who stayed active through the cold winter months actually lost weight.

No, we're not advising you to throw caution to the wind when holidays or special occasions roll around. It's still important to make smart choices. Our point is that even a couple of weeks of eating more than usual aren't enough to topple your healthy diet. Become extra active, and you can counterbalance the extra food you eat. Even if you do gain weight, it's not likely to be that much. When you return to healthier habits as the holidays end, you'll regain your balance and steadily lose any weight you might have added.

Top 10 *ChangeOne* Weight-Loss Tactics

This week, as you set out on your own to enjoy what you've achieved, let these simple but powerful directives of *ChangeOne* be your guide:

1. Eat breakfast every day—and include at least one serving of fruit.
2. Favor foods with plenty of fiber.
3. Help yourself to two servings of vegetables at lunch.
4. Keep an eye on portion sizes. If it looks oversized, divide it in half.
5. Eat slowly, savoring every bite.
6. Stop when you're satisfied.
7. Reach for a snack if you're genuinely hungry.
8. Drink plenty of water during the day, including an eight-ounce glass at each meal.
9. Help yourself to two servings of vegetables at dinner.
10. Stay active!

Keep Your Perspective

There's one more way in which keeping your balance is important as you set off from here. You've already heard about the pitfalls of all-or-nothing thinking. It's the tendency to think that a diet is working as long as you're losing weight, and that it has failed the moment you hit a plateau or gain a pound or two. It's the tendency of some people to think, the moment they slip up, "I'm a failure." All-or-nothing thinking doesn't acknowledge anything in between and is nothing more than a skewed perspective.

One thing we hope the *ChangeOne* approach has given you is a more balanced perspective on what it takes to lose weight and keep it off. It's not an all-or-nothing proposition. It's about the choices you make every day. If you go overboard on portions one day, you have the next to restore your balance. If your weight plateaus for a while, so be it. You haven't failed. The diet hasn't failed. You can give yourself a little time-out and then make another change or two when you feel ready. If you gain a few pounds when things at work or home are stressful, no big deal. You know what it takes to lose it again. The only way to fail is to decide that you've failed—and to give up.

Keep that in mind as you relax a little this week and move into the weeks beyond, and you'll be just fine. You've got what it takes to do almost anything you want. Just take it one step at a time. Keep your spirits up and your resolution firm. Stay positive. Have as much fun as you can. If you hit a rocky stretch, go easy on yourself. Set your sights on a new goal. Figure out the best ways to get there. And go for it.

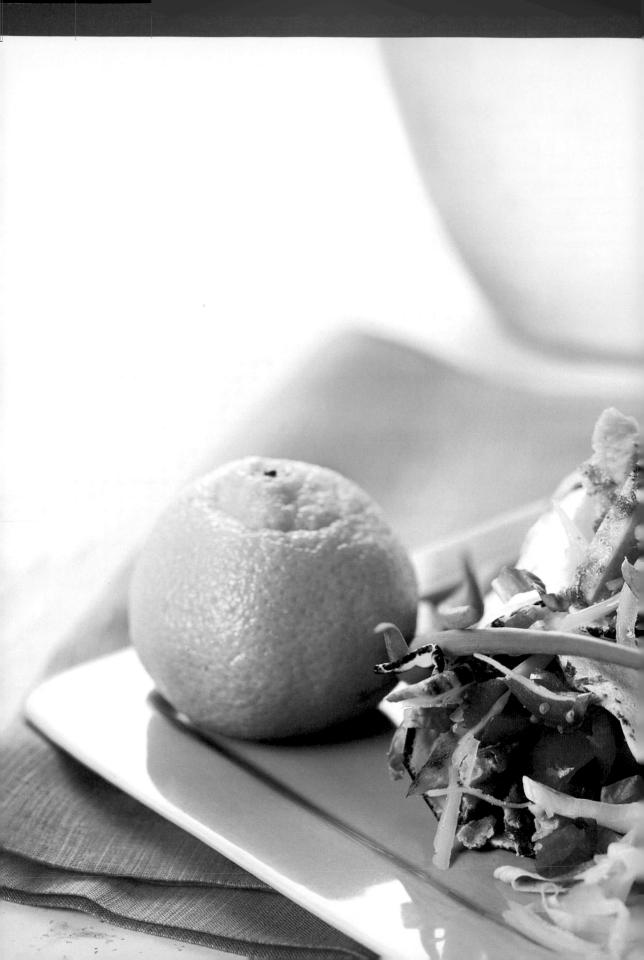

Part 2

Change
One
Resources

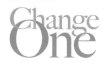
Change
One

Fitness

... is the secret to lasting weight-loss success. It's that simple.

When researchers analyze the differences between dieters who keep the weight off and those who regain it, they find—time and time again—that exercise is crucial.

Was that a groan?

Okay, okay, so it's not always easy to find time to exercise during the day. And not all of us want to be gym rats. But that shouldn't keep you from enjoying the considerable benefits of getting up and moving. You don't have to fit in a long workout session, after all; you can do a little exercise here, a little there. If you've always thought you weren't the exercise type, you may be surprised. A lot of people who lose weight discover that they like being active. It's natural to feel uneasy about exercising when you're overweight. But as you slim down, becoming physically active is a wonderful way to enjoy your new, trimmer body. And there are many payoffs.

True Rewards

Nothing else you do for yourself has more benefits than regular exercise. Exercise burns calories. And it tones muscles, tightens up arms, and cinches in that waistline. While you've heard a lot of convincing reasons to start exercising, there are so many more. Here are five of our favorites:

1. More Energy

This one may be hard to believe, but exercising will make you feel more energetic. When scientists at the University of New Orleans asked 42 volunteers to assess their moods before and after a 50-minute aerobics class, most of them said they felt less tense and less tired after breaking a sweat. And in a 1997 study, researchers found that a brisk 10-minute walk gave people more energy than eating a candy bar. How can that be? Exercise boosts a hormone that increases energy. And it takes just a few workouts to improve strength and lung capacity, which in turn increase stamina. All of which means you have more energy.

2. Less Stress

Just one simple workout can ease stress and anxiety. In a study at Indiana University, researchers used psychological tests to gauge anxiety levels in 15 volunteers before and after a 20-minute session on an exercise bicycle. The volunteers all reported feeling significantly less anxious during the hour or two after the workout. Exercise enhances the flow of brain chemicals like serotonin that are related to positive moods. Because it also increases core body temperature, it can be as relaxing as a good soak in a hot tub.

3. A Sharper Mind

Exercise can even spark creativity. Researchers at England's Middlesex University tested the creative thinking of 63 volunteers in two settings: after they'd done an aerobic workout and after they'd sat around watching a video. Volunteers in the experiment felt more positive and scored higher on creativity following the workout.

4. Healthier Arteries

Physical activity boosts levels of high-density lipoproteins, or HDL—the so-called "good cholesterol"—by as much as 20 percent. HDL helps rid the body of low-density lipoproteins, or LDL—the artery-clogging kind. Studies show that HDL can even pick up bad cholesterol deposited in arteries and move it to where it won't do harm. Another benefit for the arteries: the level of fat particles in the blood, called triglycerides, falls by as much as 40 percent after a vigorous workout. Exercising helps to convert triglycerides into fatty acids—the form in which fat can be burned for energy. You burn stored fat each and every time you work out—the key to keeping weight off. You also lower your level of triglycerides in the blood. And the lower your triglyceride level, studies show, the lower your risk of heart disease.

Staying Active on the Road

Don't let vacations or business travel sideline your exercise routine. Physical activity is a great way to relieve stress and adjust to a new time zone when you're traveling. Here are some ideas to help you stay active while you're away:

- **Find fitness-friendly accommodations.** Call ahead to make sure the hotel you're considering has a good fitness facility—or at least a place where you'll feel safe and comfortable going for a walk.
- **Take advantage of the local attractions.** Many places offer their own unique exercise opportunities—trails through beautiful parks or forests, beach walks, boat rides on the lake, or bike rides out of town, for example. Check the travel section of your bookstore or look on the Internet for information before you travel.
- **Pack what you'll need.** Walking shoes, gym shorts, a T-shirt, resistance bands—make a checklist of all the things you'll need to get a good workout while you're away. And be sure to pack them all.
- **Use every opportunity.** Too busy to set aside a block of time for activity? Be creative with your time and use every chance you get to be active. Walk whenever you can—between meetings, while you're waiting at the airport, or simply on your way from here to there.
- **Be realistic.** If you're on a hectic business trip, don't add to the stress by trying to do too much. Tallying up just 15 minutes of brisk walking, along with climbing a few flights of stairs instead of taking the elevator, should hold you until you get home and back to your regular routine.

5. Better Defenses

The moment you begin exercising, your heart starts pounding and your surging blood sends disease-fighting immune cells throughout your body, where they're able to detect troublemakers like cold or flu viruses. Studies show that people who exercise have about half as many sick days as those who sit on the sidelines.

Eight Weeks to a Better Body

A walking program is a great start. But you'll see even more results by combining an aerobic exercise like walking—the kind that burns calories and gets your heart and lungs working—with a muscle-toning program. You'll look better, feel better, and boost your metabolism.

In the following pages you'll find a simple and complete fitness program guaranteed to give you all the benefits of exercise. Don't worry if you've never done a formal exercise program before. We'll walk you through things step by step. For many of the exercises all you need is a pair of comfortable shoes and a place where you can stretch out. Once you hit your stride, kick your workout up another notch by adding a jump rope and a set of resistance bands.

The *ChangeOne* Fitness Program

Not sure where to begin? It's easy with the *ChangeOne* plan. Each week you'll make just one change to your activity routine. By the end of eight weeks you'll be doing all the exercise you need to keep the pounds off. By tightening up lax muscles and giving your heart and lungs a workout, you'll be trimmer, slimmer, and fitter.

Here's how to get with the program:
- *If you're new to exercise,* start at Week 1.
- *If you already walk at least 15 minutes most days of the week,* start at Week 4.
- *If you walk at least 30 minutes most days,* start at Week 6.

The *ChangeOne* eight-week program is based on walking. If you enjoy another form of aerobic exercise like bicycling or swimming, go for it. What's important is doing activities that increase your breathing rate and heart rate.

Read on for details of the program, sample schedules, and a visual guide that will lead you through easy but effective exercise and stretching routines.

Change One Eight-Week Fitness Program

As with the rest of *ChangeOne,* we're only asking you to make one change a week as you progress through this eight-step road map to a regular exercise routine. Before any session make sure you do 2 minutes of easy walking to warm up, and then 2 minutes more to cool down when you finish. And remember, you should check with your doctor before starting any exercise program.

Week 1

Aerobic: 4 sessions. Walk for at least 15 minutes four days this week. If you can't find the time or don't have the stamina to do a 15-minute walk, do two or three shorter walks that add up to 15 minutes. Walk at a pace that has you breathing hard but still able to talk.

Week 2

Aerobic: 4 sessions. Fit in a 15-minute walk four days this week. Schedule the time so that you can walk for a full 15 minutes—in the morning, over the lunch hour, or after dinner, for instance. If you can't find that much uninterrupted time, do several shorter walks that add up to 15 minutes.

This weekend: Schedule a leisure-time activity that involves at least 30 minutes of physical activity. Hiking, bicycling, working in the garden, playing catch with the kids, swimming—whatever sounds like fun.

Week 3

Aerobic: At least 4 sessions. Increase your walks to 20 minutes. Start at an easy pace for the first 3 to 5 minutes to get your muscles loose, then walk briskly for the rest of the time. Keep a record of when you walk and how long each session takes.

This weekend: Schedule a leisure-time activity that involves at least 45 minutes of physical activity.

Week 4

Aerobic: At least 4 sessions. Increase your walks to 25 minutes; 10 minutes before you stop, pick up your pace for 5 minutes, and then slow down for the last 5 minutes.

This weekend: Schedule a 45-minute leisure-time activity.

Stretching: 2 sessions. Try the eight-step stretching routine that you'll find on pages 243–246. Take your time completing the routine, and be sure to hold each stretch as long as directed.

Week 5

Aerobic: **At least 4 sessions.** Increase your walks to 30 minutes. As you did last week, push yourself a little harder just before you finish. Schedule at least 45 minutes of weekend activity.

Stretching: **2 sessions.** Take 10 minutes after your walk—or any time that's convenient—to do the stretching exercises you practiced last week. Feel free to add as many stretching sessions as you like.

Strengthening: **1 session.** This week work in the five muscle-toning exercises on pages 240–242. You don't need special equipment—just enough space to stretch out and a comfortable carpet or mat on the floor. Warm up your muscles before starting by doing some stretches or taking a brief stroll around the block. Give each exercise a try, but if one seems too difficult or uncomfortable, skip it and try another. You can always come back to it when you're feeling a little stronger.

Week 6

Aerobic: **At least 4 sessions.** Keep walking at least 30 minutes. If you're looking for more of a challenge, try mixing in some intervals: 10 minutes into your walk increase your pace for 1 minute, then return to your normal pace, or just a little slower, for 2 minutes. Speed up again for 1 minute followed again by 2 minutes at your regular pace or a bit slower. Do 5 repetitions of this pattern, 15 minutes total. For an alternative to intervals, buy a jump rope and set aside anywhere from 5 to 15 minutes for jumping at the end of your walk. Do some easy-paced walking afterwards to cool down. Also, continue with the weekend activity.

Stretching: **2 sessions.**
Strengthening: **2 sessions.**

Week 7

Aerobic: **At least 4 sessions.** Increase at least two of your walks to 45 minutes. This weekend plan a fun activity that involves at least 1 hour of walking.

Stretching: **2 sessions.**

Strengthening: **3 sessions.** Increase your routines to at least eight exercises. Check the additional workouts on pages 247–250 for new ideas; you'll need exercise bands and a jump rope for these.

Week 8

Aerobic: **At least 4 sessions.** Alternate 30- and 45-minute walks. You can increase your interval sets to 20 minutes total; or consider decreasing the recovery portion so that you do 1 minute of fast walking and then just 1 minute of regular walking. This weekend plan something fun that involves at least 1 hour of activity.

Stretching: **2–3 sessions.**

Strengthening: **3 sessions.** If the moves are getting easier, consider adding another set.

Change One
Eight-Week
Fitness Program
Sample Activity Schedule

	MONDAY	**TUESDAY**	**WEDNESDAY**	
Week 1	• Walk, 15 minutes	Off	• Walk, 15 minutes	
Week 2	• Walk, 15 minutes	• Walk, 15 minutes	• Walk, 15 minutes	
Week 3	• Walk, 20 minutes	• Walk, 20 minutes	• Walk, 20 minutes	
Week 4	• Walk, 25 minutes • Stretching routine	• Walk, 25 minutes	• Walk, 25 minutes • Stretching routine	
Week 5	• Walk, 30 minutes • Stretching routine	• Walk, 30 minutes	• Walk, 30 minutes • Strength workout, 5 steps	

Week 6	• Walk, 30 minutes
	  with intervals
	• Stretching routine
		• Walk, 30 minutes
		• Strength workout,
		  5 steps
			• Walk, 30 minutes
			  with intervals
			• Stretching routine	

Week 7	• Walk, 45 minutes
	• Strength workout,
	  8 steps
		• Walk, 30 minutes
		  with intervals
		• Stretching routine
			• Walk, 45 minutes
			• Strength workout,
			  8 steps	

Week 8	• Walk, 45 minutes
	• Strength workout,
	  8 steps
		• Walk, 30 minutes
		  with intervals
		• Stretching routine
			• Walk, 45 minutes
			• Strength workout,
			  8 steps	

We've made it even easier! Here's a sample schedule for the *ChangeOne* fitness program. Give it a try as suggested here, or adjust it to your own timetable. In either case, it's important *not* to try to follow the program by memory. Copy this schedule and post it on the refrigerator with your changes penciled in, or better still, make workout appointments on your daily calendar. Scheduling a specific time for exercise greatly increases the likelihood of your making it happen. Finally, if you don't feel ready to make the step to the next week's activity levels, no problem. Just repeat your current week's activities and move ahead when it feels right.

THURSDAY	FRIDAY	SATURDAY	SUNDAY
• Walk, 15 minutes	Off	• Walk, 15 minutes	Off
• Walk, 15 minutes	Off	• Leisure-time activity, 30 minutes	Off
• Walk, 20 minutes	Off	• Leisure-time activity, 45 minutes	Off
• Walk, 25 minutes	Off	• Leisure-time activity, 45 minutes	Off
• Walk, 30 minutes • Stretching routine	Off	• Leisure-time activity, 45 minutes	Off
• Walk, 30 minutes • Strength workout, 5 steps	Off	• Leisure-time activity, 45 minutes	Off
• Walk, 30 minutes with intervals • Stretching routine	Off	• Leisure-time activity, 1 hour	• Stretching routine • Strength workout, 8 steps
• Walk, 30 minutes with intervals • Stretching routine	Off	• Leisure-time activity, 1 hour	• Stretching routine • Strength workout, 8 to 12 steps

Muscle-Toning

Losing weight is only half of what it takes to win the battle of the bulge. The other half is building muscle. No, we're not talking about becoming the Incredible Hulk, and you don't have to join a gym and start pumping iron. The simple exercises in this section are all you need to get started. By tightening up sagging muscles, you'll look better. Just as important, you'll boost your metabolism. Muscle tissue requires more calories for maintenance than fat does. And by strengthening your muscles, you'll increase the number of calories your body burns even while sitting still.

In this section you'll find five simple muscle-toning exercises you can do anywhere you have some open space. Take your time to get the feel of each exercise. Do 8 to 15 repetitions of each. When you can do 15 easily, wait 30 seconds and do another set. (For the wall sit, start by holding the move for 20 to 30 seconds, and then increase the amount of time as you get stronger.) Do each move slowly, steadily, and consistently. Don't try to be a superhero at the beginning. It's better to start slow and build up to more repetitions or sets. That way you'll avoid becoming too sore.

1. Abdominal crunches

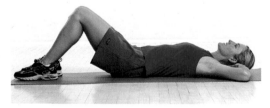

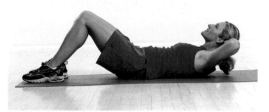

Lie on your back with your knees slightly bent and your lower back as flat against the floor as possible. Lightly clasp your hands behind your head, fingers loosely interlocked, and elbows pointing out. If you want to start with an easier approach, cross your arms over your chest.

Slowly curl your shoulders up until your upper back is off the ground; the small of your back should remain on the ground. Use your abdominal muscles to pull you up—don't pull your head with your arms or strain your neck. Keep your eyes on the ceiling. Pause at the top of your lift, then steadily lower yourself back to the floor using your abdominals.

2. Dry swimming

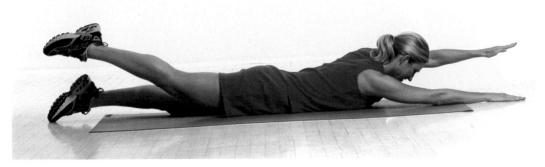

Lie on your stomach, arms extended in front of you. Keeping your hips on the floor, lift your left arm and right leg at the same time.

Hold for a count of three. Return to resting position. Repeat with the right arm and left leg. If you have back trouble, skip this move.

3. Push-ups

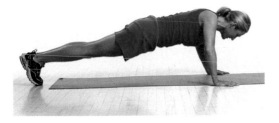

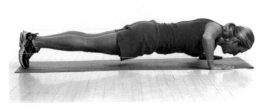

Lie face down, with your hands on the floor, pointing forward and directly under your shoulders. Your feet should be resting on your toes. Straighten your arms as you push your entire body off the floor. Make sure that your back and legs are straight, and that you aren't bending at the waist.

Lower yourself back down until your nose almost touches the floor. Pause, then slowly straighten your arms.

If you're having trouble, push off from your knees instead of your toes.

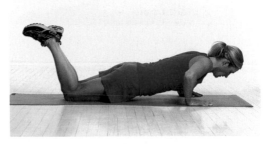

4. Wall sit

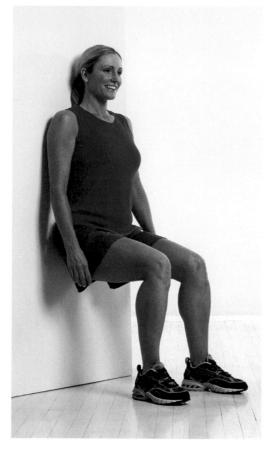

Put your back up to a wall, placing your feet shoulder-width apart and your heels about 18 inches from the wall. Slowly slide down the wall until your knees are bent at almost a 90-degree angle, as if you are sitting in an imaginary chair.

5. Kneeling leg curl

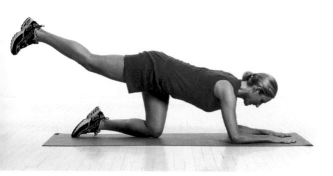 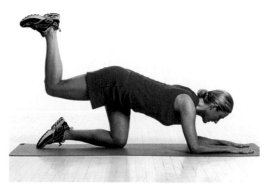

Start on your elbows and knees, hands and forearms flat on the floor. Extend your right leg straight back, pointing your toe down.

Raise your right foot until your leg forms a 90-degree angle. Keep your neck and shoulders relaxed. Hold the pose for a moment. Return to starting position. Do 8 to 15 reps, then repeat with your left leg.

Stretching

Eight Simple Moves

Stretching keeps muscles and joints limber. It's also a great way to relax yourself and release tension. The program on the following pages combines simple stretching exercises with modified yoga poses.

This series of stretches is designed to be done in sequence. But if any part feels too difficult or uncomfortable, skip it and go to the next.

1. Side stretch

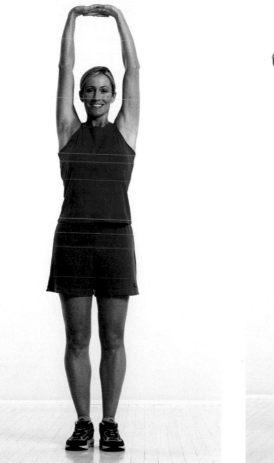

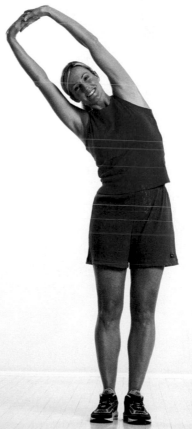

Stand up straight with your feet together, arms at chest level, and fingers interlaced. Turn your palms out and raise your arms overhead. Stretch your arms, torso, and legs. Relax your neck and hold for a count of five.

Now bend slowly to the right and hold for a count of five. Return to the overhead position, then gently bend to the left and hold for a count of five.

2. Forward bend

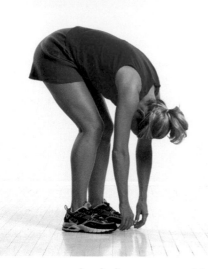

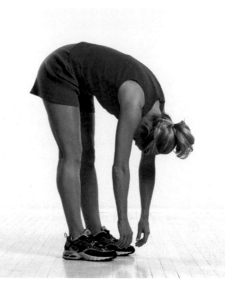

Bring your arms back down to your sides and pause. Now bend your knees and place your feet about 6 inches apart. Then bend slowly at the waist until your chest is touching your thighs. Let your arms dangle in front and hold the position for about 20 seconds.

Slowly straighten your legs as much as is comfortably possible (your hands can raise up higher). Keep your upper body and arms relaxed and in roughly the same position, and hold again for about 20 seconds. If you need a little extra support, place your hands on a stool or block of wood.

3. Downward-facing dog

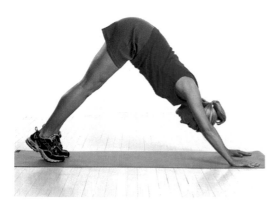

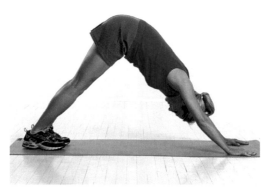

From the last position, bend your knees again and place your hands on the floor. Now walk your hands forward until you're on all fours. Tuck your toes under so the balls of your feet are on the ground. Contracting your abdominal muscles, slowly lift your hips to form an upside down V with your body.

Keeping your back straight, gently straighten your knees and press your heels toward the floor. Hold for 20 seconds.

244

4. Quad stretch

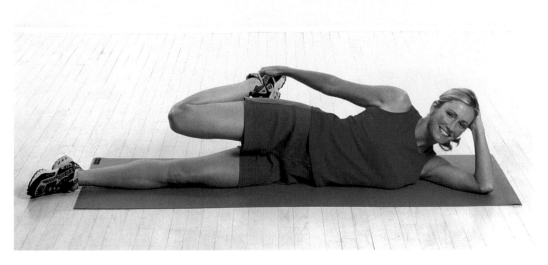

Now lower yourself to the floor and lie on your left side, your left arm supporting your head. With your right hand grasp the top of your right foot and gently pull toward your buttocks, feeling the muscles in the front of your thigh stretch. Your right knee should be in line with your left. Hold for 20 seconds. Roll over and repeat the stretch with your left leg.

5. Cobra

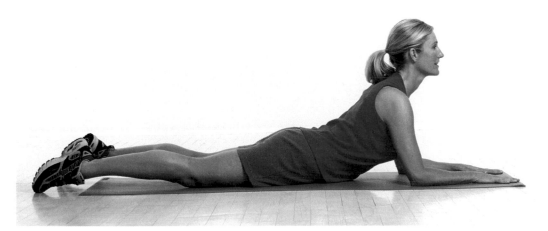

Roll over to a resting position, face down on the floor with your legs together and the tops of your toes touching the mat or carpet. Place your hands palm down on the floor, shoulder-width apart, and just in front of your head. Press up, raising your shoulders and resting on your forearms. Gaze forward or slightly up. Feel your lower back stretch. Hold for 20 seconds.

6. Child's pose

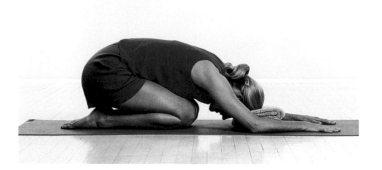

From the Cobra position, raise your midsection off the floor and slowly walk your hands back until you're sitting on your heels. The tops of your feet should be flat against the floor, and your arms should be stretched flat on the floor in front of you. Lower your shoulders and your forehead to the ground and hold for 20 seconds.

7. Hip stretch

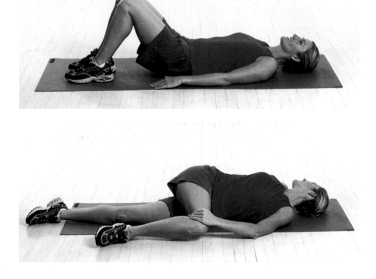

Roll over onto your back and bend your knees, keeping your feet flat on the floor.

Straighten your left leg and roll your pelvis to the right, gently lowering your right knee as close to the floor as you can. Hold for 20 seconds, then bring your knees back to center and repeat on the other side.

8. Corpse pose

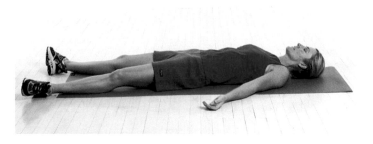

Slowly slide your feet out until your legs are flat on the floor. Put your arms about 45 degrees from your side, palms up. Place your legs about 1 to 2 feet apart, and let your feet fall to the sides. Close your eyes and relax. Concentrate on releasing tension from the center of your body outward to your fingertips and toes.

Exercising On-the-Go
The Eight-Step Workout for Anywhere

Who needs a gym membership? With a jump rope and resistance bands you can get a full gym-style strength and cardio-vascular workout. And you can do it anywhere—at home or on the road. Again, do 8 to 15 repetitions of each exercise, and add a set when 15 gets easy. Once you add these exercises to the previous ones, you'll have a workout that tones every part of your body.

When you buy resistance bands, get a pack that has several lengths and thickness. You can find a good set for less than $20 at most sporting goods stores.

1. Arm curl

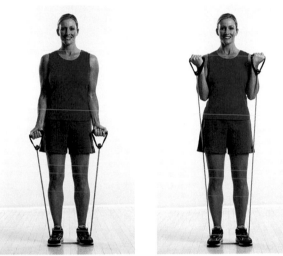

Stand on the band with your feet shoulder-width apart. Grasp one end of the band in each hand, arms at your sides, palms facing forward.

Lift your forearms, bending at the elbow with your upper arms against your body. Hold for a moment, then return to starting position.

2. Resistance rowing

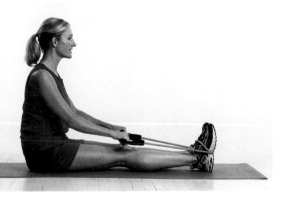

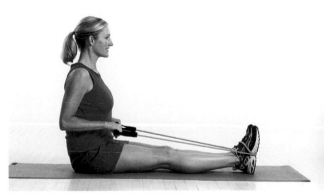

Sit on the floor with your legs straight in front of you and knees slightly bent. Loop the resistance band around your feet.

Keeping your back straight but relaxed, pull both handles of the bands back to your sides, palms facing down. Hold for a moment then straighten your arms.

3. Chest press

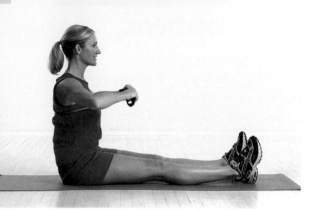 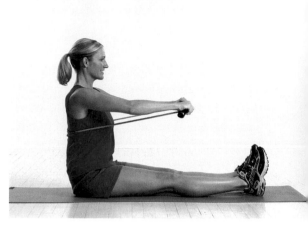

Sit down and place the resistance band around your back and under your armpits. Hold one end in each hand.

Keeping your upper arms parallel to the floor and your hands about shoulder-width apart, extend arms out in front of your body and hold for a moment. Ease your arms back toward your body.

4. Band squat

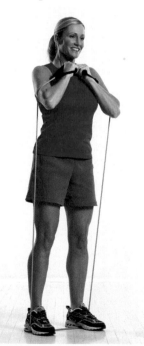 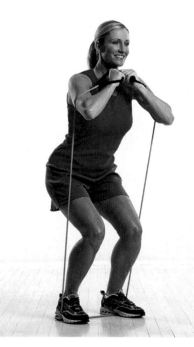

Hold the end of a resistance band in each hand and stand on top of the center of the band, with feet hip-width apart. Bring your hands together in front of your chest so that your elbows point down and the bands wrap over your upper arms. Be sure to stand tall.

Ease your body down as if sitting on a chair. Lower yourself as far as you can without leaning your upper body more than a few inches forward. Be sure not to move past the point at which your thighs are parallel to the floor. Keep your head up throughout the motion. Slowly return to the starting position.

5. Tricep extension

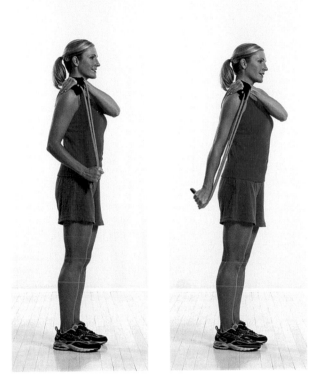

Hold both ends of resistance band with your left hand and the doubled-up middle of the band with your right hand, feet hip-width apart. Place your left hand over the front of your right shoulder. Bend your right elbow so that your right hand is by your hip, palm facing inward. Make sure the band isn't too loose; if it is, grab the band higher up.

With your elbow stationary, straighten your right arm out behind you so that the band gets tighter as you go. Don't allow your elbow to lock. Hold for a moment. Slowly return to starting position. Switch sides, and alternate arms.

6. Calf press

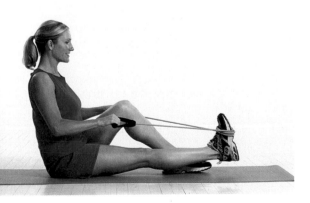

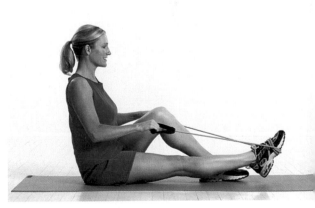

Hold one end of the resistance band in each hand and sit on the floor with your legs straight in front of you. Wrap the band around the top of your right foot. Bend your right knee slightly and lift it in the air. Sit up straight. Bend your left knee for comfort if needed.

Point your toe forward as you pull back on the band. Hold this position a moment, and while maintaining your pull on the band, straighten your foot and then pull your toes back to your body. Repeat until your set is complete, and then switch feet.

7. Shoulder press

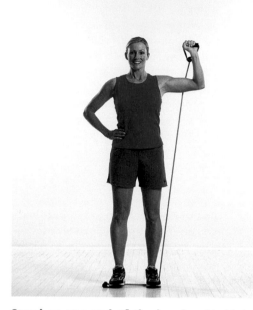

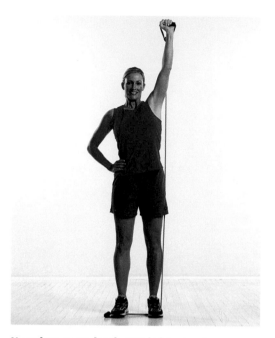

Stand on one end of the band and hold the handle at the other end in your left hand. Your right hand should be resting gently on your hip.

Keeping your back straight, slowly press your left arm up above your head, as if you were volunteering to answer a question. Hold for a moment, then slowly lower your arm to the starting position. Repeat until the set is complete, then switch to your right arm.

8. Jump rope

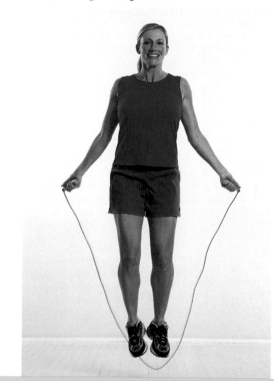

Jumping rope is a fabulous way to burn calories fast. It's also a great alternative to walking when the weather is foul. Make sure to wear a good pair of exercise shoes and jump on a surface with a little "give," like a wooden floor or an exercise mat. Keep your shoulders relaxed. Jumping rope is strenuous, so go easy at first. If you find yourself out of breath or sweating heavily, you are overdoing it. Start with just 5 minutes of uninterrupted jumping, and then work your way up.

When buying a jump rope, make sure the rope is the right length for you. Gauge this by standing on the center of the rope; the handles should reach to your armpits. For most adults, a jump rope 9 to 10 feet long is adequate.

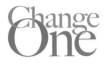

Meals
& Recipes

We hope you've had a chance to try the recipes contained in the first 12 weeks of *ChangeOne*, and that you enjoyed them. Because we have lots more for you.

In the coming pages you'll discover a delicious mix of ideas for breakfast, lunch, dinner, and snacks.

You'll also find tips, recipes, substitutions, and other guidance you need to bring these foods to life in your own kitchen, with your own sense of style and taste.

Here's the lineup:

- Quick Breakfasts, pages 252–258.
- Smart Lunches, pages 259–267.
- Delicious Dinners, pages 268–283.
- Snacks & Desserts, pages 284-292.

Muffins and Scones

What's more inviting than a basket of muffins or scones on the breakfast table? Piping hot, they're delicious as is, or with a thin spread of butter or jam.

Café-Style Breakfast

1 Blueberry Muffin with Lemon Glaze

1 cantaloupe wedge (about ⅛)

¾ cup steaming latte (½ cup skim milk plus ¼ cup strong coffee)

Calories 290, fat 6 g, saturated fat 3.5 g, cholesterol 50 mg, sodium 330 mg, carbohydrate 48 g, fiber 2 g, protein 11 g, calcium 350 mg.

BLUEBERRY MUFFINS WITH LEMON GLAZE

Makes 12

2 **cups all-purpose flour**
1 **tablespoon baking powder**
½ **teaspoon salt**
½ **cup granulated sugar**
1 **cup plus 1 tablespoon skim or low-fat milk**
2 **eggs**
4 **tablespoons butter or margarine, melted**
⅓ **cup reduced-fat sour cream**
2 **teaspoons vanilla extract**
1½ **cups fresh or frozen blueberries**
½ **cup sifted confectioners' sugar**
2 **teaspoons lemon zest (grated peel)**

1. Preheat oven to 400ºF. Put paper liners in 12-cup muffin pan. Mix flour, baking powder, salt, and granulated sugar in large bowl. In separate bowl, blend 1 cup milk, eggs, butter, sour cream, and vanilla.

2. Make well in center of flour mixture. Pour in milk mixture and stir with fork until just blended; don't overmix. Fold in 1 cup blueberries.

3. Spoon batter into muffin cups and sprinkle evenly with remaining blueberries. Bake until toothpick inserted in center comes out clean, about 20 minutes. Cool muffins on wire rack for 10 minutes.

4. To make glaze, mix confectioners' sugar, lemon zest, and enough remaining milk in small bowl so that the glaze is liquid enough to drizzle over muffins after they have cooled.

Instead of	Try
Sour cream	Lemon yogurt
Blueberries	Sliced strawberries
	1 cup banana slices, ½ cup walnuts (eliminate glaze)
	1 cup diced apple, ½ cup pecans (eliminate glaze)
	1 cup pumpkin, 1 teaspoon pumpkin pie spice (eliminate glaze)

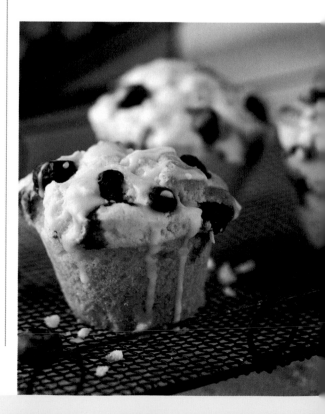

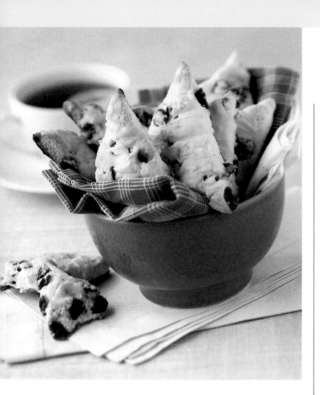

the 18 triangles 1 inch apart on lined baking sheets. Bake until golden, about 15 minutes.

4. Set wire rack on piece of waxed paper, parchment, or foil. Stir confectioners' sugar, orange zest, and juice in small bowl. When scones are cool, transfer in batches to wire rack and drizzle glaze over them with a small spoon.

Time-Saver

Buy or bake a batch of muffins and freeze in a sealable plastic bag. Pull one out in the morning for a quick breakfast.

ABOUT MUFFINS AND SCONES

Muffins are really just a quick bread (like banana bread) baked in a muffin tin. Scones, a kissing cousin to biscuits, are drier and flakier than muffins. *ChangeOne* muffins should fill a standard paper cupcake liner. Store-bought or diner muffins can creep up to double that size, so share one of those with a friend, or save half for another serving.

TIPS FOR BAKING SMART

- Cut the amount of butter, margarine, or oil in half, and add that amount of plain nonfat yogurt, reduced-fat sour cream, or applesauce.
- Switch from sour cream to reduced-fat sour cream.
- Cut down sugar amount by one-third.

DRIED CRANBERRY SCONES WITH ORANGE GLAZE

Makes 18

3	cups all-purpose flour
1½	teaspoons baking powder
½	teaspoon salt
¼	cup sugar
1¼	cups plain nonfat yogurt
3	tablespoons butter plus 3 tablespoons margarine, melted
1	egg, lightly beaten
1	cup sweetened dried cranberries
½	cup sifted confectioners' sugar
1	teaspoon orange zest (grated peel)
1	tablespoon fresh orange juice

1. Preheat oven to 400ºF. Line 2 baking sheets with parchment paper. Stir flour, baking powder, salt, and sugar in large bowl. In a separate bowl, mix yogurt, butter, margarine, and egg.

2. Make well in center of flour mixture. Pour in yogurt mixture. Stir with fork until moistened, and then stir in cranberries. Flour your hands and gently knead dough in bowl just until it comes together.

3. Turn out dough onto floured work surface and pat into 9-inch square, about 1 inch thick; cut that into 9 squares with small knife. Cut each square into 2 triangles. Place

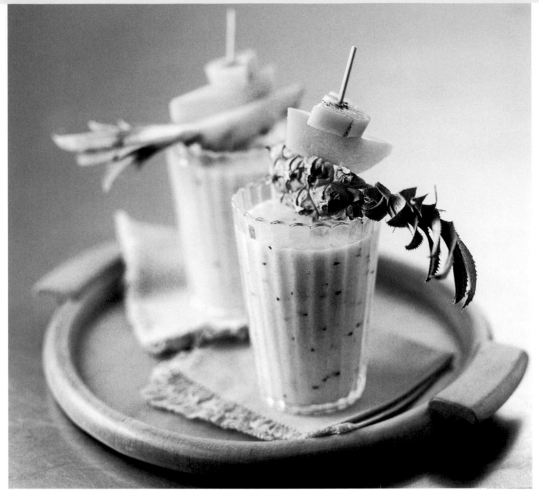

Smoothie Breakfast

Shakes, batidas, smoothies—no matter what you call them, these frosty combos of fruit and milk or yogurt refresh and nourish.

1 Tropical Smoothie, about 2 cups

1 toasted English muffin half, with
   1 teaspoon (thumb tip) peanut butter

Calories 260, fat 4 g, saturated fat 1 g, cholesterol 0 mg, sodium 250 mg, carbohydrate 47 g, fiber 4 g, protein 11 g, calcium 300 mg.

TROPICAL SMOOTHIE

Serves 4

   1 **mango, cut into cubes**
   1 **banana, cut into large chunks**
   1 **cup pineapple chunks**
   1 **kiwifruit, peeled and sliced**
   2 **cups plain nonfat yogurt**
   1 **cup ice cubes**

1. Combine mango, banana, pineapple, kiwi, yogurt, and ice cubes in a blender. Puree until smooth and thick.

2. Pour into 4 tall glasses. Freeze leftovers in sealable plastic containers. To defrost, microwave for 30–60 seconds and stir.

HEALTH TIP

When at a restaurant, order the smallest smoothie available—12 ounces is ideal. And be sure to request that they use nonfat yogurt or skim or low-fat milk.

The Hearty Frittata

This no-fuss Italian egg dish is baked in the pan, so don't worry about mastering omelet-flipping skills—you put the filling on top.

1 Vegetable Frittata wedge (checkbook)

½ cup fresh blueberries (2 golf balls)

1 slice wheat toast

Calories 280, fat 10 g, saturated fat 4 g, cholesterol 275 mg, sodium 490 mg, carbohydrate 28 g, fiber 4 g, protein 19 g, calcium 150 mg.

VEGETABLE FRITTATA

Serves 4

- 4 ounces white mushrooms, cleaned, trimmed, and thinly sliced
- ⅓ cup sliced red onion
- 5 eggs plus 4 egg whites
- 1 teaspoon chopped fresh herbs (thyme, oregano, or basil)
- ¼ teaspoon salt
- ¼ teaspoon black pepper
- 4 small plum tomatoes, thinly sliced
- 8 tablespoons shredded part-skim mozzarella cheese

1. Preheat broiler. Coat 10-inch nonstick, oven-proof skillet with cooking spray and set over medium-high heat on the stove. Sauté mushrooms and onion until tender, about 5 minutes. Transfer to plate. Wipe out skillet, coat again with cooking spray, and return to medium-high heat.

2. Whisk eggs, whites, herbs, salt, and pepper in medium bowl; pour into hot skillet. Cook until eggs begin to set, about 2 minutes; don't stir, but lift edge of eggs with heat-proof rubber spatula as you tilt skillet to let uncooked portion flow underneath.

3. Arrange tomato slices and sautéed vegetables in concentric circles on top. Continue cooking frittata until eggs are golden-brown on bottom and almost set on top, 2 to 3 minutes longer.

4. Sprinkle mozzarella around edge of frittata. Transfer skillet to broiler and broil until cheese melts and begins to brown, about 2 minutes. Cut frittata into quarters. A serving equals 1 of the quarters.

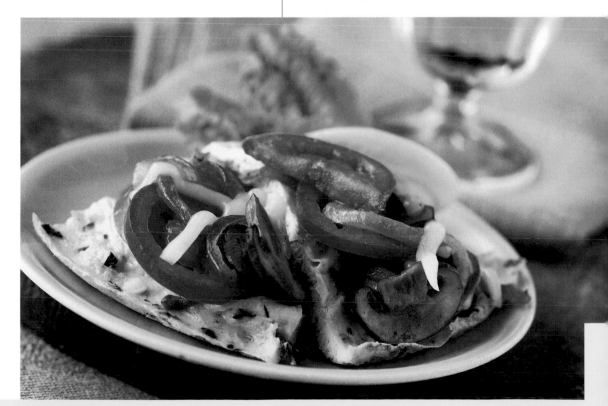

Quick Bread Delight

Every bit as enjoyable as muffins, quick breads are a natural partner for a cup of tea and a leisurely morning.

1 slice Peach Quick Bread, about ½-inch thick

½ cup fresh raspberries (2 golf balls)

1 glass (8 ounces) skim milk

1 cup coffee or tea

Calories 250, fat 3.5 g, saturated fat 0.5 g, cholesterol 20 mg, sodium 300 mg, carbohydrate 44 g, fiber 6 g, protein 13 g, calcium 350 mg.

PEACH QUICK BREAD

Makes 16 slices

- 2 medium peaches
- 1½ cups all-purpose flour
- ¾ cup whole wheat flour
- ¼ cup toasted wheat germ
- ¾ cup sugar
- 1 teaspoon baking soda
- ½ teaspoon salt
- ½ cup plain nonfat yogurt
- 1 egg plus 2 egg whites
- 2 tablespoons canola oil
- 1 teaspoon almond extract

1. Preheat oven to 350ºF. Coat 9-by-5-inch loaf pan with cooking spray.

2. Blanch peaches in medium saucepan of boiling water for 20 seconds. Peel, pit, and finely chop peaches (you should have about 1 cup).

3. Combine all-purpose flour, whole wheat flour, wheat germ, sugar, baking soda, and salt in large bowl.

4. Combine yogurt, egg, egg whites, oil, and almond extract in separate small bowl. Make well in dry ingredients, pour in yogurt mixture, and stir just until combined. Do not overmix. Fold in peaches.

5. Spoon batter into pan, smoothing top. Bake until toothpick inserted in center comes out clean, about 1 hour. Cool in pan on rack for 10 minutes, then turn out onto rack to cool completely.

6. Cut into 16 equal slices. A serving equals 1 slice.

HEALTH TIP

When you have banana bread or other quick breads at a coffee shop or bakery, your slice should be about the thickness of a deck of cards—if it's more, share it.

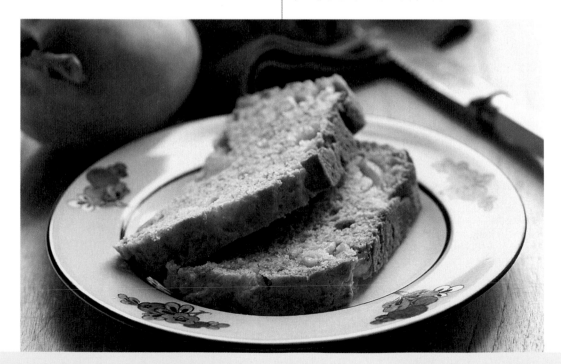

Yogurt Parfait

This simple breakfast treat is also healthy and delicious

- ¾ **cup plain or artificially sweetened nonfat yogurt**
- ¼ **cup berries** (golf ball)
- ¼ **cup mango** (golf ball)
- ¼ **cup low-fat granola** (golf ball)
- 1 **tablespoon shredded coconut** (thumb)

In a tall parfait glass, layer: one-third of the yogurt; half of the fruit; all of the granola; another one-third of the yogurt; the rest of the fruit; and the rest of the yogurt. Top with the coconut.

Calories 250, fat 4 g, saturated fat 2.5 g, cholesterol 5 mg, sodium 210 mg, carbohydrate 44 g, fiber 4 g, protein 13 g, calcium 400 mg.

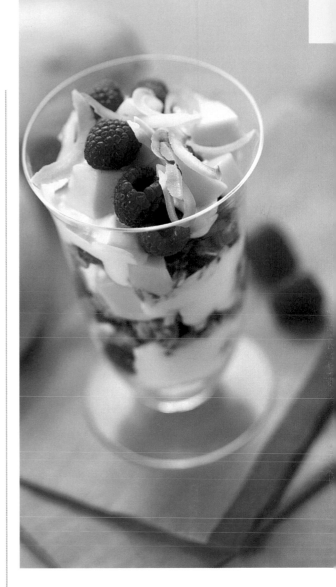

Instead of	Try
Low-fat granola	½ cup flake cereal (about 80 calories), or 1 cup puffed cereal
Berries and mango	½ cup sliced peaches, or ½ cup unsweetened applesauce
Coconut	1 tablespoon chopped nuts

Time-Saver
Stock up on frozen unsweetened berries and other frozen fruit. No need to wash or defrost ahead of time.

HEALTH TIP

In a recent University of Kentucky study, volunteers who ate a serving of yogurt every day lowered their blood cholesterol levels by as much as 3 percent. That corresponds to a cut in the risk of heart disease by as much as 10 percent.

Cottage Cheese Melba

Don't think of cottage cheese as diet food. Combined with tasty sides like these, it's a wonderful breakfast treat.

½ cup (2 golf balls) low-fat cottage cheese topped with:

    ½ cup peach slices
    1 teaspoon raspberry jam*

1 slice raisin bread toast

¾ cup Vanilla Steamer*

Calories 290, fat 2.5 g, saturated fat 1 g, cholesterol 10 mg, sodium 730 mg, carbohydrate 42 g, fiber 3 g, protein 23 g, calcium 300 mg.

VANILLA STEAMER

    ¾ cup skim or low-fat milk
    ½ teaspoon vanilla extract
    Artificial sweetener of choice, or
    1 teaspoon sugar (adds 16 calories)

1. Place milk in a microwave-safe mug. Stir in vanilla extract and sweetener.

2. Heat in microwave until warm.

For variety, use different fruits and jams with the cottage cheese; and use other extracts—almond or hazelnut, for instance—in the steamed milk.

ABOUT COTTAGE CHEESE

Cottage cheese is "fresh," meaning that its curds have not been aged or ripened. Its moist, loose texture and mild flavor make it ideal for all sorts of accompaniments, including fruits and jams, cereals, nuts, spices, and vegetables. It comes with different amounts of fat, ranging from none to 4 percent. *ChangeOne* recommends the medium range: low-fat. It tastes richer than fat-free and has fewer calories than regular 4-percent fat cottage cheese. Ricotta cheese, a fresh cousin made from whey (the liquid drained off from the semi-solid curds that make up cottage cheese), is smoother and creamier, but higher in fat. Farmer and pot cheeses are drier than cottage cheese.

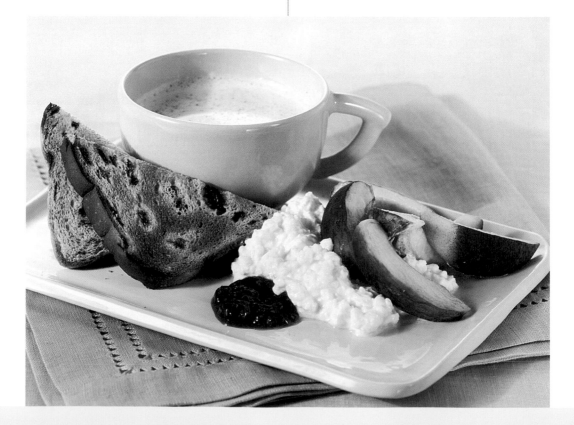

Well-Dressed Baked Potato

With the right toppings, potatoes go from side dish to a tasty, healthy entrée.

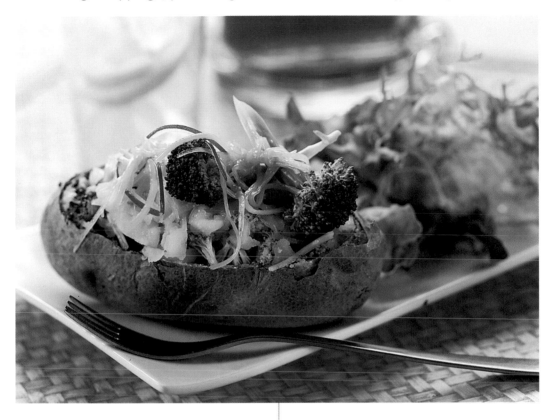

1 medium baked potato, about
   6 ounces (tennis ball) **topped with:**
   ¼ cup grated cheddar cheese (palmful)
   Steamed broccoli, unlimited

1 green salad with 2 tablespoons fat-
   free dressing (2 salad dressing caps),
   or reduced-fat dressing—adds about
   30 calories

½ cup berries in season (2 golf balls)

Calories 350, fat 10 g, saturated fat 6 g, cholesterol 30 mg,
sodium 420 mg, carbohydrate 54 g, fiber 8 g, protein 14 g,
calcium 300 mg.

Instead of	Try
Steamed broccoli	Diced tomatoes
	Chopped onions
	Steamed spinach
	Grilled mushrooms
Grated cheddar	½ cup canned beans
	½ cup 1-percent cottage cheese
	⅓ cup chili

Vegetable stuffings for your potato are
unlimited—they carry so few calories that
you can pile on as much as you wish.

Soups

A cup of soup at lunchtime, paired with a simple sandwich and fruit, makes a hearty meal. Here are two options—an old standard and a delicious departure.

Soup and Sandwich

1½ cups Hearty Split-Pea Soup

1   Bavarian Sandwich, open face

1   piece of fruit—orange, apple, peach

Calories 350, fat 8 g, saturated fat 4 g, cholesterol 30 mg, sodium 1,050 mg, carbohydrate 50 g, fiber 11 g, protein 21 g, calcium 250 mg.

HEARTY SPLIT-PEA SOUP

Serves 6

- 1   **teaspoon olive oil**
- 1   **tablespoon broth or stock**
- 1   **large onion, finely chopped**
- 3   **cloves garlic, minced**
- 2   **carrots, halved lengthwise and thinly sliced crosswise**
- ¾   **cup split peas**
- 2   **tablespoons tomato paste**
- ½   **pound smoked turkey breast, diced**
- ½   **teaspoon salt**
- ½   **teaspoon black pepper**
- ½   **teaspoon rubbed or ground sage**
- 4½ **cups water**
- ⅓   **cup small pasta shapes**
- ¼   **cup grated parmesan**

1. Heat oil and broth in nonstick Dutch oven over medium heat. Add onion and garlic to pan and cook, stirring frequently, until onion is golden-brown, about 7 minutes. Add carrots to pan and cook, stirring frequently, until crisp-tender, about 5 minutes.

2. Stir in split peas, tomato paste, turkey breast, salt, pepper, sage, and water, and bring to a boil. Reduce to a simmer, cover, and cook 30 minutes.

3. Uncover, add pasta, and cook until pasta and split peas are tender, about 15 minutes. Divide into 6 equal portions. (Unused portions will keep for 3 to 4 days in the refrigerator, 2 to 3 months in the freezer.) Sprinkle with parmesan and serve.

For the Bavarian Sandwich:
Spread honey mustard on 1 thin slice of black bread. Top with ½ ounce sharp cheddar cheese—cut into curls with a vegetable peeler—and lettuce. Serve open face, or add a second slice of bread.

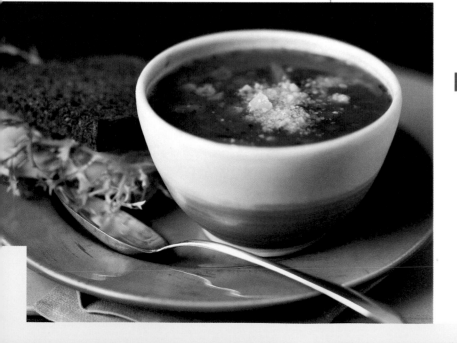

HEALTH TIP

At a restaurant or lunch counter, always ask how a soup is made so that you can keep an eye out for high-calorie ingredients.

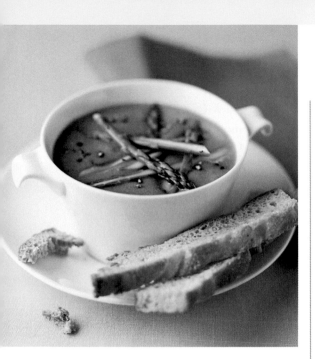

CREAM OF ASPARAGUS SOUP

Serves 4

- 1¼ **pounds asparagus, tough ends trimmed**
- 1½ **teaspoons olive oil**
- 4 **scallions, thinly sliced**
- 8 **ounces all-purpose potatoes, peeled and thinly sliced**
- 1¾ **cups water**
- 1 **teaspoon tarragon**
- ¾ **teaspoon salt**
- ¼ **teaspoon ground black pepper**
- ½ **cup low-fat (1 percent) milk**

1. Cut 10 thin asparagus stalks into 3 pieces each to use as garnish. Cut remaining asparagus into ½-inch lengths.

2. Heat oil in medium nonstick saucepan over low heat. Add scallions and cook, stirring frequently, until tender, about 2 minutes. Add potatoes and cut-up asparagus to pan and stir to combine.

3. Add water, tarragon, salt, and pepper to pan and bring to a boil. Reduce to a simmer, cover, and cook until potatoes and asparagus are tender, about 10 minutes.

4. Transfer mixture to food processor and puree. Return to saucepan and stir in milk and reserved asparagus. Cook over low heat until soup is heated through and asparagus pieces are tender, about 3 minutes.

5. Divide into 4 equal portions.

ABOUT SOUPS

Want a soup that's substantial enough to be a meal in itself? Try one made from legumes (split peas, beans, lentils) and include vegetables and pasta. On the other hand, if you prefer a broth-based soup—chicken noodle or miso, for example—you'll want to pair it with a sandwich or salad. And what about "cream of" soups? Unless you're certain they're similar to our *ChangeOne* recipe at left, assume that they are indeed made with cream and thus high in calories.

TIPS FOR CREAMY SOUPS WITHOUT THE CREAM

Try these variations (one at a time) for a soup that tastes creamy and still stays faithful to your *ChangeOne* plan:

- Add two peeled, finely diced potatoes when cooking the other ingredients.
- Add up to 1 cup evaporated skim milk and heat soup until just warmed.
- Stir in ½ cup plain yogurt or reduced-fat sour cream immediately before serving.
- Dice 2 slices American cheese and stir into soup shortly before serving.

Instead of	Try
Split peas	Black beans
Smoked turkey	Ham
Asparagus	Broccoli
All-purpose potatoes	Carrots and sweet potato

Caesar Salads

Now wildly popular, Caesar salads are readily available with all sorts of toppings—chicken breast, grilled tuna, tuna salad, and here, grilled turkey.

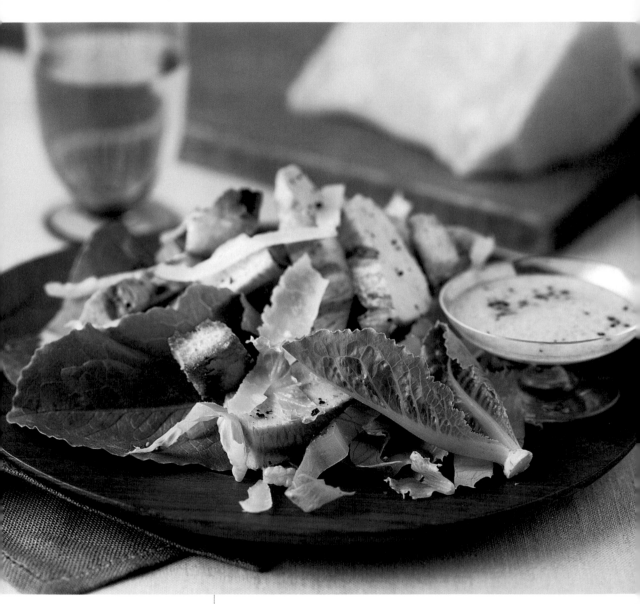

Time-Saver

Wrap and refrigerate leftover grilled meat or fish for your next day's Caesar salad.

Turkey Caesar Lunch

2 cups Grilled Turkey Caesar Salad (2 baseballs)

3 Ak-Mak flatbread crackers

½ cup fresh fruit salad (2 golf balls)

Calories 310, fat 8 g, saturated fat 2 g, cholesterol 40 mg, sodium 1,270 mg, carbohydrate 39 g, fiber 5 g, protein 23 g, calcium 150 mg.

GRILLED TURKEY CAESAR SALAD

Serves 4

- 2 **garlic cloves, peeled**
- 3 **tablespoons fresh lemon juice**
- 2 **tablespoons plain nonfat yogurt**
- 1 **tablespoon olive oil**
- ¾ **pound boneless, skinless turkey breast**
- ¼ **teaspoon salt**
- ½ **teaspoon ground black pepper**
- 8 **cups romaine lettuce torn into bite-size pieces**
- ½ **cup garlic croutons**
- 1 **ounce parmesan cheese**

1. Preheat grill. With a mini-processor or side of chef's knife, mash garlic cloves until paste-like. Put garlic paste, lemon juice, yogurt, and oil into jar with tight-fitting lid and shake until blended.

2. Sprinkle turkey with salt and pepper and lightly coat with cooking spray. Grill until cooked through, 4 to 5 minutes on each side. Cut across grain into ½-inch thick slices.

3. Toss together romaine, croutons, and turkey until mixed.

4. Shake dressing again, drizzle on salad, and toss lightly.

5. Divide salad evenly among four plates.

6. Shave strips of parmesan with a vegetable peeler evenly over each portion.

Instead of	Try
Grilled turkey breast	Grilled chicken breast
	Grilled marinated tuna
	Canned (water-packed) tuna
	Tofu cubes
	Grilled salmon
	Grilled steak
	Steamed or grilled shrimp
Use 3-ounce servings for all	

ABOUT CAESAR SALAD

Legend has it that the Caesar salad was invented by Caesar Cardini, a Tijuana, Mexico, restaurant owner, for a group of visiting movie stars. Others credit Caesar's brother Alex with the concoction. Whoever dreamed it up, the salad has become a classic. It originally featured romaine lettuce with a dressing of raw egg, lemon juice, Worcestershire sauce, garlic, and olive oil, and was adorned with parmesan cheese and croutons. Today variations abound, so in the spirit of the Cardinis, be sure to add your own.

TIPS FOR CROUTONS

- Use croutons sparingly unless you're willing to skip your bread or roll for the meal.
- When buying croutons, compare packages and portions to find brands that are lowest in calories.
- To make your own croutons: brush day-old bread lightly with olive oil (or coat with cooking spray), cut into ½-inch cubes, dust with dried basil, and bake on baking sheet at 250°F until crisp, about 20 minutes. Store croutons in an airtight container to keep them crisp.

Chili

Whether born in the American Southwest or borrowed from Mexico, this standard delivers a stick-to-your-ribs combination of beans, meat, peppers, and any other ingredients on hand. With meat or without, it makes a tasty and popular lunch.

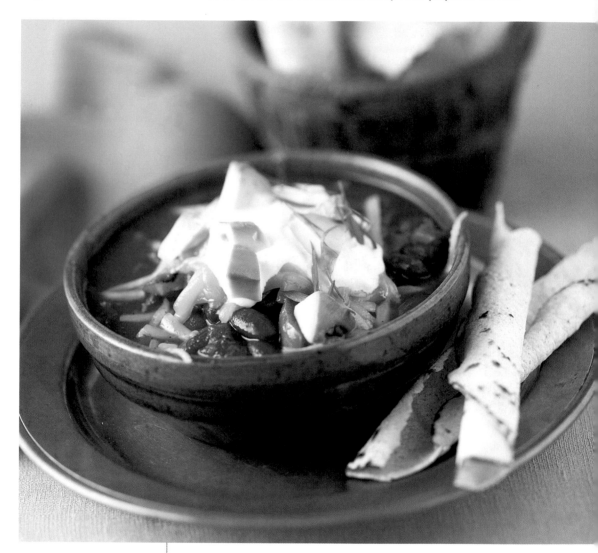

Meatless Chili and Salad

2 cups Meatless Chili Pots Con Queso (2 baseballs)

1 corn tortilla

1 green salad with 2 tablespoons fat-free dressing (2 salad dressing caps), or reduced-fat dressing—adds about 30 calories

Calories 250, fat 8 g, saturated fat 2.5 g, cholesterol 10 mg, sodium 1,000 mg, carbohydrate 58 g, fiber 13 g, protein 18 g, calcium 300 mg.

MEATLESS CHILI POTS CON QUESO

Serves 4

- 1 medium green bell pepper, finely chopped
- 1 medium onion, finely chopped
- 2 large garlic cloves, minced
- 2 cans (15 ounces each) red kidney beans, drained and rinsed
- 1 can (28 ounces) no-salt-added crushed tomatoes in puree
- ½ teaspoon chili powder
- ½ teaspoon ground black pepper
- ½ teaspoon ground cumin
- ¼ teaspoon ground cinnamon
- ½ cup shredded reduced-fat cheddar cheese
- ¼ cup plain yogurt
- ½ cup diced avocado

1. Lightly coat large nonstick skillet with cooking spray and set over medium-high heat. Sauté green pepper, onion, and garlic until onion is browned, about 5 minutes.

2. Stir in beans, tomatoes and puree, chili powder, black pepper, cumin, and cinnamon. Simmer 5 minutes.

3. Dish into four bowls, and sprinkle each with 2 tablespoons cheese. Garnish with yogurt and avocado.

Instead of	Try
Green pepper	Chopped carrots
Red kidney beans	Black beans
	Lean ground beef
Crushed tomatoes	Fresh diced tomatoes
Reduced-fat cheddar	Reduced-fat pepper jack

ABOUT CHILI

Classic chili contains beans and ground beef in a seasoned tomato sauce. Texas chili is all meat and chili peppers, no beans or tomatoes. Cincinnati chili is served on a bed of spaghetti and covered in cheddar cheese. White chili has white beans, chicken or turkey breast, and no tomatoes.

TIPS FOR USING CANNED AND DRIED BEANS

- Canned beans cut down preparation time by several hours. Use just one type, or mix and match varieties.
- Drain and rinse canned beans to reduce their saltiness before adding to your chili. No need to buy low-sodium beans—they often lack flavor, can be mushy, and are more expensive.
- To soak dry beans, place in a large pot covered with water. Bring water to a boil. Remove from heat and allow beans to soak for several hours, or overnight. Discard water.
- One cup dry beans yields three cups cooked.

ABOUT CHILI TOPPINGS

Smart chili toppings add tons of flavor without tons of calories. You can enjoy unlimited amounts of chopped onions, diced tomato, chopped cilantro, salsa, diced green chilis, and hot peppers.

Wrap Sandwiches

Mexico's burrito takes on new meaning—and becomes a hearty, diet-friendly lunch—when you amend it with a variety of fillings and wrap it with flavored tortillas.

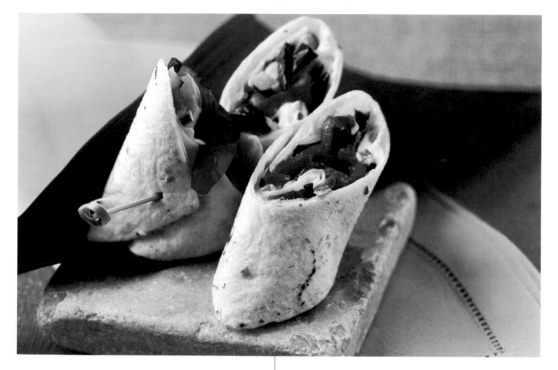

1 Roasted Vegetable Wrap with Chive Sauce

1 green salad with 2 tablespoons fat-free dressing (2 salad dressing caps), or reduced-fat dressing—adds about 30 calories

½ cup honeydew melon (2 golf balls), topped with a mint leaf

Calories 320, fat 8 g, saturated fat 1.5 g, cholesterol 0 mg, sodium 770 mg, carbohydrate 55 g, fiber 7 g, protein 11 g, calcium 250 mg.

ROASTED VEGETABLE WRAPS WITH CHIVE SAUCE

Serves 4

  1 **tablespoon olive oil**
  1 **tablespoon rice vinegar**
  1 **teaspoon chopped fresh rosemary**
  1 **garlic clove, minced**
  ¼ **teaspoon salt**
  2 **medium zucchini, total 1 pound**
  2 **large red bell peppers**
  1 **large red onion**
  4 **7-inch flour tortillas**
    Yogurt cheese from ¾ cup plain nonfat yogurt (see page 29)
  ¼ **teaspoon onion salt**
  1 **tablespoon snipped fresh chives**

1. Preheat oven to 450°F. Lightly coat jelly-roll pan or shallow-sided baking pan with cooking spray. Whisk oil, vinegar, rosemary, garlic, and salt in a small bowl. Cut each zucchini crosswise in half, then lengthwise into ¼-inch slices. Cut each red pepper into 8 strips. Cut onion into 16 wedges.

2. Heat oil mixture in pan and add vegetables. Cook, tossing frequently, until brown and tender, about 30 minutes. Sprinkle the 4 tortillas with a little water, wrap in foil, and place in oven during the last 5 minutes.

3. Combine yogurt cheese, onion salt, and chives in small bowl. Spread evenly on each tortilla and top with vegetables. Fold in sides of tortillas and roll up. A serving is 1 wrap.

Chopped Salads

Chopped salads are light—yet filling—and versatile. Swap ingredients and add different seasonings, and you have a whole new dish.

1 cup Pete's Chopped Salad (baseball)

1 medium whole wheat pita

½ cup grapes (2 golf balls)

Calories 330, fat 5 g, saturated fat 1 g, cholesterol 0 g, sodium 510 mg, carbohydrate 67 g, fiber 10 g, protein 11 g, calcium 40 mg.

PETE'S CHOPPED SALAD

Serves 6

 ½ cup chopped red pepper
 ½ cup chopped green pepper
 ½ cup chopped cucumber
 ½ cup diced red onion
 1½ cups diced tomato
 1 cup fresh, canned, or frozen corn kernels
 1 cup canned black beans, drained
 2 tablespoon red wine vinegar
 1 tablespoon olive oil
 1 tablespoon lime juice
 2 tablespoons minced cilantro
 1 jalapeno pepper, finely minced (optional)

Combine all ingredients in a large bowl and divide into 6 equal portions.

ABOUT CHOPPED SALADS

A chopped salad can be made from just about any vegetables in your fridge (see below). Chop up at least four cups of veggies (more if you wish), add a cup of beans, fish, or meat, and season to taste. Try international flavorings: cilantro and lime for Mexican; basil for Italian; lemon and garlic for continental; and soy sauce and sesame seeds for Asian.

Instead of	Try
Red and green peppers	Green and yellow zucchini
Cucumber	Celery
Black beans	Baby shrimp, Diced ham, Smoked turkey breast, Chickpeas
Lime juice and cilantro	Lemon juice, garlic, basil

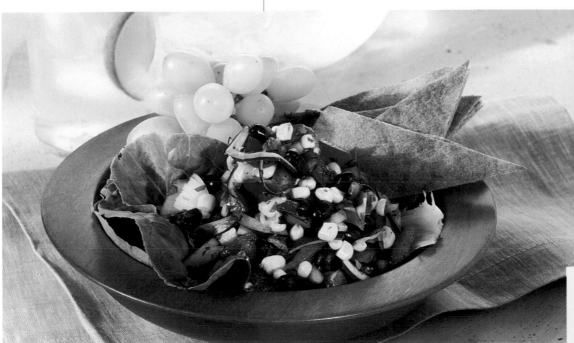

Chicken Breast

Your freezer should be stocked with boneless, skinless chicken breast halves—the most convenient cut of chicken you can buy. Slice while frozen for stir-frying, defrost and use whole, or pound into cutlets. Pair it with a sauce to keep it moist.

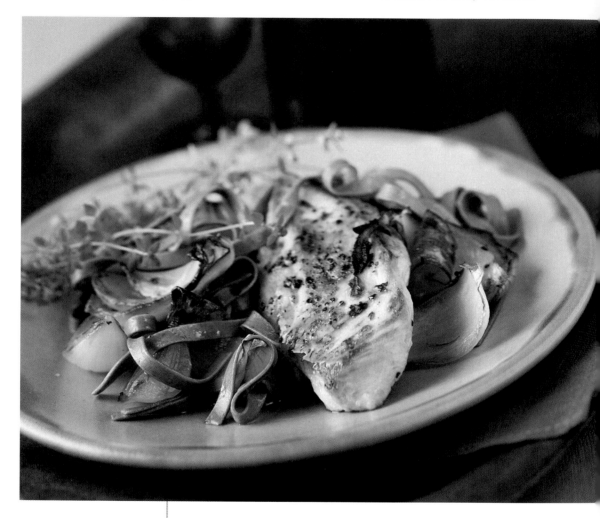

Sautéed Chicken Dinner

1 piece Sautéed Chicken with Caramelized Onions

2/3 cup spinach fettuccine (tennis ball)

1 green Mediterranean salad: unlimited romaine and assorted lettuces topped with tomato wedges, fresh ground pepper, 1/2 teaspoon olive oil, and unlimited balsamic vinegar

Calories 430, fat 10 g, saturated fat 1.5 g, cholesterol 75 mg, sodium 420 mg, carbohydrate 49 g, fiber 8 g, protein 37 g, calcium 100 g.

SAUTÉED CHICKEN WITH CARAMELIZED ONIONS

Serves 4

- 1½ pounds medium onions
- 4 boneless, skinless chicken breast halves, about 4 to 5 ounces each
- ½ teaspoon salt
- ½ teaspoon black pepper
- 4 teaspoons olive oil
- 2 tablespoons sugar
- ⅓ cup reduced-sodium chicken broth
- 1 teaspoon chopped fresh rosemary
- 1 teaspoon chopped fresh thyme
- 1 tablespoon red wine vinegar

1. Cut onions into 6 wedges each. Sprinkle chicken with ¼ teaspoon salt and ¼ teaspoon pepper.

2. Coat large nonstick skillet with cooking spray. Add 2 teaspoons olive oil and heat over medium-high heat for about 30 seconds. Add chicken and sauté until browned, about 3 minutes on each side; transfer to plate.

3. Reduce heat to medium and add remaining oil. Sauté onions, 1 tablespoon sugar, and remaining salt and pepper until onions turn golden-brown and caramelize, about 8 minutes. Stir frequently, breaking onions apart as they cook. Add broth and boil until it evaporates, about 2 minutes.

4. Stir in rosemary, thyme, and remaining sugar. Return chicken to skillet and sprinkle with vinegar. Cook uncovered until juices of chicken run clear, about 4 minutes.

5. Divide into 4 portions. One serving equals one chicken breast topped with about ½ cup onions.

Instead of	Try
Onions	Leeks, scallions, or shallots for similar flavor but a different look.

ABOUT CHICKEN AND OTHER POULTRY

Chicken is our most popular and least expensive type of poultry. In 1999 (the most recent year for these statistics), the average American ate more than 77 pounds of chicken, compared to 18 pounds of turkey. Turkey is lowest in fat—followed by farm-raised ducks that are bred to be lean. Here is a calorie and fat comparison, based on a 3-ounce cooked portion, without skin:

	Calories	Fat (grams)
Turkey breast	114	0.6
Duck breast	119	2.1
Chicken breast	140	3.0
Duck leg meat	151	5.1
Turkey leg meat	159	6.1
Chicken leg meat	174	8.2
Goose	202	10.8

ABOUT SKIN

Skin off: Boneless, skinless chicken breasts are a perfect match for dishes that are cooked with other ingredients; there's no fatty chicken skin to drip onto the accompaniments, altering flavor and adding calories.

Skin on: Chicken in its skin is perfect for roasting. The skin helps keep the chicken moist, and a thin membrane between the skin and the flesh keeps the fat from getting into the meat. It's best not to eat the skin—it adds almost a teaspoon of fat per 3-ounce serving.

Barbecue Beef

Where's a better place to be than standing next to your trusty grill on a warm summer evening? While the dish below is not technically a barbecue—that takes many hours of work—it tastes of pure summer fun.

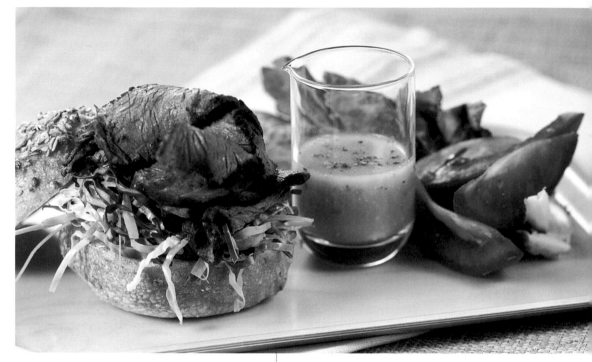

Barbecue Beef Picnic Dinner

1 Barbecue Beef on a Bun

1 cup Colorful Cole Slaw (palmful)

Calories 460, fat 14 g, saturated fat 4 g, cholesterol 50 mg, sodium 940 mg, carbohydrate 61 g, fiber 5 g, protein 27 g, calcium 100 mg.

BARBECUE BEEF ON A BUN

Serves 4

⅓	**cup ketchup**
1	**tablespoon red wine vinegar**
2	**teaspoons brown sugar**
½	**teaspoon ground ginger**
½	**teaspoon yellow prepared mustard**
12	**ounces sirloin steak**
4	**medium (2 ounces each) rolls**

1. Preheat grill. Combine ketchup, vinegar, sugar, ginger, and mustard. Brush on one side of sirloin steak.

2. Broil the steak 6 inches from heat for 4 minutes. Turn over, brush with sauce, and broil for an additional 3 to 4 minutes.

3. Slice thinly, divide into 4 equal portions (refrigerate extra), and serve on buns.

See tips on next page for ideas on preparing this using indirect heat.

ABOUT BARBECUE SAUCE

Barbecue sauce adds way more taste than calories. Our recipe is Kansas City-style, but you can choose your favorite. Lowest in calories are the vinegar-based sauces popular in North Carolina and the Memphis dry seasoning combo of paprika, onion powder, garlic powder, and dry mustard.

COLORFUL COLE SLAW

Serves 4

- 1 **cup shredded green cabbage**
- 1 **cup shredded red cabbage**
- ½ **cup shredded Napa cabbage, or other cabbage as available**
- ½ **cup shredded carrots**
- ¼ **cup low-fat mayonnaise**
- ½ **tablespoon deli or Dijon mustard**
- 1 **tablespoon red wine vinegar**
- ½ **tablespoon sugar**
  Salt and pepper to taste

1. Combine all ingredients and mix well. Refrigerate for at least 1 hour.

2. Before serving, divide into 4 equal portions and refrigerate extra. (Cabbage wilts and "shrinks" down when marinated.)

3. Cole slaw can be served separately, or on the sandwich (as pictured). To save a few calories keep dressing on the side and use a small amount as a condiment on the sandwich, or drizzled on top of the shredded vegetables.

Portion bonus: Increase all ingredients except mayonnaise.

Instead of Beef

Chicken and pork stand up well to the zestiness of barbecue sauce. To make these sandwiches with chicken:

- ■ Use about 1 pound of skinless, boneless chicken breast or thigh meat.
- ■ Cut into strips and combine with the sauce.
- ■ Heat in a 350°F oven or simmer on the stove until the sauce bubbles and the chicken is cooked, about 15 minutes.

To make the sandwiches with pork—a meat that is leaner (about one-third fewer calories) than it was 10 years ago:

- ■ Choose a lean cut, like tenderloin.
- ■ Cook as you would beef, brushing with sauce and broiling until done.

ABOUT BARBECUE

What many Americans call barbecuing—cooking meat, chicken, or fish over gas or charcoal in the backyard—is not true barbecue; it's actually grilling. Whether you're barbecuing or grilling, you win by cooking in a way that allows extra fat—with its calories—to drip off the meat. If you're lucky enough to live in a barbecue state like North Carolina or Texas, you know that barbecue refers to slow-cooking pork, chicken, or beef that is basted with sauce over indirect heat in a special barbecue pit. It's not cooked right on top of the coals or wood. While the smoky juiciness of barbecued meat is unique, you can enjoy a replica of barbecue flavor by basting your meat with your favorite sauce and cooking it under the broiler or on the grill.

TIPS FOR THE GRILL

Meat and chicken that are burned on the outside and barely done on the inside are all too common. They're also unhealthy. The undercooked meat can harbor harmful bacteria, and the charred parts of the skin contain cancer-causing compounds. The culprit is direct heat—the hot coals or gas flame of the outdoor grills. The solution: cook with indirect heat.

- ■ On a gas grill, turn on only one or two burners, leaving part of the grill top unheated.
- ■ On a charcoal grill, arrange the coals along the "wall" of the grill.
- ■ Place meat or chicken on the unlit side of a gas grill or in the center of a charcoal grill. You may want to place a drip pan under the meat. If desired, follow your grill's directions for adding wood chips.
- ■ Cover and cook until done (but open lid to baste frequently), about 150°F for beef, 150°F to 160°F for pork, 160°F for chicken breast, and 170°F for chicken thighs.

Pot Roast

Say the words "pot roast" and you can almost smell its savory aroma and see a warm, homey kitchen filled with family or friends. Save this recipe for a rainy afternoon that has the several hours needed for the roast to cook to perfection.

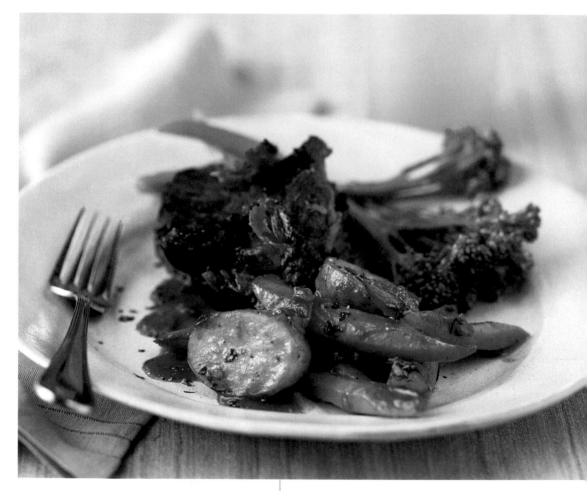

Sunday Roast Dinner

3 ounces All-American Pot Roast (deck of cards)

¾ cup Braised Vegetables (tennis ball)

1 small slice crusty sourdough bread

Calories 500, fat 20 g, saturated fat 8 g, cholesterol 75 mg, sodium 800 mg, carbohydrate 44 g, fiber 6 g, protein 28 g, calcium 60 mg.

ALL-AMERICAN POT ROAST WITH BRAISED VEGETABLES

Serves 12

1 **boneless beef chuck pot roast, about 3 pounds, fat trimmed**

1½ **teaspoons salt**

1½ **teaspoons ground black pepper**

8 **large carrots, peeled and cut into 2-inch chunks**

2 **medium onions, coarsely chopped**

4 **garlic cloves, crushed**

1 **can (28 ounces) whole tomatoes in puree**

1 **cup chopped fresh basil**

2 cups dry red wine or reduced-sodium beef broth

2 pounds small red-skinned or Yukon Gold potatoes, scrubbed

2 teaspoons cornstarch dissolved in 2 tablespoons water

1. Preheat oven to 325ºF. Tie roast. Rub roast with 1 teaspoon salt and 1 teaspoon pepper. Sear in Dutch oven over medium-high heat until browned on all sides, about 8 minutes. Transfer to plate. Sauté carrots, onions, and garlic in pan drippings until onions are browned, about 8 minutes. Stir in tomatoes, ½ cup basil, and remaining salt and pepper. Cook 5 minutes, breaking tomatoes up with spoon.

2. Return meat to pot. Add wine or broth and enough water to come 2 inches up side of pot. Bring to a boil. Cover with foil then with lid to create tight seal. Transfer to oven and roast 1 hour, turning meat once.

3. Add potatoes and remaining basil to pot, adding water if needed to come 2 inches up side of pot. Roast until meat and vegetables are tender, 1 hour longer. Cut meat into small chunks and arrange on platter with vegetables. Strain braising liquid into saucepan and bring to a simmer. Whisk dissolved cornstarch into liquid and bring to a boil. Cook until gravy thickens, about 1 minute. Ladle over roast and vegetables.

4. Cover and refrigerate leftovers for 1 to 2 days, or divide into individual portions and freeze for up to 1 month.

Portion bonus: Add extra vegetables to your pot roast to enhance the flavor and fill out your plate. Your portion of cooked beef should be about the size of a deck of cards.

TIPS FOR ORDERING

At a restaurant, size up your meat portion before you start eating. Keep the *ChangeOne* visual guide of a deck of cards for meat servings in mind. If your portion is bigger than that, set the rest aside to share or take home.

TIPS FOR TENDER MEAT

- Keep liquid in the cooking pot at all times.
- Cover pot and lid with foil to create a tighter seal.
- Roast meat in the oven at a low (325ºF) temperature or on the stove on low heat.
- Allow enough time for cooking; don't turn up heat to cut down cook time.
- Cook until "fork tender." Take a double-pronged grill fork and insert into the thickest part of the pot roast. If the fork goes in easily and pulls out easily, the roast is done.

ABOUT BUYING POT ROAST MEAT

Lower-fat, muscular cuts of meat like chuck and round require moist roasting, as in this recipe, to make them more tender. The best cuts to buy for pot roast are round rump roast, bottom round roast, eye round roast, and round tip roast. For freshness, choose roasts that feel firm to the touch, not soft.

TIPS FOR GREAT GRAVY

Pot roast and other meats cooked with moist heat create delicious cooking juices that you can use for gravy. After removing the roast and vegetables from the pan, gently pour the cooking juices into a gravy separator or measuring cup so that you can pour off the fat. Or use a turkey baster to suction off the liquid from under the thin layer of fat. Thicken by adding cornstarch or flour (about 1 to 2 tablespoons) and gently simmering until the gravy thickens. For *au jus* gravy, skip the thickening.

Meat Loaf

There are almost as many different types of meat loaf as there are people who love eating it. Traditionally a low-budget dish, meat loaf can make ground meat grand with an endless assortment of fillers and flavors.

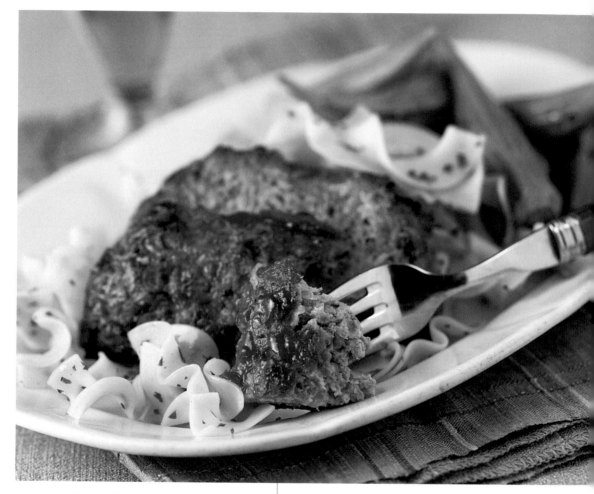

Heartland Dinner

1 slice Heartland Meat Loaf, about 1-inch thick

⅔ cup Parsleyed Egg Noodles (tennis ball)

Steamed baby zucchini, unlimited, drizzled with 1 teaspoon (thumb tip) olive oil

Calories 390, fat 10 g, saturated fat 3 g, cholesterol 120 mg, sodium 560 mg, carbohydrate 45 g, fiber 6 g, protein 32 g, calcium 60 mg.

HEARTLAND MEAT LOAF

Serves 8

2 large onions, chopped

2 large celery ribs, chopped

1 large green bell pepper, chopped

3 garlic cloves, minced

2 pounds 90-percent lean ground beef

1 cup fresh whole wheat bread crumbs (about 2 slices)

1 egg

½ teaspoon fresh ground black pepper

2 cups chopped canned tomatoes in puree

¼ cup ketchup

1. Preheat oven to 350ºF. Lightly coat 13-by-9-inch baking dish and large nonstick skillet with cooking spray. Set skillet over medium-high heat. Sauté onions, celery, green pepper, and garlic until soft, about 5 minutes. Transfer vegetables to large bowl.

2. Add beef, bread crumbs, egg, and pepper to vegetables in bowl and mix with your hands. Combine tomatoes and ketchup in small bowl. Add half to meat loaf mixture, and mix again.

3. Transfer meat loaf mixture to baking dish and shape into a loaf about 10 inches by 7 inches, mounding slightly in center. Make lengthwise groove down center and pour remaining tomato mixture into groove. Bake meat loaf until instant-read thermometer inserted in center reaches 165ºF, about 75 minutes. Let stand 10 minutes before slicing into 8 equal pieces.

4. Cover and refrigerate leftovers for tomorrow's dinner, or wrap in foil and freeze for up to 1 month.

To make Parsleyed Egg Noodles:
Cook a 12-ounce bag of egg noodles according to package directions. Drain, reserving ¼ cup of cooking water. Place noodles in a bowl, add reserved cooking water plus ¼ cup chopped parsley. Toss to mix. A serving equals ⅔ cup.

Instead of	Try
Ground beef	Ground pork
	Freshly ground sirloin steak
	Equal parts beef, pork, and veal
	Ground lamb
	Ground turkey
	Soy crumbles

TIPS FOR STRETCHING MEAT LOAF

Meat loaf is designed to be "stretched" to serve more people. You can make it go farther with one or two of the following per 2 pounds of ground meat:
- 1 cup of fresh or dried bread crumbs, preferably whole wheat.
- 1 cup grated carrots or diced potatoes, or both.
- ½ cup oats.
- ¼ cup quick-cooking rice.

ABOUT BABY VEGETABLES

Baby vegetables are miniature versions of zucchini, yellow squash, eggplant, and several other varieties. Some truly are young, while others are bred to be tiny when full grown. Select baby veggies that feel firm to the touch; softness can mean a vegetable is past its prime. To steam, place in a steamer basket for about 5 minutes, or in the microwave for about 2 minutes, until tender. Drizzle with olive oil, dust with a touch of salt and fresh ground pepper, and add fresh herbs if you like.

TIPS FOR COOKING MEAT LOAF

Meat loaf should be moist but not overly greasy, filling but not too high in calories. Start with ground meat that is at least 90-percent lean, or ground from a lean cut by the butcher. Add ingredients that moisten the mixture like ketchup or tomato sauce, as well as ingredients that hold moisture—for example, bread or cracker crumbs. If possible bake in a double meat loaf pan—an inner pan with holes that fits into an outer pan to catch the drippings. If using a standard loaf pan, gently pour off the drippings after the meat loaf is cooked.

Pork

Hogs have been on a diet, and while they're losing, we're winning. Today's pork is leaner and more flavorful than ever.

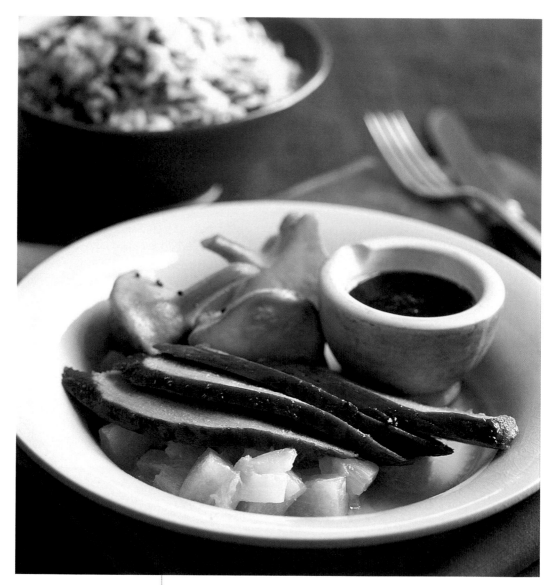

Sweet-and-Sour Pork

3 ounces Sweet-and-Sour Glazed Pork with Pineapple (deck of cards)

²⁄₃ cup basmati rice (tennis ball)

Steamed pattypan squash, unlimited

Calories 440, fat 6 g, saturated fat 1.5 g, cholesterol 65 mg, sodium 750 mg, carbohydrate 70 g, fiber 3 g, protein 29 g, calcium 60 mg.

SWEET-AND-SOUR GLAZED PORK WITH PINEAPPLE

Serves 4

- 1 **can (16 ounces) pineapple chunks packed in juice**
- 1/3 **cup red currant jelly**
- 2 **tablespoons plus 2 teaspoons Dijon mustard**
- 3/4 **teaspoon salt**
- 1 **tablespoon lemon juice**
- 1 **pound well-trimmed pork tenderloin**

1. Preheat oven to 400°F. Drain pineapple, reserving juice. Combine pineapple juice, currant jelly, 2 tablespoons of mustard, and 1/4 teaspoon of salt in small saucepan. Cook over medium heat, stirring frequently, until jelly has melted and mixture is slightly syrupy and reduced to 2/3 cup, about 5 minutes. Cool to room temperature. Measure out 1/2 cup of mixture and set aside to be used as a sauce. Reserve mixture in saucepan for basting.

2. Place pork in 7-by-11-inch baking dish. Sprinkle with lemon juice and remaining 1/2 teaspoon salt. Brush pork with basting mixture. Roast pork, basting every 10 minutes with pan juices, until cooked through, about 30 minutes.

3. Meanwhile, combine diced pineapple with remaining 2 teaspoons mustard in small bowl. Let cooked pork stand 10 minutes before slicing into 3-ounce portions. Serve sliced pork with reserved sauce and pineapple-mustard mixture on the side.

TIPS FOR ORDERING

Many restaurant menus now include pork tenderloin, an extremely lean cut. Chefs are careful with this piece, so it usually arrives at the table juicy and flavorful. Portions vary, so keep your serving to about the size of a deck of cards.

ABOUT PORK

Pork loin, chops, and tenderloin are the leanest cuts. But what's good news for lowering calories can be bad news for taste. Lean cuts are easy to overcook because they have very little fat to keep them moist. Best to buy thicker cuts that are less apt to dry out during cooking.

TIPS ON SQUASH

If you can't find pattypan squash, any summer-type squash with a thin skin will work—zucchini, yellow, scallop, crook-neck, or straight-neck. Pick medium-sized squash that feels firm to the touch. Super-sized summer squash can be dry. Wash well. Cut into 1/2-inch slices, then cut each slice into thirds or quarters. Measure about 1 cup per person—about half a medium zucchini. Place squash chunks in a microwave-safe bowl, cover with a plate, and microwave for 2 minutes. Uncover, stir, re-cover, and microwave for an additional minute. If not yet fully cooked (a fork won't go in easily), microwave in 1-minute intervals until done.

ABOUT BASMATI RICE

Basmati rice is a fragrant, traditional rice of India. Both basmati rice and texmati rice, its American cousin, are widely available in markets, health-food stores, and gourmet stores. Cook as you would other types of long-grain white rice.

Fish

Fish is growing in popularity, and for good reason. The American Heart Association and others recommend enjoying a fish meal at least twice a week. The best news: fish and seafood are among your lowest-calorie entrée options.

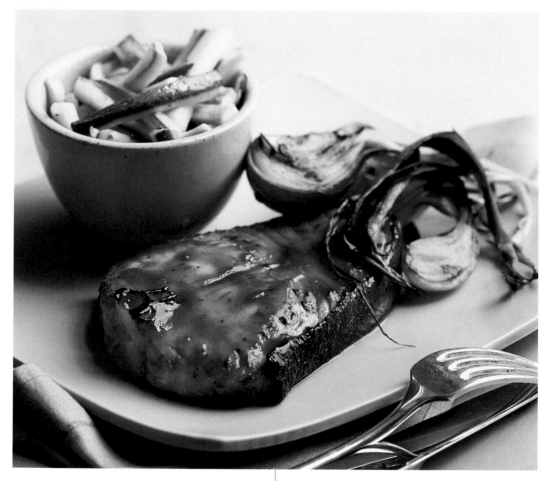

Fish on the Grill

1 Barbecued Halibut Steak,
about 5 ounces (checkbook)

1 serving Grilled Onions and Scallions:
1 onion and 2 scallions

1½ cups Ziti and Zucchini (2 tennis balls)

Calories 440, fat 7 g, saturated fat 1.5 g, cholesterol 45 mg, sodium 1,170 mg, carbohydrate 55 g, fiber 5 g, protein 38 g, calcium 200 mg.

BARBECUED HALIBUT STEAKS

Serves 4

   3 **small scallions**
  ¼ **cup reduced-sodium soy sauce**
  ⅓ **cup reduced-sugar apricot jam**
   3 **tablespoons ketchup**
   1 **tablespoon red wine vinegar**
   4 **halibut steaks (5 ounces each)**

1. Preheat broiler or ready the grill. Thinly slice scallions on diagonal and set aside.

2. Combine soy sauce, jam, ketchup, and vinegar in small bowl. Measure out ⅓ cup of mixture and set aside as a sauce.

3. Place halibut steaks on broiler rack and brush with remaining sauce mixture. Broil 4 inches from heat until browned and cooked through, about 5 minutes. Or grill on 1 side only until cooked, about 10 minutes.

4. Spoon reserved sauce over fish. A serving equals 1 steak.

5. Pass a small bowl of sliced scallions at table for sprinkling over fish.

To make Grilled Onions and Scallions:
Slice 4 small onions in half lengthwise. Place onion halves and 8 scallions on a baking sheet coated with cooking spray or brushed lightly with olive oil. Broil 4 inches from heat until browned; turn over and broil other side. If grilling, place directly on the grill grate, or use a grill basket. Grill until soft. Divide into 4 portions.

ZITI AND ZUCCHINI

Serves 4

- 6 ounces dry ziti pasta
- 2 medium zucchini
- 2 teaspoons olive oil
- 2 tablespoons slivered basil
- 2 tablespoons grated parmesan cheese

1. Cook ziti according to package directions; drain.

2. While ziti cooks, slice each zucchini in half crosswise, then slice each half into eighths lengthwise.

3. Place zucchini in a medium bowl and microwave until just soft, about 3 minutes.

4. Toss zucchini with cooked ziti, oil, basil, and cheese.

TIPS FOR COOKING FISH

With the exception of grilled tuna, which often is served rare, most fish should be cooked until just done, with flaky but moist flesh. The 10-minute rule is helpful: cook fish a total of 10 minutes per inch of thickness. Steaks and large filets may take longer, while thin filets will cook in a matter of minutes. Be sure to match fish to a cooking method appropriate to its texture. Here are a few guidelines:

Steaks: Grilling is good for fish steaks like halibut, salmon, shark, swordfish, and tuna, which hold together well when you turn them.

Filets: Higher-fat fish filets like salmon, sea bass, and trout won't fall apart on the grill, especially if you invest in a special grill basket for fish. Baking or pan-sautéing is best for thin filets like sole, flounder, red snapper, mahi mahi, tilapia, and other varieties. They are more apt to fall apart on the grill.

Whole fish, large filets: These can be grilled, steamed in a wok or fish steamer, baked, or poached.

TIPS FOR ORDERING

Feel free to order any type of fish at restaurants. Even though higher-fat fish like salmon are higher in calories, they're also packed with heart-healthy omega-3 fatty acids. The health benefits are worth the extra calories. Grilled, steamed, and blackened (coated in paprika, pepper, and other spices) cooking methods all involve little or no extra fat. Baked or sautéed fish may be cooked with butter or served with a high-fat sauce, so be sure to ask before ordering.

Pot Pies

Mom, a fire crackling in the fireplace, and pot pies simmering in the oven. What could be more warm and welcoming? Enjoy the *ChangeOne* version of chicken pot pie, a comfort food favorite.

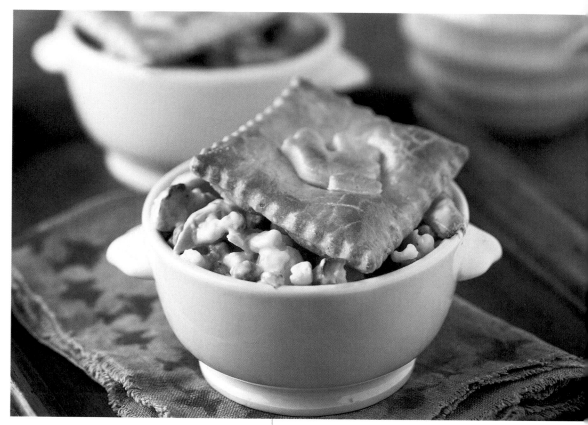

Pot Pie Dinner

1 cup One-Crust Chicken Pot Pie (baseball)

1 green salad with 2 tablespoons fat-free dressing (2 salad dressing caps), or reduced-fat dressing—adds about 30 calories

Calories 420, fat 12 g, saturated fat 5 g, cholesterol 80 mg, sodium 520 mg, carbohydrate 43 g, fiber 5 g, protein 35 g, calcium 150 mg.

ONE-CRUST CHICKEN POT PIE

Serves 4

  1 **pound boneless, skinless chicken breasts**

  ¼ **teaspoon salt**

  ½ **of 1 crust from 15-ounce package of refrigerated piecrust**

  1 **egg white, lightly beaten with 1 teaspoon water**

  2 **medium carrots, peeled and thinly sliced**

  1 **cup frozen corn kernels**

  1 **cup frozen green peas**

  1 **cup frozen small white onions**

  ½ **cup evaporated skim milk**

  3 **tablespoons all-purpose flour**

  ½ **tablespoon butter**

  ¼ **teaspoon ground black pepper**

1. Bring chicken breasts, ⅛ teaspoon salt, and enough water to cover to a simmer in large saucepan over medium-high heat. Reduce heat to low and gently poach chicken until juices run clear, about 15 minutes. Transfer chicken to cutting board; cool and cut into bite-size pieces. Reserve 1 cup poaching liquid.

2. Preheat oven to 425°F. Lightly coat baking sheet and four 1-cup oven-proof dishes with cooking spray.

3. Dust work surface lightly with flour. Unfold piecrust on surface and cut in half. Wrap the other half in foil or plastic wrap and refrigerate or freeze. Roll out crust ⅛ inch thick. Cut out 4 squares to fit on top of pies. Brush tops of squares with egg white mixture. Transfer to baking sheet and bake until crisp and golden-brown, about 12 minutes. Transfer to wire rack to cool.

4. Meanwhile, cook carrots in boiling water until tender, about 5 minutes; drain. Rinse frozen vegetables with hot water; drain. Whisk evaporated milk and flour in small bowl until smooth. Melt butter in medium saucepan over medium heat. Whisk in milk mixture, then reserved poaching liquid.

Cook until sauce thickens and boils, about 5 minutes. Stir in chicken, carrots, corn, peas, onions, pepper, and remaining salt. Cook until heated through, about 3 minutes; divide among the 4 dishes and bake until filling is bubbling, about 15 minutes. Top each with a pastry square.

ABOUT POT PIES

Pot pies are perfect for *ChangeOne* because they're already portioned into individual servings. They're also easy to adapt. You can change the chicken to turkey, tuna, or even tofu without changing the wonderful flavor of the dish. The recipe calls for frozen vegetables—available year-round—so pot pies always are in season. And if you're serving a crowd, double the recipe and bake in a casserole dish. Skip the pot pie, however, when dining out or purchasing ready-made dishes. Traditional pot pies are made with cream in the filling and crust, pushing them well beyond 500 calories per serving.

Instead of	Try
Chicken breast	Boneless, skinless chicken thighs, ¾ pound
	Turkey breast chunks, 1 pound
	Canned tuna in water, 3 cans, drained
	Firm tofu, ¾ pound
Piecrust	Refrigerated biscuit dough (½ biscuit per pie)
Frozen peas	Frozen edamame (soybeans), without shell
	Mixed frozen vegetables
Frozen corn	Fresh corn
	Fresh or frozen lima beans
Evaporated skim milk	Nonfat half-and-half

Super Sides

The beauty of *ChangeOne* is its adaptability: you can interchange main courses and side dishes for a wide variety of meal combinations.

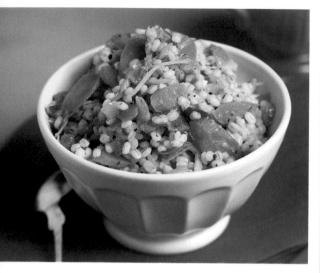

BARLEY PILAF WITH HERBS

Serves 4

- 1½ teaspoons olive oil
- 2 slices turkey bacon, coarsely chopped
- 1 medium onion, finely chopped
- 2 cloves garlic, minced
- 2 carrots, thinly sliced
- ½ cup pearled barley
- ½ teaspoon salt
- ½ teaspoon rubbed sage
- ½ teaspoon thyme
- 2¼ cups water
- ½ teaspoon lemon zest (grated peel)
- ½ teaspoon fresh ground pepper
- ¼ cup grated parmesan cheese

1. Heat oil in medium saucepan over medium heat. Add bacon and cook for 2 minutes. Add onion and garlic to pan and cook until onion is tender and golden-brown, about 5 minutes.

2. Add carrots to pan and cook until tender, about 5 minutes.

3. Add barley, stirring to combine. Add salt, sage, thyme, and water to pan and bring to a boil. Reduce to a simmer and cook, stirring frequently, until barley is tender, about 45 minutes.

4. Stir in lemon zest, pepper, and parmesan until evenly combined.

5. Divide into 4 portions. A serving equals approximately ⅔ cup (tennis ball).

Calories 170, fat 5 g, saturated fat 1.5 g, cholesterol 10 mg, sodium 490 mg, carbohydrate 26 g, fiber 6 g, protein 6 g, calcium 100 mg.

SUMMER RATATOUILLE

Serves 4

- 1 medium eggplant (about 1½ pounds)
- ¾ teaspoon salt
- 1 small fennel bulb
- 2 teaspoons olive oil
- 2 small yellow squash (6 ounces each), chopped
- 1 small onion, cut into thin wedges
- 2 tablespoons reduced-sodium chicken broth
- 2 large garlic cloves, minced
- 1 can (16 ounces) no-salt-added whole tomatoes
- 1 tablespoon chopped fresh oregano
- 1 teaspoon chopped fresh rosemary, plus sprigs for garnish
- 1 green bell pepper, chopped

1. Slice eggplant crosswise. Sprinkle on both sides with ½ teaspoon salt. Set on double layer of paper towels. Let stand 15 minutes. Rinse, pat dry, and cut into cubes.

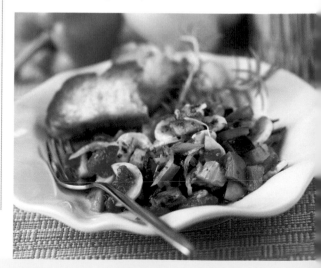

2. Trim and chop fennel bulb.

3. Heat 1 teaspoon oil in large nonstick skillet over medium-high heat. Sauté squash and onion until onion is soft, about 5 minutes. Transfer to large bowl. Add ½ teaspoon oil and broth to skillet. Stir in eggplant and reduce heat to medium. Cook covered, stirring occasionally, until eggplant is tender, about 12 minutes. Add to vegetables in bowl.

4. Add remaining oil and garlic to skillet and cook 30 seconds. Stir in tomatoes, fennel, oregano, and chopped rosemary, breaking up tomatoes with spoon. Cover and simmer 5 minutes. Stir in green pepper. Cover and simmer 7 minutes longer. Return vegetables to skillet. Sprinkle with remaining salt and bring to a boil. Cook uncovered 3 minutes, stirring occasionally. Serve warm or at room temperature, garnished with sprigs of rosemary.

5. Divide into 4 portions. A serving equals approximately 1 cup (baseball).

Calories 130, fat 3 g, saturated fat 0 g, cholesterol 0 mg, sodium 340 mg, carbohydrate 25 g, fiber 8 g, protein 4 g, calcium 100 mg.

ASPARAGUS WITH CONFETTI VINAIGRETTE

Serves 4

1½ **pounds asparagus**
1¼ **teaspoons salt**
2 **large red bell peppers, finely chopped**
2 **large yellow bell peppers, finely chopped**
4 **scallions, thinly sliced**
2 **teaspoons fresh thyme or ½ teaspoon dried**
⅓ **cup reduced-sodium chicken broth**
3 **tablespoons white wine vinegar**
½ **teaspoon pepper**

1. Bring ½ inch of water to a simmer in large skillet over medium-high heat. Add asparagus and 1 teaspoon salt. Simmer until asparagus is tender, 3 to 4 minutes. Transfer to platter. Keep warm.

2. Wipe skillet dry. Coat with cooking spray and set over medium-high heat. Sauté red and yellow peppers until tender, about 4 minutes. Stir in scallions and thyme and

cook 1 minute longer.

3. Stir in broth and vinegar and bring to a simmer. Sprinkle with pepper and remaining salt and pour over asparagus.

4. Divide into 4 portions. One serving equals approximately 5 spears.

Calories 80, fat 1 g, saturated fat 0 g, cholesterol 0 mg, sodium 750 mg, carbohydrate 17 g, fiber 4 g, protein 4 g, calcium 60 mg.

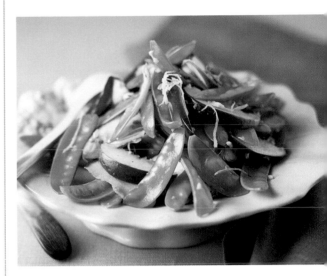

SNOW PEAS AND APPLES WITH GINGER

Serves 4

2 **teaspoons olive oil**
2 **tablespoons finely slivered fresh ginger (peeled)**
3 **cloves garlic, minced**
1 **pound snow peas, strings removed**
2 **crisp red apples (unpeeled), cut into thin wedges**
½ **teaspoon salt**

1. Heat oil in large nonstick skillet over low heat. Add ginger and garlic, and cook until tender, about 2 minutes.

2. Add snow peas, apples, and salt to skillet and cook, stirring frequently, until peas are crisp-tender, about 7 minutes.

3. Divide into 4 portions. A serving equals approximately ⅔ cup (tennis ball).

Calories 110, fat 2.5 g, saturated fat 0 g, cholesterol 0 mg, sodium 300 mg, carbohydrate 20 g, fiber 5 g, protein 3 g, calcium 60 mg.

Chocolate

Who doesn't love chocolate? Its unique flavor has been a favorite for centuries. Not only is it sweet, it contains plant chemicals that actually promote good health. Used judiciously, chocolate can be a tasty part of your *ChangeOne* program.

CHOCOLATE SNACKING CAKE

Makes 36

- 1 1/3 **cups all-purpose flour**
- 1 1/2 **teaspoons baking powder**
- 1/2 **teaspoon salt**
- 1 **cup plus 2 teaspoons unsweetened cocoa powder**
- 1/4 **cup nonfat buttermilk**
- 1 **tablespoon instant espresso powder**
- 1 **cup granulated sugar**
- 1/2 **cup packed light brown sugar**
- 1/2 **cup unsweetened applesauce**
- 2 **teaspoons vanilla**
- 2 **egg whites**
- 1/2 **cup semisweet mini chocolate chips**
- 1 **tablespoon confectioners' sugar**

1. Preheat oven to 325°F. Line 8-inch square baking pan with foil, leaving 1-inch overhang. Sift flour and 1 cup cocoa together into small bowl, and add baking powder and salt. Heat buttermilk and espresso in small saucepan over low heat until espresso is dissolved.

2. Mix granulated and brown sugars, applesauce, buttermilk mixture, and vanilla in medium bowl. Stir in flour mixture just until blended. Beat egg whites in large bowl with electric mixer at high speed just until soft peaks form. Fold egg whites into batter. Stir in chocolate chips.

3. Scrape batter into pan. Bake 35 minutes or just until set; do not overbake. Cool in pan on wire rack 15 minutes. Lift out cake and set on rack to cool completely. Sift confectioners' sugar and remaining cocoa over cake. Cut into 36 squares of a little more than 1 inch. A serving is 1 square.

4. Wrap leftover cake in heavy foil and freeze for up to 1 month.

TIPS FOR LIGHTENING UP BAKED DESSERTS

- If adapting your own recipe, replace just half the oil in the recipe with applesauce. The batch may not turn out well if you replace more than that.
- Use buttermilk or plain yogurt in recipes that call for sour cream.
- To keep the texture light, mix just until ingredients are blended. Avoid overmixing, which makes dough tough and ropy.
- Look for recipes that call for applesauce or prune butter. They can replace most of the oil or other fat in the recipe.

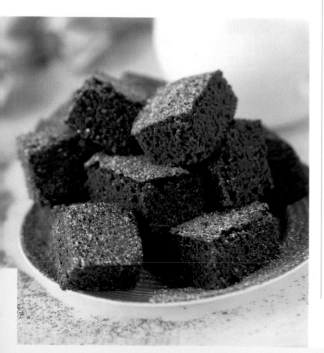

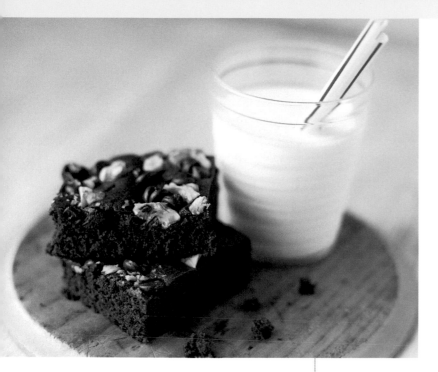

BROWNIE BITES

Makes 16

- ²/₃ **cup flour**
- ¹/₃ **cup unsweetened cocoa powder**
- 2 **tablespoons cornstarch**
- 1 **teaspoon baking powder**
- ¹/₄ **teaspoon baking soda**
- ¹/₄ **teaspoon salt**
- 1 **cup packed light brown sugar**
- ¹/₄ **cup prune butter**
- 2 **tablespoons plain nonfat yogurt**
- 2 **tablespoons canola or other vegetable oil**
- 1 **egg**
- 3 **tablespoons semisweet mini chocolate chips**
- ¹/₂ **cup coarsely chopped walnuts**

1. Preheat oven to 350°F. Coat an 8-inch square baking pan with cooking spray.

2. Stir together flour, cocoa powder, cornstarch, baking powder, baking soda, and salt in medium bowl. Set aside.

3. Beat together brown sugar, prune butter, yogurt, oil, and egg in large bowl with electric mixer. Stir in flour mixture just until combined.

4. Pour batter into pan. Scatter chocolate chips and walnuts on top of batter. Bake 18 to 20 minutes or until a toothpick inserted in center comes out with some crumbs sticking to it and sides of brownie begin to pull away from pan. Cool in pan on a wire rack. Cut into 16 squares of about 2 inches each. A serving is 1 brownie.

5. Wrap leftover brownies in heavy foil and freeze for up to 1 month.

CHOCOLATE-DIPPED STRAWBERRIES

- 1 **pint strawberries, rinsed and dried completely**
- 4 **ounces (²/₃ cup) semisweet chocolate chips**

1. Spread baking sheet with parchment.

2. Melt chips in microwave on medium for about 30 seconds, or until melted into a thick liquid. Stir well.

3. Using a fork or strawberry stem, dip each strawberry into the chocolate. Allow excess chocolate to drip off. Gently place dipped strawberry on baking sheet.

4. When all strawberries have been dipped, place baking sheet in refrigerator until chocolate hardens, about 30 minutes. A serving is 1 strawberry.

5. Store leftovers in refrigerator for up to a day.

Cookies

Cookies are always a favorite. And in *ChangeOne* there's no need to give them up. In fact, you can enjoy cookies guilt free if you limit them to one or two small ones—about a few inches each. Here we've put together some of our favorites for you. For each, one serving equals a *ChangeOne* snack or dessert portion.

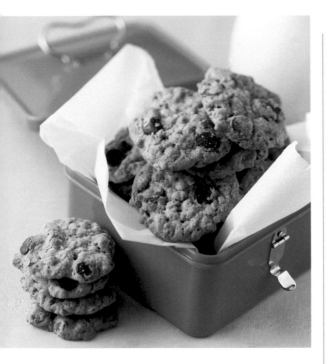

CHOCOLATE CHIP OATMEAL COOKIES

Makes 36

1 **cup all-purpose flour**
1/2 **teaspoon baking soda**
1/2 **teaspoon salt**
1 **cup old-fashioned oats**
4 **tablespoons butter**
2/3 **cup packed light brown sugar**
1/2 **cup granulated sugar**
1 **egg**
1 1/2 **teaspoons vanilla**
1/3 **cup reduced-fat sour cream**
3/4 **cup semisweet chocolate chips**

1. Preheat oven to 375ºF. Line two large baking sheets with parchment paper. Whisk flour, baking soda, and salt in medium bowl. Stir in oats.

2. Cream butter, brown sugar, and granulated sugar in large bowl with electric mixer at high speed until well blended. Add egg and vanilla and beat until light and creamy, about 3 minutes. Blend in sour cream with wooden spoon, then flour mixture all at once until combined. Don't overmix or the cookies may become tough. Stir in chocolate chips.

3. Drop heaping teaspoonfuls of dough 2 inches apart onto baking sheets. Bake until cookies are golden, about 10 minutes. Cool on baking sheets 2 minutes, then transfer to wire racks and cool completely. A serving is 1 cookie.

4. Store remaining cookies in airtight container for up to 2 weeks, or freeze for up to 3 months.

TIPS FOR HIGH-CALORIE INGREDIENTS

Ingredients like chocolate chips, nuts, and butter make cookies delicious. But just because they're high in calories doesn't mean you have to avoid them.

- Use semisweet mini chocolate chips—they scatter throughout the dough and deliver a stronger chocolate flavor than milk chocolate does.
- Just a few finely chopped nuts can go a long way. To bring out their flavor, toast them first in a skillet, or in the microwave for 1 to 2 minutes.
- A tablespoon of butter adds rich flavor without too many extra calories per cookie—but keep it to 1 tablespoon.

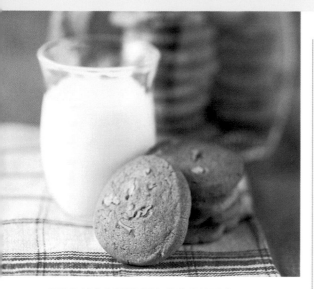

PECAN ICEBOX COOKIES

Makes 72

- 1¾ **cups all-purpose flour**
- ½ **teaspoon cinnamon**
- ¼ **teaspoon salt**
- ¼ **teaspoon baking soda**
- ¼ **cup (half stick) butter, softened**
- ⅔ **cup granulated sugar**
- ⅓ **cup packed light brown sugar**
- 1 **egg**
- 1 **tablespoon vanilla**
- ⅓ **cup reduced-fat sour cream**
- ⅓ **cup chopped pecans, toasted**

1. Whisk flour, cinnamon, salt, and baking soda in medium bowl. Cream butter, granulated sugar, and brown sugar in a separate large bowl with electric mixer at high speed until light and fluffy, about 4 minutes. Add egg and vanilla and beat until well blended. Using a wooden spoon, stir in flour mixture, and then sour cream and pecans.

2. Tear off 20-inch sheet of plastic wrap and sprinkle lightly with flour. Transfer dough to plastic wrap and shape into 15-inch log. Tightly roll in plastic and refrigerate until firm, about 2 hours.

3. Preheat oven to 375ºF. Cut dough into rounds ¼ inch thick, making about 72 cookies. Working in batches, place ½ inch apart on ungreased baking sheets. Bake just until crisp and golden brown around edges, about 8 minutes. Transfer cookies to wire racks to cool completely. A serving is 2 cookies.

4. Store cookies in airtight container for up to 2 weeks or freeze for up to 3 months.

MERINGUE NUT COOKIES

Makes 36

- ⅓ **cup walnuts**
- ½ **cup plus 2 tablespoons confectioners' (powdered) sugar**
- 4 **teaspoons unsweetened cocoa powder**
- ¼ **teaspoon cinnamon**
- 2 **egg whites**
- ⅛ **teaspoon salt**

1. Preheat oven to 300ºF. Line 2 baking sheets with parchment paper. Toast walnuts in small skillet, stirring frequently until crisp and fragrant, about 7 minutes. When cool enough to handle, chop coarsely.

2. Sift together ½ cup confectioners' sugar, cocoa powder, and cinnamon on sheet of waxed paper.

3. With electric mixer, beat egg whites and salt in large bowl until stiff peaks form. With rubber spatula, gently fold cocoa mixture into egg whites, then fold in nuts.

4. Drop batter by generous teaspoonfuls onto baking sheets, spacing them 1 inch apart. Bake until set, about 20 minutes. Remove and cool on wire rack. Dust with remaining 2 tablespoons confectioners' sugar just before serving. A serving is 4 or 5 cookies.

5. Store leftovers at room temperature in a tightly sealed container.

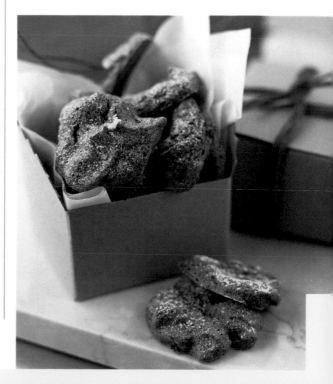

Snack Sensations

Here are four smart snacks that will help you keep hunger at bay between meals. Some, like the soft pretzels, can be quite a project, but also interesting and fun— exactly what food is all about. And you'll be impressed by the results.

RUBY-STUDDED TRAIL MIX

Makes 3 cups

- 1 1/2 **cups corn cereal squares**
- 3/4 **cup thin pretzel sticks**
- 2 **tablespoons hulled sunflower seeds**
- 1/4 **teaspoon salt**
  Cooking spray
- 1/4 **cup grated parmesan cheese**
- 3/4 **cup dried cranberries, coarsely chopped**

1. Preheat oven to 350ºF. Combine cereal, pretzels, sunflower seeds, and salt in large bowl. Lightly spray with cooking spray. Add parmesan and toss to combine.

2. Transfer mixture to jelly-roll pan and bake, stirring occasionally, until crisp and slightly crusty, about 15 minutes.

3. Let cool to room temperature. Transfer to large bowl. Add dried cranberries and toss to combine. A serving is 1/2 cup (2 golf balls).

4. Store leftovers in the refrigerator in an airtight container.

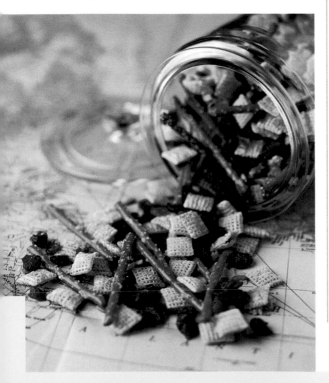

ROASTED-PEPPER PINWHEELS

Makes 8 pieces

- 1 **red bell pepper, cut lengthwise into flat panels (about 4, depending on shape of pepper)**
- 1/2 **cup canned chickpeas, rinsed and drained**
- 1 **tablespoon plain nonfat yogurt**
- 1/2 **teaspoon dark sesame oil**
- 1/2 **teaspoon lemon zest (grated peel)**
- 2 **teaspoons fresh lemon juice**
- 2 **teaspoons water**
  Pinch salt
- 1 **spinach-flavored flour tortilla, about 8 inches**
- 1 **cup mixed salad greens**

1. Preheat broiler. Broil pepper pieces, skin side up, 4 inches from heat, until charred, about 10 minutes. Transfer to a plate. When cool enough to handle, peel and cut into 1/2-inch-wide strips.

2. Combine chickpeas, yogurt, sesame oil, lemon zest, lemon juice, water, and salt in food processor and puree until smooth.

3. Spread mixture evenly over one side of the tortilla, leaving 1/2-inch border all around. Top with salad greens and roasted peppers. Roll up jelly-roll fashion.

4. Wrap tightly in foil or plastic wrap and refrigerate for at least 1 hour and no more than 4 hours. The roll will get softer and easier to slice as it sits in the refrigerator before serving. Unwrap and slice crosswise into 8 pieces (1 inch wide) to serve. A serving is 2 pieces.

5. Send leftovers home with friends to eat that day—these pinwheels do not keep well.

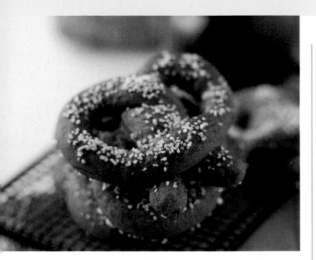

MULTIGRAIN SOFT PRETZELS

Makes 12 pretzels
- ¾ cup old-fashioned rolled oats
- 1¾ cups all-purpose flour
- 1 cup whole wheat flour
- ½ cup toasted wheat germ
- 1 packet (¼ ounce) rapid-rise yeast
- 5 teaspoons sugar
- 1½ teaspoons table salt
- 1½ cups very warm water (120°F to 130°F)
- 3 tablespoons baking soda
- 1 tablespoon coarse or kosher salt

1. Toast oats in small skillet over low heat, stirring frequently until golden brown, about 5 minutes. Transfer to large bowl.

2. To large bowl add all-purpose flour, whole wheat flour, wheat germ, yeast, 3 teaspoons of sugar, and the table salt. Stir in water. Transfer to floured work surface and knead until smooth, about 5 minutes. Transfer dough to ungreased bowl. Cover and let rise in warm spot until doubled, about 45 minutes.

3. Line 2 large baking sheets with parchment paper. Punch dough down and cut into 12 equal portions. With your hands roll each portion into a 16- to 18-inch rope. Twist each rope into pretzel shape. Place on baking sheets, cover, and let rise until almost doubled, about 20 minutes.

4. Preheat oven to 425°F. Bring large skillet of water to simmer and add remaining 2 teaspoons sugar and baking soda. Slide pretzels into simmering water, 3 at a time. Cook 15 seconds, turn pretzels over, and cook another 15 seconds. Blot dry on paper towels.

5. Transfer to baking sheets. Sprinkle kosher salt over pretzel tops and bake 18 to 20 minutes, or until crisp and golden. Cool on wire rack. Serve pretzels warm or at room temperature. A serving is 1 pretzel.

6. Allow leftovers to cool completely before storing in an airtight container.

SWEET AND SPICY SNACK MIX

Makes 8 cups
- ½ cup walnut halves
- 5 cups air-popped popcorn
- 1½ cups unsalted mini pretzel twists (about 2 ounces)
- ½ cup sugar
- 1 tablespoon lemon juice
- 3 tablespoons hulled pumpkin seeds
- ½ tablespoon ground cumin
- ½ teaspoon salt
- ¼ teaspoon cayenne pepper

1. Preheat oven to 350°F. Bake walnuts until lightly crisp and fragrant, about 7 minutes. Chop coarsely.

2. Spray large heat-proof bowl with cooking spray. Add popcorn and pretzels and toss well to combine.

3. Stir together sugar and lemon juice in large heavy skillet. Cook over medium heat, stirring until sugar has dissolved, about 5 minutes. Add walnuts, pumpkin seeds, cumin, salt, and cayenne. Cook and stir until nuts are well coated.

4. Transfer to bowl with popcorn and pretzels. Stir quickly to combine. Let cool to room temperature. A serving is ½ cup (2 golf balls).

5. Store in an airtight container in the refrigerator.

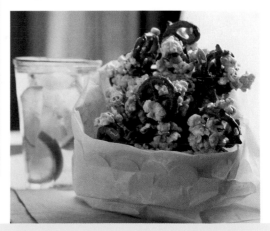

Fruit Desserts

What could be more refreshing than a fruit-based dessert to cap off dinner? Fruit adds color, flavor, and texture to your meal, along with weight-controlling fiber, vitamins, and a whole host of beneficial nutrients. Don't tell your guests that you've lightened up dessert—they'll never know.

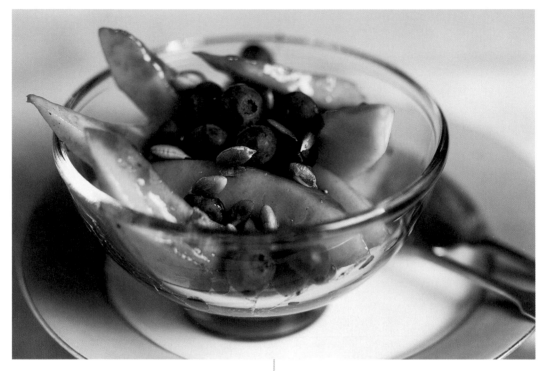

CANTALOUPE SALAD WITH RASPBERRY VINAIGRETTE

Serves 4

- 1 tablespoon hulled pumpkin seeds
- ¼ cup seedless raspberry all-fruit spread
- 1 tablespoon balsamic vinegar
- 2 teaspoons fresh lemon juice
- ¼ teaspoon cinnamon
- 1 large cantaloupe cut into 8 wedges
- 1 cup blueberries

1. Toast pumpkin seeds in small, heavy skillet over medium heat until they begin to pop, about 5 minutes. Set aside to cool.

2. Whisk together raspberry spread, vinegar, lemon juice, and cinnamon in large bowl.

3. Add cantaloupe and blueberries to bowl and toss to combine. Sprinkle with toasted pumpkin seeds.

4. A serving equals 2 cantaloupe wedges, ¼ cup (golf ball) blueberries, and 1 teaspoon (thumb tip) pumpkin seeds.

ABOUT MELON

Melons—cantaloupe, honeydew, Crenshaw, watermelon, and a growing number of gourmet varieties—are among the lowest-calorie fruits. They have a high water content and less sugar than other fruits. Cantaloupe is a standout for its vitamin C and vitamin A, two important nutrients that you get mainly from fruits and vegetables. A cup of melon contains between 45 and 60 calories.

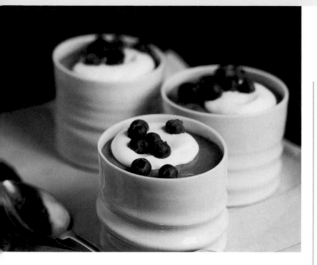

BLUEBERRY BONANZA

Serves 4

- ½ **cup low-fat (1-percent) milk**
- 2 **tablespoons fat-free dry milk**
- 1 **package (12 ounces) frozen blueberries, thawed**
- ¼ **cup plus 1 teaspoon sugar**
- ⅛ **teaspoon salt**
- ½ **cup plain nonfat yogurt**
- ½ **packet unflavored gelatin**
- 2 **tablespoons cold water**
- ½ **cup fresh blueberries**

1. Combine milk and dry milk in small bowl and whisk until well blended. Place in freezer for up to 30 minutes.

2. Combine frozen blueberries, ¼ cup sugar, and salt in medium saucepan over low heat. Bring to a simmer and cook until sugar has dissolved, berries have broken up, and mixture has reduced to 1 cup, about 10 minutes. Let cool to room temperature. Stir in ⅓ cup yogurt.

3. Sprinkle gelatin over cold water in heat-proof measuring cup. Let stand 5 minutes to soften. Set measuring cup in saucepan of simmering water until gelatin has melted, about 2 minutes. Let cool.

4. With a hand mixer, beat chilled milk until thick, soft peaks form. Beat in remaining teaspoon sugar. Beat in gelatin mixture. Fold milk mixture into blueberry mixture.

5. Spoon into 4 dessert bowls or glasses. Chill until set, about 2 hours. At serving time, top each with a dollop of remaining yogurt and the fresh blueberries. A serving is 1 bowl or glass.

ABOUT FAT-FREE AND REDUCED-FAT DAIRY

Fat-free and reduced-fat dairy products can be used to make creamy desserts with fewer calories than recipes made with cream. In this recipe, low-fat milk and fat-free dry milk are combined, chilled, and whipped to a fluffy consistency. The gelatin helps keep the whipped milk firm. A cup of the whipped milk combo supplies about 58 calories; a cup of whipped cream has over 400. Try fat-free or part-skim ricotta cheese in this recipe for a thicker consistency, but more calories.

TIPS FOR USING GELATIN

- Gelatin helps thicken desserts and adds texture when lower-fat dairy products are used instead of heavy cream.
- Use only the amount called for in the recipe. More is not better—you may end up with a rubbery dessert.
- Stir gelatin mixtures well until all granules dissolve. Undissolved gelatin gives desserts a grainy texture.
- Refrigerate desserts made with gelatin, but do not freeze; freezing will cause your dessert to separate.

ABOUT BERRIES

You can make this dessert with your favorite berry—blueberry, strawberry, raspberry, blackberry, or any combination. All berries pack a healthful punch. Blueberries supply the most antioxidants: naturally occurring plant compounds that help protect the body's cells from damage by guarding against cancer and keeping blood vessels sound. Strawberries are lowest in calories and richest in vitamin C. Raspberries and blackberries supply the most fiber.

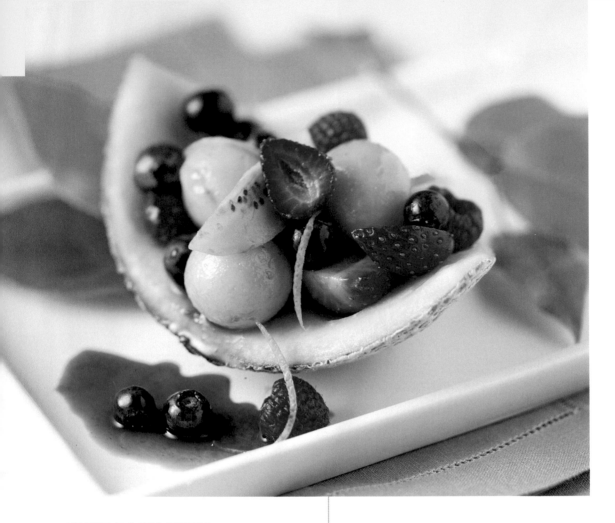

FRUIT BOATS WITH
ORANGE-BALSAMIC GLAZE

Serves 4

- ¼ **cup balsamic vinegar**
- ¼ **teaspoon orange zest (grated peel)**
- 2 **tablespoons fresh orange juice**
- 2 **teaspoons brown sugar**
- 1 **large cantaloupe**
- 1 **pint strawberries, hulled and quartered**
- ½ **pint blueberries**
- ½ **pint raspberries**
- 2 **kiwifruits, peeled, halved, and cut into thin wedges**

1. To make glaze, combine vinegar, orange zest, juice, and brown sugar in microwave-safe dish. Microwave on high until syrupy, 2 to 3 minutes; or cook over medium-high heat in a small saucepan, 4 to 5 minutes. Set glaze aside.

2. Make melon balls and prepare cantaloupe boats by cutting melon into quarters and scooping out balls, leaving a thin layer of flesh on the rind that you'll use for the boats. Put cantaloupe balls, strawberries, blueberries, raspberries, and kiwis in large bowl.

3. Drizzle fruit with glaze. Toss to coat. Spoon into the 4 cantaloupe boats and serve immediately. A serving equals 1 boat.

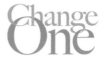

Meal Plans & Shopping Guide

It's a vicious circle: if you don't know what you're going to be cooking this coming week, you can't shop for food effectively. And if you're not shopping effectively, it's awfully hard to cook and eat well. As we've said a few times, eating the *ChangeOne* way takes a little planning.

We're here to help. This section includes detailed weekly meal plans, plus strategies to buy and stock food.

Following a rigid eating plan may seem unappealing, but give it a look. At worst you'll get a quick overview of the *ChangeOne* program in action. And you may even stumble on a day or week that's worth a try.

Each day's meal plan falls right around our 1,300-calorie target. For those in the 1,600 Club, remember as you look at these plans that you can double your starch or grain at breakfast; and you can double your protein at lunch or dinner, *or* add an extra serving of starch or grain at dinner.

And don't forget to check out the shopping strategies that follow the meal plans. You'll find tips and advice that will improve even the savviest kitchen.

Week 1	MONDAY	TUESDAY	WEDNESDAY	
Breakfast	**Yogurt Parfait** (page 257) • Yogurt layered with granola, fruit, and coconut	**Bagel Delight** (page 29) • Mini-bagel topped with jam and reduced-fat cream cheese • Yogurt with sliced ripe peach	**Breakfast on the Run** (page 30) • Cereal bar • Yogurt topped with blueberries	
Lunch	**Chef's Salad** (page 44) • Green salad topped with sliced turkey breast, ham, and cheese • Medium whole grain roll • Cantaloupe cubes	**Soup and Sandwich** (page 260) • Hearty Split-Pea Soup • Open-face Bavarian Sandwich • Seasonal fruit	**DINING OUT** **Friendly Fast-Food** (page 50) • Regular hamburger with lettuce, tomato, and condiments • Green salad	
Snack	Baked tortilla chips and salsa	Hot cocoa made with skim milk	Baked Apple (page 72)	
Dinner	**Barbecued Halibut Steak** (page 278) • Barbecued Halibut Steak • Grilled Onions and Scallions • Ziti and Zucchini	**Beef Stew** (page 92) • Beef Stew • Egg noodles	**Sweet-and-Sour Pork** (page 276) • Sweet-and-Sour Glazed Pork with Pineapple • Basmati rice • Steamed pattypan squash	
Snack/ Dessert	Blueberry Bonanza (page 291)	Fudgsicle	Yogurt smoothie	

THURSDAY	FRIDAY	SATURDAY	SUNDAY
A Perfect Bowl of Cereal (page 32) • Bran flakes topped with raisins and chopped nuts • Skim or low-fat milk	**Cottage Cheese Melba** (page 258) • Cottage cheese with peach slices • Raisin bread toast • Vanilla Steamer	**Pancakes to Start** (page 24) • Silver Dollar Pancakes topped with light syrup and sliced strawberries • Skim or low-fat milk	Streusel-Top Coffee Cake (page 227) Skim or low-fat milk # Brunch Hummus and pita Crudité platter **The Sunday Omelet** (page 130) • Vegetable-Cheddar Omelet • Whole wheat toast with butter and jam • Cantaloupe wedge
The Perfect Deli Lunch (page 52) • Turkey and Swiss on wheat bread • Italian pickled vegetable salad • Melon salad	**Soup and Salad** (page 40) • Vegetable soup with breadsticks • Green salad topped with grilled chicken • Green or red grapes	**Pizza and Salad** (page 39) • Pita Pizza • Green salad • Apple	
Frozen yogurt	Corn tortilla with melted cheese	Cup of yogurt topped with fruit	
DINING OUT **Italian Restaurant** (page 112) • Minestrone soup • Chicken breast cacciatore with pasta • Sautéed spinach and garlic • Fresh berries	**Kitchen Sink Stew** (page 156) • Kitchen Sink Stew • Garlic bread	**DINING OUT** **Chinese Restaurant** (page 114) • Wonton soup • Egg roll • Chicken chow mein • Steamed Chinese vegetables • Pineapple chunks	**Heartland Meat Loaf** (page 274) • Heartland Meat Loaf • Parsleyed Egg Noodles • Steamed baby zucchini
Brownie Bites (page 285)	Skim or low-fat latte	Air-popped popcorn	

Week 2	MONDAY	TUESDAY	WEDNESDAY	
Breakfast	**Smoothie Breakfast** (page 254) • Tropical Smoothie • Toasted English muffin half with peanut butter	**A Perfect Bowl of Cereal** (page 32) • Bran flakes topped with raisins and chopped nuts • Skim or low-fat milk	**Egg on a Roll** (page 23) • Scrambled egg on a whole wheat roll • Fresh fruit salad • Skim or low-fat milk	
Lunch	**Tuna Salad Sandwich** (page 224) • Tuna Salad Sandwich • Carrot and celery sticks • Banana	**Turkey Caesar Lunch** (page 262) • Grilled Turkey Caesar Salad • Ak-Mak flatbread crackers • Fresh fruit salad	**Well-Dressed Baked Potato** (page 259) • Baked potato stuffed with broccoli and cheese • Green salad • Seasonal berries	
Snack		Chocolate Chip Oatmeal Cookie (page 286) with skim or low-fat milk	Frozen yogurt	
Dinner	**Sautéed Chicken Dinner** (page 268) • Sautéed Chicken with Caramelized Onions • Spinach fettuccine • Green salad	**Sunday Roast Dinner** (page 272) • All-American Pot Roast • Braised Vegetables • Crusty sourdough bread	**Pasta Primavera** (page 98) • Pasta Primavera • Italian Salad	
Snack/ Dessert	Fruit Boats with Orange-Balsamic Glaze (page 292)	Apple	Pineapple chunks	

THURSDAY	FRIDAY	SATURDAY	SUNDAY
Café-Style Breakfast (page 252) • Blueberry Muffin with Lemon Glaze • Cantaloupe wedge • Steaming latte	**Breakfast on the Run** (page 30) • Cereal bar • Yogurt topped with blueberries	**Yogurt Parfait** (page 257) • Yogurt layered with granola, fruit, and coconut	**Pancakes to Start** (page 24) • Silver Dollar Pancakes topped with light syrup and sliced strawberries • Skim or low-fat milk
Chopped Salad (page 267) • Pete's Chopped Salad • Whole wheat pita • Grapes	**The Perfect Deli Lunch** (page 52) • Turkey and Swiss on wheat bread • Italian pickled vegetable salad • Melon salad	**Burrito to Go** (page 55) • Chicken and bean burrito with condiments • Orange	**Wrap Sandwich** (page 266) • Roasted Vegetable Wrap with Chive Sauce • Green salad • Honeydew melon
Peanut butter on a rice cake	Strawberry smoothie	Graham crackers with skim or low-fat milk	Pretzel sticks and reduced-fat string cheese
DINING OUT **Mexican Restaurant** (page 120) • Ceviche • Steak soft tacos with condiments	**Pot Pie Dinner** (page 280) • One-Crust Chicken Pot Pie • Green salad	**Weekend Grilling** (page 138) • Crudité platter • Stand-Up Chicken • Grilled Summer Vegetables • German Potato Salad with Dijon Vinaigrette • Sesame breadsticks	**Barbecue Beef Picnic Dinner** (page 270) • Barbecue Beef on a Bun • Colorful Cole Slaw
Almond-flavored milk	Brownie Bites (page 285)	Chocolate Snacking Cake (page 284)	Blueberry Bonanza (page 291)

Week 3	MONDAY	TUESDAY	WEDNESDAY	
Breakfast	**Quick Bread Delight** (page 256) • 1 slice Peach Quick Bread • Fresh raspberries • Skim or low-fat milk	**Café-Style Breakfast** (page 252) • Blueberry Muffin with Lemon Glaze • Cantaloupe wedge • Steaming latte	**Yogurt Parfait** (page 257) • Yogurt layered with granola, fruit, and coconut	
Lunch	**Soup and Sandwich** (page 260) • Hearty Split-Pea Soup • Open-face Bavarian Sandwich • Seasonal fruit	**Meatless Chili** (page 264) • Meatless Chili Pots Con Queso • Corn tortilla • Green salad • Banana	**DINING OUT** **Friendly Fast-Food** (page 50) • Regular hamburger with lettuce, tomato, and condiments • Green salad • Orange	
Snack	Crackers with peanut butter	Graham crackers and hot cocoa with skim milk	Edamame (steamed soybeans)	
Dinner	**Red Snapper and Spanish Rice** (page 100) • Snapper and Snaps in a Packet • Spanish Rice	**DINING OUT** **Diner** (page 118) • Chicken noodle soup • Green salad • Half a hot roast beef sandwich • Mashed potatoes • Cooked carrots • 2 butter cookies	**Italian-Style Stir-Fry** (page 90) • Chicken and Broccoli Stir-Fry • Orzo	
Snack/ Dessert	Brownie Bites (page 285)		Frozen yogurt	

THURSDAY	FRIDAY	SATURDAY	SUNDAY
Breakfast on the Run (page 30) • Cereal bar • Yogurt topped with blueberries	**Bagel Delight** (page 29) • Mini-bagel topped with jam and reduced-fat cream cheese • Yogurt with sliced ripe peach	**Hearty Frittata** (page 255) • Vegetable Frittata wedge • 1 slice wheat toast • Fresh blueberries	**Pancakes to Start** (page 24) • Silver Dollar Pancakes topped with light syrup and sliced strawberries • Skim or low-fat milk
Pizza and Salad (page 39) • Pita Pizza • Green salad • Apple	**The Perfect Deli Lunch** (page 52) • Turkey and Swiss on wheat bread • Italian pickled vegetable salad • Melon salad	**Soup and Salad** (page 40) • Vegetable soup with breadsticks • Green salad topped with grilled chicken • Green or red grapes	**Crab Cakes** (page 132) • Chesapeake Crab Cakes • Green salad • Crusty roll • Seasonal berries • Pecan Icebox Cookies (page 287)
Mixed dried fruit	Ruby-Studded Trail Mix (page 288)	Container of nonfat yogurt	Mixed nuts
Quick Black Beans and Rice (page 159) • Grilled Chicken Breast Filet • Quick Black Beans and Rice • Green salad	**Noodles and Greens** (page 102) • Thai Noodle Salad with greens	**Casserole Dinner** (page 162) • Homestyle Tuna Noodle Casserole • Arugula salad	**DINING OUT** **Italian Restaurant** (page 112) • Green salad • Spaghetti with red clam sauce • Sautéed broccoli
Frozen yogurt	Fresh fruit	Air-popped popcorn	Fresh fruit salad

Shopping Smartly

Putting *ChangeOne* into action at the grocery store is a snap with our guide to sensible shopping lists that will ensure you're never without the essentials.

Chances are you already have many of the ingredients for the meals in the three weekly sample plans on the previous pages. They're drawn from the basic provisions—the pantry supplies and refrigerator items—that we detailed back in Week 7. As you think about shopping strategies, take some time to look back at that list of Kitchen Essentials on page 157, and keep it handy. You'll be referring to it often as you get comfortable with stocking a *ChangeOne* kitchen.

A well-planned list allows you to keep fresh foods on hand.

Our meals call for lots of perishable foods, especially fruits, vegetables, meats, and dairy products, so it's important to have a checklist to track these items and avoid waste. We've included two sample *ChangeOne* shopping lists on the next page that will help you track perishables.

Grocery stores stock produce separately from dairy, meats, and seafood, so start your list with that in mind. It's also helpful to divide the perishables into two groups: long-life items and short-life items.

Long-life items are those that can be stored in a cool pantry or in the refrigerator and will keep for a few weeks. Plan to check these items and restock as needed about twice a month. Short-life items will keep only a few days in the refrigerator and are best bought and used for a specific recipe. Check these once a week and restock as needed.

Okay, now it's time to tackle the whole store. Use the following shopping guidelines to stay on top of the master list on page 157, and to stay timely with perishable items.

Monthly: Around the same time every month check and restock your kitchen staples.

Twice monthly: Check and replenish long-life produce, dairy, meats, and seafood as needed.

Weekly: Pick up short-life items for that week's meals.

A few more general guidelines can simplify your shopping strategy even further:

■ Plan a week's recipes, then check your pantry and refrigerator for items you will need that week and make sure they're on your list.

■ You're the best judge of how much you'll need of each item, based on the number of people you're cooking for and the substitutions you make.

■ You can substitute just about any fruit or vegetable for another, so buy the ones you like or those that are in season.

■ If you find you're not going to use fresh meat, poultry, or fish within a day after you buy it, freeze it.

Twice-Monthly List

QTY	PRODUCE
	Apples
	Oranges
	Lemons and limes
	Melons, uncut
	Kiwifruit
	Cabbage
	Carrots
	Celery
	Garlic
	Onions
	Potatoes
	Scallions
	Squash in season

QTY	DAIRY, MEAT, SEAFOOD
	Butter
	Cheeses, hard and dry (parmesan)
	Yogurt
	Beef (freezer)
	Chicken parts (freezer)
	Salami, hard Italian
	Salmon (freezer)

Weekly List

QTY	PRODUCE
	Berries in season
	Grapes
	Bananas
	Peaches
	Pears
	Mangoes
	Cucumbers
	Edamame (soybeans)
	Lettuce and salad greens
	Red and green peppers
	Tomatoes
	Zucchini

QTY	DAIRY, MEAT, SEAFOOD
	Cheeses, medium (cheddar, jack)
	Cheeses, soft (ricotta, cottage)
	Milk
	Deli meats
	Meats, uncooked
	Seafood, uncooked

Essential Tools

Well-chosen kitchen tools are a dieter's friend. Here are some top choices:

1. Quality knives: Any professional chef will tell you that good knives are crucial. If yours won't cut butter, it's time to sharpen them up or invest in a new set.

2. Kitchen scissors: Removing chicken skin, trimming string-bean tips—you'll be surprised how often these come in handy.

3. Measuring cups: Essential tools to prevent portion creep.

4. Adjustable measuring spoon: This simple tool will replace the clutter of spoons on your counter when baking or making a dish with lots of ingredients.

5. Kitchen scale: Another great way to keep portions in check. If you do a lot of cooking at home, a scale will also be handy for recipes that list ingredients in ounces or grams.

6. Wok: If you love stir-fries, this is essential. By distributing heat evenly over the cooking surface, woks allow you to cook very fast. A nonstick wok will let you go easy on cooking oil.

7. Nonstick frying pan or skillet: Here, too, the nonstick surface cuts down on the amount of oil needed for sautéing.

8. Grill pan: When you cook moist foods like fish filets or vegetables on the grill, they tend to stick or break apart—but not when you use a grill pan. Consider a grill wok as well.

9. Skewers: Skewers are wonderful tools for grilling, of course, but they're useful other ways, from testing the doneness of cakes and muffins to tenderizing meat.

10. Salad spinner: A must for salad lovers. A spinner makes it easy to rinse and dry salad leaves without bruising them.

11. Vegetable steamer: Try a collapsible metal steamer rack that will fit into a saucepan, or buy a dedicated steamer. Make sure you have one big enough to handle a variety of vegetables.

12. Blender: With a decent blender you can whip up yogurt smoothies, fruit ices, savory sauces, and homemade soups.

13. Timers: Accurate timers with loud alarms will keep watch over what's cooking and remind you when you're needed.

14. Microplane grater: Super sharp, these graters make easy work out of grating high-flavor ingredients like hard cheese or choco-late. Thy're also perfect for zesting citrus.

Clockwise from top left: rice steamer, grill pan, adjustable measuring spoon, squeeze bottle, microplane grater, skewers, and kitchen scissors.

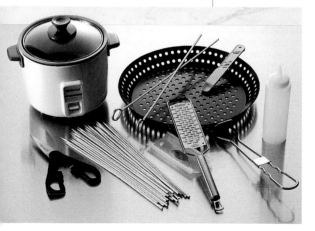

15. Crock pot: Put together a simple meal early and let it cook all day. Perfect for chilis, stews, and other slow-cook items.

16. Rice steamer: Automatic rice steamers make it easy to prepare perfect rice every time.

17. Plastic squeeze bottles: Fill with your favorite sauces to squirt on foods; it's how professional chefs decorate dishes.

18. Erasable chalkboard: A great way to keep track of what you're running low on so that you won't be caught short.

Tips for Storing Food

In our *ChangeOne* recipes, we often suggest you dish out a meal's servings and then immediately package and refrigerate leftovers. That keeps you from serving unnecessary second helpings and guarantees you have correctly portioned meals available at any time.

The trick to smart storage is to get food sealed quickly and thoroughly to minimize bacteria on the food, and just as quickly refrigerate the food to prevent bacteria from growing (generally, bacteria hate cold).

Here are more storage tips, along with safe refrigeration times for everyday foods:

■ Make sure your containers have a tight seal. The less air around the food, the less chance of bacteria finding it.

■ Use a shallow container for hot leftovers to help them cool more rapidly. Don't worry about putting warm containers in the refrigerator; rapid cooling doesn't affect the food. The only issue is that the container will warm the refrigerator very slightly.

■ If you know you're not going to eat leftovers within the time specified in this table, freeze them. Freezing means zero bacteria growth, but also "freezer burn," which occurs when the moisture in the food gets drawn out by the dry environment. To minimize freezer burn, place the sealed container in a second sealed container (freezer bags work fine).

Food	Use within
Yogurt, cottage cheese	7 days
Hard cheese	6–12 weeks unopened; 1 week opened
Cheese spreads	3–4 weeks
Eggs, in shell	3 weeks
Eggs, hard-boiled	1 week
Beef or pork roasts, steaks, chops, uncooked	3–5 days
Beef or pork roasts, steaks, chops, cooked	3–4 days
Ground beef, uncooked	1–2 days
Stew meat, uncooked	1–2 days
Poultry, uncooked	1–2 days
Poultry, cooked	3–4 days
Fresh sausage, uncooked	1–2 days
Ham slices, cooked	3–4 days
Luncheon meats	3–5 days
Fresh fish, uncooked	1–2 days
Live crab, lobster	Same day
Shucked mussels, clams	1–2 days
Scallops, crabmeat, shrimp	2–3 days

And remember:
Many foods are stamped with a suggested last date of sale; that isn't necessarily the last day you can safely eat them. Once opened, refrigerated food may spoil before the date on the package, so use caution.

Personal Tools

Throughout *ChangeOne* we've asked you to write things down. How's the weight loss progressing? What are your current goals? What did you eat today? How active are you?

But truth is, few of us are in the habit of writing down such things. So we've tried to make it easier for you.

On the following pages are all the guides you need to progress through *ChangeOne*.

Each of these forms was conceived to be as simple to use as possible. They'll ask the tough questions, but they'll also lead to clear, concise answers. So give them a try; each one will take just a few minutes. Make as many copies of each form as you need to track your progress.

Here's what you'll find:

- The *ChangeOne* Contract
- Hunger Profile
- Daily Food Diary
- Daily Activity Log
- Personal Time Analyzer
- Progress Log
- Your Healthy Weight Calculator

And remember, for these and other interactive weight-loss tools, subscribe to our Web site, **changeone.com/special**.

Change One Contract

ChangeOne begin date: _____

I VOW TO MYSELF that over the next three months I will learn and practice the eating habits necessary to lose weight and improve my health. I put forth the following goals:

Intermediate weight target: _____

Ultimate weight target: _____

HOW I EXPECT MY LIFE TO IMPROVE: _____

_____

_____

_____

HOW I EXPECT MY HEALTH TO IMPROVE: _____

_____

_____

_____

IN ADDITION to weekly weigh-ins on a scale, I will track my progress by the two methods I will list below (for example, clothing size, appearance, energy, notches in a belt, or self-confidence):

1. _____

2. _____

I HEREBY AFFIRM that the goals I have set meet the TRIM test. Each one is Time-bound, Realistic, Inspiring, and Measurable.

I agree to review my progress and reevaluate my strategies for reaching my goals every two weeks during the program.

I agree to keep this contract as a reminder of my commitment.

Signed: _____

Witnessed by (optional): _____

Date:

Hunger Profile

Instructions: Make a copy of this form and carry it with you during the day. Every time you get hungry, record the time, how you felt (tired, bored, ravenous, stressed-out, just plain hungry), what you ate, or what you did instead of eating (took a walk, distracted myself with work). This will help you determine your eating habits—both good and bad— and make it easier to adjust your meal and snack times for healthy weight loss.

	TIME	HOW I FELT	WHAT I ATE	WHAT I DID
MORNING				
AFTERNOON				
EVENING				

Date: _____

Daily Food Diary

Instructions: First, write down what you eat. Next, estimate portions as carefully as you can based on what you've learned throughout *ChangeOne*. For example, if one egg is the recommended portion at breakfast and you eat two, write in "two portions." Keep a copy of the form with you and fill it in as soon as you can after a snack or meal.

Tallying calories is optional. We don't recommend that *ChangeOne* participants worry too much about calories—managing portion sizes should take care of that. But if you really want to see how you are doing, here's how to find calorie information:

- For *ChangeOne* meals, use calorie counts that we provide.
- For *ChangeOne* snacks and desserts, estimate 100 calories per portion.
- For other snacks and prepared foods, use nutrition labels.
- For all other foods, visit **changeone.com/calorie** for a link to a calorie counter.

	WHAT I ATE	ESTIMATED PORTIONS	CALORIES
BREAKFAST			
LUNCH			
DINNER			
SNACKS			
		TOTAL CALORIES (optional):	

Date:

Daily Activity Log

Instructions: Use this form to track daily exercise. Include all activities of 5 minutes or more in duration and estimate their intensity. As general guidelines, light activities could be dusting, ironing, or playing croquet; moderate activities could be playing golf, raking the lawn, walking, or washing the car; and strenuous activities could be aerobic dance, jogging, bicycling, swimming, hiking, or playing tennis. When you're done, add up the number of minutes you spent doing light, moderate, and strenuous activities.

TIME	WHAT I DID	TIME SPENT IN MINUTES PER INTENSITY		
		Light	Moderate	Strenuous
AM				
6:00				
7:00				
8:00				
9:00				
10:00				
11:00				
PM				
12:00				
1:00				
2:00				
3:00				
4:00				
5:00				
6:00				
7:00				
8:00				
9:00				
10:00				
11:00				
AM				
12:00				
1:00				
2:00				
3:00				
4:00				
5:00				
TOTAL MINUTES:				

Date: _____

Personal Time Analyzer

Instructions: On at least one weekday and one weekend day, keep track of how you spend your time. Make copies of this form and keep one with you on the day of focus. In the two columns to the right, estimate in minutes how much time you spent being active and how much time you spent being inactive. "Active" covers anything that requires you to get up and move around. "Inactive" includes sitting, lying down, or standing.

TIME	ACTIVITIES/TASKS	ACTIVE	INACTIVE
AM			
6:00			
7:00			
8:00			
9:00			
10:00			
11:00			
PM			
12:00			
1:00			
2:00			
3:00			
4:00			
5:00			
6:00			
7:00			
8:00			
9:00			
10:00			
11:00			
AM			
12:00			
1:00			
2:00			
3:00			
4:00			
5:00			
	TOTAL MINUTES:		

Progress Log

Instructions: Once a week record your weight and estimate how much time you spend being active. Jot down notes on any problems or issues you're facing. Try to schedule the same time each week to weigh yourself and fill in the form.

Week of: _____ **Weight:** _____

AVERAGE DAILY ACTIVITY
- ❑ 45 minutes or more
- ❑ 30 minutes
- ❑ Less than 30 minutes

HOW I'M FEELING
- ❑ Great
- ❑ Okay
- ❑ Stressed out
- ❑ Discouraged
- ❑ _____

NOTES
_____
_____
_____
_____
_____

Week of: _____ **Weight:** _____

AVERAGE DAILY ACTIVITY
- ❑ 45 minutes or more
- ❑ 30 minutes
- ❑ Less than 30 minutes

HOW I'M FEELING
- ❑ Great
- ❑ Okay
- ❑ Stressed out
- ❑ Discouraged
- ❑ _____

NOTES
_____
_____
_____
_____
_____

Week of: _____ **Weight:** _____

AVERAGE DAILY ACTIVITY
- ❑ 45 minutes or more
- ❑ 30 minutes
- ❑ Less than 30 minutes

HOW I'M FEELING
- ❑ Great
- ❑ Okay
- ❑ Stressed out
- ❑ Discouraged
- ❑ _____

NOTES
_____
_____
_____
_____
_____

Week of: _____ **Weight:** _____

AVERAGE DAILY ACTIVITY
- ❑ 45 minutes or more
- ❑ 30 minutes
- ❑ Less than 30 minutes

HOW I'M FEELING
- ❑ Great
- ❑ Okay
- ❑ Stressed out
- ❑ Discouraged
- ❑ _____

NOTES
_____
_____
_____
_____
_____

At the end of each week use the graph at right to chart weight changes; track it for four weeks.

	WEEK 1	WEEK 2	WEEK 3	WEEK 4
+8 lbs				
+6 lbs				
+4 lbs				
+2 lbs				
_____ STARTING WEIGHT				
-2 lbs				
-4 lbs				
-6 lbs				
-8 lbs				

Your Healthy Weight Calculator

What's your ideal weight? The answer depends on your body type. Researchers use a scale called Body Mass Index, or BMI, which assigns a number based on a combination of height and weight. Essentially, the number indicates whether you are carrying a healthy or unhealthy level of body fat.

To find your BMI on the chart below, locate your height in inches in the column on the left. Then scan the horizontal row of numbers to find your weight. Finally, move up to locate the number directly above the column where your weight appears, in the row marked "BMI" at the top of the chart. (If you don't see your weight or height on the chart below, visit **changone.com** to calculate your place on the BMI.)

You'll notice that the BMI chart gives a wide range of weights that fall within the normal category. The normal BMI weight range for someone who is 5 foot 7 inches (67 inches) is between 121 and 153 pounds, for instance. The reason for the 32-pound range: people have different body types, some slender, some stocky, some small-boned, some large.

The BMI index isn't foolproof. It tends to overestimate body fat in athletes and people with very muscular builds. And it tends to underestimate body fat in older people, who have usually lost muscle mass.

			NORMAL						OVERWEIGHT								OBESE				
BMI	**19**	**20**	**21**	**22**	**23**	**24**	**25**	**26**	**27**	**28**	**29**	**30**	**31**	**32**	**33**	**34**	**35**	**36**	**37**	**38**
HEIGHT (INCHES)									BODY WEIGHT IN POUNDS											
58	91	96	100	105	110	115	119	124	129	134	138	143	148	153	158	162	167	172	177	181
59	94	99	104	109	114	119	124	128	133	138	143	148	153	158	163	168	173	178	183	188
60	97	102	107	112	118	123	128	133	138	143	148	153	158	163	168	174	179	184	189	194
61	100	106	111	116	122	127	132	137	143	148	153	158	164	169	174	180	185	190	195	201
62	104	109	115	120	126	131	136	142	147	153	158	164	169	175	180	186	191	196	202	207
63	107	113	118	124	130	135	141	146	152	158	163	169	175	180	186	191	197	203	208	214
64	110	116	122	128	134	140	145	151	157	163	169	174	180	186	192	197	204	209	215	221
65	114	120	126	132	138	144	150	156	162	168	174	180	186	192	198	204	210	216	222	228
66	118	124	130	136	142	148	155	161	167	173	179	186	192	198	204	210	216	223	229	235
67	121	127	134	140	146	153	159	166	172	178	185	191	198	204	211	217	223	230	236	242
68	125	131	138	144	151	158	164	171	177	184	190	197	203	210	216	223	230	236	243	249
69	128	135	142	149	155	162	169	176	182	189	196	203	209	216	223	230	236	243	250	257
70	132	139	146	153	160	167	174	181	188	195	202	209	216	222	229	236	243	250	257	264
71	136	143	150	157	165	172	179	186	193	200	208	215	222	229	236	243	250	257	265	272
72	140	147	154	162	169	177	184	191	199	206	213	221	228	235	242	250	258	265	272	279
73	144	151	159	166	174	182	189	197	204	212	219	227	235	242	250	257	265	272	280	288
74	148	155	163	171	179	186	194	202	210	218	225	233	241	249	256	264	272	280	287	295
75	152	160	168	176	184	192	200	208	216	224	232	240	248	256	264	272	279	287	295	303
76	156	164	172	180	189	197	205	213	221	230	238	246	254	263	271	279	287	295	304	312

Remember that losing even a few pounds when you're overweight will make you healthier, reducing your risk of heart disease and diabetes. Trying to bring your weight down to the normal range in the BMI is a terrific goal. But if you have a long way to go to get there, set some milestones for the road ahead. Reward yourself at each step, and don't get discouraged. Every little bit helps.

changeone.com Makes Losing Weight Even Easier

You've been reading about the *ChangeOne* program—now let us help you customize it to the way *you* live.

Increase your chances of weight-loss success with *ChangeOne* Online. Here are five great reasons to join today:

■ You'll have access to hundreds of additional healthy, mouthwatering meals and recipes. We'll design you a meal plan with your weight-loss goals and preferences in mind.

■ You'll get around-the-clock encouragement and advice from a caring community of other *ChangeOne* dieters to help you reach your weight-loss goals.

■ You can use our calculators, tools, and interactive features to track your progress and get personalized feedback.

■ You'll find the latest articles, news, and expert advice to keep you up to date on health, food, and fitness information.

■ You'll receive weekly e-mail newsletters packed with delicious recipes, proven weight-loss tips, and lots more.

Sign up now: point your browser to **changeone.com/special** and get a *ChangeOne* program made for you.

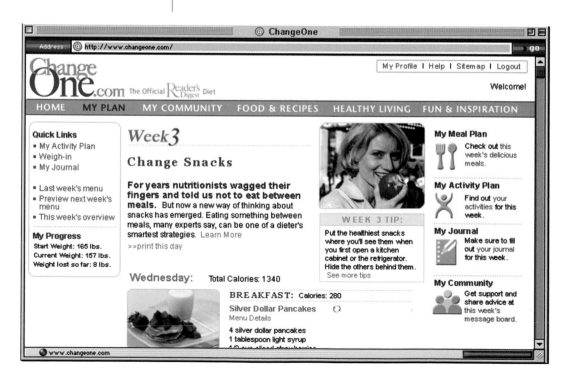

John Hastings is the senior staff editor for health at *Reader's Digest*, the world's largest consumer magazine. He has worked as a journalist covering medicine, nutrition, and fitness for 14 years. Over the years Hastings has written and edited for a variety of magazines and electronic publications, including *Health, Men's Journal, Town & Country, EcoTraveler,* MyLifePath.com, and BabyCenter.com.

Mindy Hermann is a registered dietitian who speaks and consults on weight loss and nutrition. She is also a writer and editor, and her articles have appeared in *Family Circle, Ladies' Home Journal, Men's Health, Woman's Day, Fitness,* and *New York* magazines. Hermann co-authored *Live Longer & Better* and she was the nutrition writer for the American Medical Association *Family Health Cookbook*, which won a James Beard cookbook award.

Peter Jaret is a frequent contributor to *Reader's Digest, Health, Eating Well, National Wildlife,* and other magazines. His work also has appeared in *National Geographic, Newsweek, Vogue, Glamour, Men's Journal, Remedy, Harper's Bazaar,* and *Self.* The author of Reader's Digest *Heart Healthy for Life*, Jaret is also the recipient of an American Medical Association award for medical reporting and a James Beard journalism award.

Recipe Index

Beef
All-American pot roast with braised vegetables **272**
Barbecue beef on a bun **270**
Beef stew **92**
Heartland meat loaf **274–75**
Tacos **220–21**

Beverages
Tropical smoothie **254**
Vanilla steamer **258**

Breads
Bagel delight **29**
Blueberry muffins with lemon glaze **252**
Dried cranberry scones with orange glaze **253**
Garlic bread **156**
Multigrain soft pretzels **289**
Peach quick bread **256**
Streusel-top coffee cake **227**

Breakfast
22–37, 252–58
Bagel delight **29**
Blueberry muffins with lemon glaze **252**
Breakfast on the run **30**
Cottage cheese melba **258**
Dried cranberry scones with orange glaze **253**
Egg on a roll **23**
Lox and bagels **133**
Peach quick bread **256**
Perfect bowl of cereal **32**

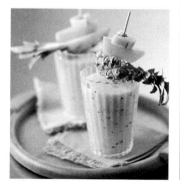

Silver dollar pancakes **24**
Streusel-top coffee cake **227**
Tropical smoothie **254**
Vanilla steamer **258**
Vegetable-cheddar omelet **130**
Vegetable frittata **255**
Yogurt parfait **257**
Zesty cheddar-asparagus quiche **131**

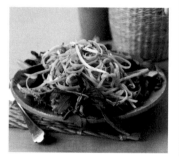

Dinner
82–107, 268–83
All-American pot roast with braised vegetables **272**
Barbecue beef on a bun **270**
Barbecued halibut steaks **278–79**
Beef stew **92**
Chicken and broccoli stir-fry **90**
Grilled chicken breast filet **159**
Heartland meat loaf **274–75**
Homestyle tuna noodle casserole **162**
Kitchen sink stew **156**
Mediterranean treats **217**
One-crust chicken pot pie **280**
Pasta primavera **98–99**
Sautéed chicken with caramelized onions **269**
Shrimp and pepper kebabs **88**
Snapper and snaps in a packet **100**
Sweet-and-sour glazed pork with pineapple **277**
Tacos **220–21**
Tuna salad sandwich **224**

Ziti and zucchini **279**

Eggs
Egg on a roll **23**
Vegetable-cheddar omelet **130**
Vegetable frittata **255**
Zesty cheddar-asparagus quiche **131**

Fowl
Apple-stuffed turkey breast with orange marmalade glaze **141**
Beer-can chicken **139**
Burrito to go **55**
Chicken and broccoli stir-fry **90**
Grilled chicken breast filet **159**
Grilled turkey caesar salad **263**
One-crust chicken pot pie **280**
Sautéed chicken with caramelized onions **269**
Tacos **220–21**

Lunch
38–57, 259–67
Bavarian sandwich **260**
Burrito to go **55**
Chef's salad **44**
Cream of asparagus soup **261**
Grilled turkey caesar salad **263**
Hearty split-pea soup **260**
Meatless chili pots con queso **265**
Pete's chopped salad **267**
Pita pizza **39**
Roasted vegetable wraps with chive sauce **266**
Tuna salad sandwich **224**
Turkey and swiss cheese sandwich **52**
Well-dressed baked potato **259**

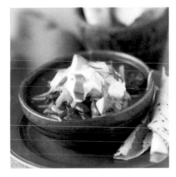

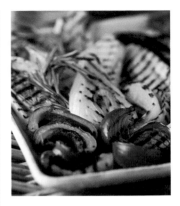

General Index

Metric Conversions

Length

When you know:	If you multiply by:	You can find:
inches	25	millimeters
inches	2.5	centimeters
feet	30	centimeters
yards	0.9	meters
miles	1.6	kilometers
millimeters	0.04	inches
centimeters	0.4	inches
meters	3.3	feet
meters	1.1	yards
kilometers	0.6	miles

Volume

When you know:	If you multiply by:	You can find:
teaspoons	4.9	milliliters
tablespoons	14.8	milliliters
fluid ounces	29.6	milliliters
cups	0.24	liters
pints	0.47	liters
quarts	0.95	liters
gallons	3.79	liters
milliliters	0.03	fluid ounces
liters	4.22	cups
liters	2.11	pints
liters	1.06	quarts
liters	0.26	gallons

Weight

When you know:	If you multiply by:	You can find:
ounces	28.4	grams
pounds	0.45	kilograms
grams	0.035	ounces
kilograms	2.2	pounds

Metric Equivalents

Linear

U.S.	Metric
1/8 in	3 mm
1/4 in	6 mm
1/2 in	1.3 cm
3/4 in	1.9 cm
1 in	2.5 cm
6 in	15 cm
12 in (1 ft)	30 cm
39 in	1 m

Weight

U.S.	Metric
1/4 oz	7 g
1/2 oz	14 g
3/4 oz	21 g
1 oz	28 g
8 oz (1/2 lb)	225 g
12 oz (3/4 lb)	341 g
16 oz (1 lb)	454 g
35 oz (2.2 lbs)	1 kg

Volume

U.S.	Metric
1 tbsp (1/2 fl oz)	15 ml
1/4 cup (2 fl oz)	60 ml
1/3 cup	80 ml
1/2 cup (4 fl oz)	120 ml
2/3 cup	160 ml
3/4 cup (6 fl oz)	180 ml
1 cup (8 fl oz)	235 ml
1 qt (32 fl oz)	950 ml
1 qt + 3 tbsps	1 l
1 gal (128 fl oz)	4 l

Temperature

U.S.	Metric
0°F (freezer temperature)	-18°C
32°F (water freezes)	0°C
98.6°F	37°C
180°F (water simmers*)	82°C
212°F (water boils*)	100°C
250°F (low oven)	120°C
350°F (moderate oven)	175°C
425°F (hot oven)	220°C
500°F (very hot oven)	260°C

*at sea level

All numbers have been rounded. For more exact numbers, use metric conversion chart at left.

---

mm = millimeter
cm = centimeter
m = meter
in = inch
ft = foot

ml = milliliter
l = liter
tsp = teaspoon
tbsp = tablespoon
oz = ounce

fl oz = fluid ounce
qt = quart
gal = gallon
g = gram
kg = kilogram

lb = pound
C = celsius
F = fahrenheit